Recent Advances in Acetaminophen Hepatotoxicity

Recent Advances in Acetaminophen Hepatotoxicity

Guest Editor

Hartmut W. Jaeschke

Basel • Beijing • Wuhan • Barcelona • Belgrade • Novi Sad • Cluj • Manchester

Guest Editor
Hartmut W. Jaeschke
Department of Pharmacology,
Toxicology & Therapeutics
University of Kansas
Medical Center
Kansas City, MO
USA

Editorial Office
MDPI AG
Grosspeteranlage 5
4052 Basel, Switzerland

This is a reprint of the Special Issue, published open access by the journal *Livers* (ISSN 2673-4389), freely accessible at: https://www.mdpi.com/journal/livers/special_issues/acetaminophen_hepatotoxicity.

For citation purposes, cite each article independently as indicated on the article page online and as indicated below:

Lastname, A.A.; Lastname, B.B. Article Title. *Journal Name* **Year**, *Volume Number*, Page Range.

ISBN 978-3-7258-5539-1 (Hbk)
ISBN 978-3-7258-5540-7 (PDF)
https://doi.org/10.3390/books978-3-7258-5540-7

Contents

About the Editor

Hartmut W. Jaeschke

Hartmut W. Jaeschke is a Distinguished Professor and former Chairman (2012-2024) of the Department of Pharmacology, Toxicology, and Therapeutics at the University of Kansas Medical Center, Kansas City, Kansas, USA. He is a Fellow of the Academy of Toxicological Sciences (ATS) and American Association for the Study of Liver Diseases (FAASLD). After receiving his PhD degree in toxicology from the University of Tübingen, Germany, he completed his postdoctoral research at the same institution and the Baylor College of Medicine in Houston, Texas, USA. Since 1987, he has held faculty positions at Baylor (1987–1992), the University of Arkansas for Medical Sciences, Little Rock (1999–2002), and the University of Arizona, Tucson (2002–2006). From 1992 to 1998, he worked in the pharmaceutical industry (The Upjohn Co. and Pharmacia & Upjohn Co., Kalamazoo, MI). He has published more than 530 peer-reviewed manuscripts, invited reviews, and book chapters on liver toxicology and liver pathophysiology ("h-factor 131"; >73,000 citations; Google Scholar). Moreover, Dr. Jaeschke was a standing member of the Hepatobiliary Pathophysiology NIH study section (2008–2013) and was as an ad hoc member on numerous NIH grant review committees, additionally serving on numerous editorial boards of journals related to liver and toxicology. He was an Associate Editor for *Hepatology* (2002–2006) and *Liver International* (2007–2012), and he currently serves as Editor-in-Chief of *Livers* and Associate Editor for *Toxicological Sciences* (since 2014). He is the recipient of the CSSOT John Doull Award (2015) and the Translational Impact Award (2019) from the Society of Toxicology (SOT). His research interests pertain to basic mechanisms and translational aspects of xenobiotic-induced hepatotoxicity and tissue repair, focusing on acetaminophen overdose and mechanisms of inflammatory liver injury in animal models and humans.

livers

MDPI

Editorial

Acetaminophen Hepatotoxicity: Not as Simple as One Might Think! Introductory Comments on the Special Issue—*Recent Advances in Acetaminophen Hepatotoxicity*

Hartmut Jaeschke

Department of Pharmacology, Toxicology & Therapeutics, University of Kansas Medical Center, Kansas City, KS 66160, USA; hjaeschke@kumc.edu

Acetaminophen (N-acetyl-para-aminophenol (APAP)) is one of the most-studied drugs worldwide. APAP causes liver toxicity after an overdose, with thousands of papers published on various aspects of the mechanisms of cell death and organ injury, as well as regeneration and recovery. It is also a highly popular experimental model to test the efficacy of various potential drugs and chemicals to treat or prevent acute liver injury and promote regeneration. The popularity of the APAP overdose model is derived from two main aspects: the clinical relevance of the model and the perceived simplicity of the experimental design.

Regarding the clinical relevance, APAP is present in hundreds of prescriptions and over-the-counter medicines, which are consumed daily by tens of millions of patients worldwide. Although considered safe at therapeutic doses, an overdose of APAP dose-dependently causes liver injury, which can progress to acute liver failure (ALF) and even death in patients [1,2]. In fact, APAP toxicity is the most frequent cause of ALF in the US, the UK and many other western countries [3,4]. Mitchell and coworkers [5–7] discovered that the sensitivity of mice to APAP toxicity is comparable to that of humans and defined the early steps of toxicity in the murine model. Importantly, an APAP overdose in the mouse accurately reproduces most of the mechanistic aspects of cell death and liver injury observed in patients [8] and human hepatocytes [9], with the only exception being the more delayed pathophysiology observed in humans compared to mice. Thus, the mechanistic data and therapeutic intervention strategies obtained in the mouse model translate very well to the human pathophysiology [10,11]. The only clinically approved antidote against APAP toxicity, N-acetylcysteine, was developed based on the early mechanistic insight generated by Mitchell and coworkers in the mouse model [12,13]. In addition, the most-promising new antidote under clinical development, fomepizole (4-methylpyrazole), is being advanced due to preclinical studies in the mouse model that demonstrated that the compound is an effective inhibitor of cytochrome P450 2E1 (Cyp2E1) and of c-jun N-terminal kinase (JNK) [14,15]; one aspect of this mechanism (Cyp2E1 inhibition) was confirmed in a human volunteer trial [16]. Based on this experience, APAP overdose in the mouse is the preferred experimental model to study clinically relevant mechanisms of acute drug hepatotoxicity and regeneration and evaluate potential therapeutic targets.

The second aspect that contributes to the popularity of APAP toxicity is the perceived simplicity of the model. Fed or overnight fasted mice from most mouse strains develop severe liver injury when intraperitoneally injected with a dose of 300–600 mg/kg APAP [17]. Thus, it seems simple enough to sacrifice the animals 24 h after APAP administration and measure as many parameters related to injury, modes of cell death, inflammation, oxidant stress, etc., as possible. However, this simplistic experimental design provides a substantial problem for the interpretation of the results. APAP toxicity is a complex, time-dependent process involving many different, interrelated mechanistic aspects, including drug metabolism, with the formation of a reactive metabolite, GSH depletion and protein adducts formation, an initial oxidant stress that activates a mitogen-activated protein kinase cascade leading to JNK phosphorylation, phospho-JNK translocation to mitochondria with amplification of the oxidant stress and peroxynitrite formation, and iron-dependent nitrotyrosine protein adduct formation in mitochondria, eventually leading to the mitochondrial permeability transition pore opening and collapse of the mitochondrial membrane potential [18,19]. The mitochondrial dysfunction then leads to the release of endonucleases, which cause DNA fragmentation. These are the key events leading to necrotic cell death [20,21]. However, there are many different mechanisms that can affect these central pathways of cell death, including Nrf2 activation with an impact on drug metabolism and defense mechanisms [22], autophagy and mitophagy to limit the propagation of mitochondrial damage [23], and mitochondrial biogenesis to replace damaged mitochondria, limit cell death and facilitate regeneration [24,25], and an extensive sterile inflammatory response to promote recovery. However, they may also risk aggravating the injury process under certain conditions [26,27]. In addition to these major adaptive responses to the stress of injury, there are additional aspects to consider, such as the gut microbiome, dietary effects, and genetic background, all of which could influence the pathophysiology through modulation of any of the above-mentioned effects, and thus ultimately influence cell necrosis. Although the zonation of hepatocytes has been known for many years [28], the more recent application of single-cell RNA-sequencing now allows for the response of individual hepatocytes and non-parenchymal cells to hepatotoxins such as APAP to be studied, and opens up a new dimension in the investigation of APAP hepatotoxicity [29,30]. Despite this wealth of information, there are still many open questions that need to be investigated and novel interactions that can be discovered. However, avoiding pitfalls in experimental design and mistakes in data interpretation is critical to relevant progress in this field [31].

Therefore, the objective of this Special Issue on "Recent Advances in Acetaminophen Hepatotoxicity"(https://www.mdpi.com/journal/livers/special_issues/acetaminophen_hepatotoxicity (accessed on 19 June 2022)) is to publish state-of-the-art reviews summarizing the newest developments by leading experts and attract additional reviews and original manuscripts that can further define the field, advance our understanding of the pathophysiology, and identify novel therapeutic targets.

Funding: The work discussed was supported in part by the U.S. National Institutes of Health grants R01 DK102142, P20 GM103549, and P30 GM118247.

Conflicts of Interest: The author declares no conflict of interest.

References

1. Larson, A.M. Acetaminophen hepatotoxicity. *Clin. Liver Dis.* **2007**, *11*, 525–548. [CrossRef] [PubMed]
2. Jaeschke, H. Acetaminophen: Dose-Dependent Drug Hepatotoxicity and Acute Liver Failure in Patients. *Dig. Dis.* **2015**, *33*, 464–471. [CrossRef] [PubMed]
3. Stravitz, R.T.; Lee, W.M. Acute liver failure. *Lancet* **2019**, *394*, 869–881. [CrossRef]
4. Bernal, W.; Wendon, J. Acute liver failure. *N. Engl. J. Med.* **2013**, *369*, 2525–2534. [CrossRef]
5. Mitchell, J.R.; Jollow, D.J.; Potter, W.Z.; Davis, D.C.; Gillette, J.R.; Brodie, B.B. Acetaminophen-induced hepatic necrosis. I. Role of drug metabolism. *J. Pharmacol. Exp. Ther.* **1973**, *187*, 185–194.
6. Jollow, D.J.; Mitchell, J.R.; Potter, W.Z.; Davis, D.C.; Gillette, J.R.; Brodie, B.B. Acetaminophen-induced hepatic necrosis. II. Role of covalent binding in vivo. *J. Pharmacol. Exp. Ther.* **1973**, *187*, 195–202.
7. Mitchell, J.R.; Jollow, D.J.; Potter, W.Z.; Gillette, J.R.; Brodie, B.B. Acetaminophen-induced hepatic necrosis. IV. Protective role of glutathione. *J. Pharmacol. Exp. Ther.* **1973**, *187*, 211–217.
8. McGill, M.R.; Sharpe, M.R.; Williams, C.D.; Taha, M.; Curry, S.C.; Jaeschke, H. The mechanism underlying acetaminophen-induced hepatotoxicity in humans and mice involves mitochondrial damage and nuclear DNA fragmentation. *J. Clin. Investig.* **2012**, *122*, 1574–1583. [CrossRef]
9. Xie, Y.; McGill, M.R.; Dorko, K.; Kumer, S.C.; Schmitt, T.M.; Forster, J.; Jaeschke, H. Mechanisms of acetaminophen-induced cell death in primary human hepatocytes. *Toxicol. Appl. Pharmacol.* **2014**, *279*, 266–274. [CrossRef]
10. Jaeschke, H.; Xie, Y.; McGill, M.R. Acetaminophen-induced Liver Injury: From Animal Models to Humans. *J. Clin. Transl. Hepatol.* **2014**, *2*, 153–161.

11. Ramachandran, A.; Jaeschke, H. Mechanisms of acetaminophen hepatotoxicity and their translation to the human pathophysiology. *J. Clin. Transl Res.* **2017**, *3* (Suppl. 1), 157–169. [CrossRef] [PubMed]
12. Rumack, B.H.; Bateman, D.N. Acetaminophen and acetylcysteine dose and duration: Past, present and future. *Clin. Toxicol.* **2012**, *50*, 91–98. [CrossRef] [PubMed]
13. Akakpo, J.Y.; Ramachandran, A.; Curry, S.C.; Rumack, B.H.; Jaeschke, H. Comparing N-acetylcysteine and 4-methylpyrazole as antidotes for acetaminophen overdose. *Arch. Toxicol.* **2022**, *96*, 453–465. [CrossRef] [PubMed]
14. Akakpo, J.Y.; Ramachandran, A.; Kandel, S.E.; Ni, H.M.; Kumer, S.C.; Rumack, B.H.; Jaeschke, H. 4-Methylpyrazole protects against acetaminophen hepatotoxicity in mice and in primary human hepatocytes. *Hum. Exp. Toxicol.* **2018**, *37*, 1310–1322. [CrossRef] [PubMed]
15. Akakpo, J.Y.; Ramachandran, A.; Duan, L.; Schaich, M.A.; Jaeschke, M.W.; Freudenthal, B.D.; Ding, W.X.; Rumack, B.H.; Jaeschke, H. Delayed Treatment With 4-Methylpyrazole Protects Against Acetaminophen Hepatotoxicity in Mice by Inhibition of c-Jun n-Terminal Kinase. *Toxicol. Sci.* **2019**, *170*, 57–68. [CrossRef] [PubMed]
16. Kang, A.M.; Padilla-Jones, A.; Fisher, E.S.; Akakpo, J.Y.; Jaeschke, H.; Rumack, B.H.; Gerkin, R.D.; Curry, S.C. The Effect of 4-Methylpyrazole on Oxidative Metabolism of Acetaminophen in Human Volunteers. *J. Med. Toxicol.* **2020**, *16*, 169–176. [CrossRef]
17. McGill, M.R.; Lebofsky, M.; Norris, H.R.; Slawson, M.H.; Bajt, M.L.; Xie, Y.; Williams, C.D.; Wilkins, D.G.; Rollins, D.E.; Jaeschke, H. Plasma and liver acetaminophen-protein adduct levels in mice after acetaminophen treatment: Dose-response, mechanisms, and clinical implications. *Toxicol. Appl. Pharmacol.* **2013**, *269*, 240–249. [CrossRef]
18. Ramachandran, A.; Jaeschke, H. Acetaminophen Hepatotoxicity. *Semin. Liver Dis.* **2019**, *39*, 221–234. [CrossRef]
19. Ramachandran, A.; Jaeschke, H. A mitochondrial journey through acetaminophen hepatotoxicity. *Food. Chem. Toxicol.* **2020**, *140*, 111282. [CrossRef]
20. Jaeschke, H.; Ramachandran, A.; Chao, X.; Ding, W.X. Emerging and established modes of cell death during acetaminophen-induced liver injury. *Arch. Toxicol.* **2019**, *93*, 3491–3502. [CrossRef]
21. Iorga, A.; Dara, L. Cell death in drug-induced liver injury. *Adv. Pharmacol.* **2019**, *85*, 31–74. [PubMed]
22. Bataille, A.M.; Manautou, J.E. Nrf2: A potential target for new therapeutics in liver disease. *Clin. Pharmacol. Ther.* **2012**, *92*, 340–348. [CrossRef] [PubMed]
23. Chao, X.; Wang, H.; Jaeschke, H.; Ding, W.X. Role and mechanisms of autophagy in acetaminophen-induced liver injury. *Liver Int.* **2018**, *38*, 1363–1374. [CrossRef]
24. Jaeschke, H.; Duan, L.; Nguyen, N.; Ramachandran, A. Mitochondrial Damage and Biogenesis in Acetaminophen-induced Liver Injury. *Liver Res.* **2019**, *3*, 150–156. [CrossRef]
25. Ramachandran, A.; Umbaugh, D.S.; Jaeschke, H. Mitochondrial Dynamics in Drug-Induced Liver Injury. *Livers* **2021**, *1*, 102–115. [CrossRef] [PubMed]
26. Jaeschke, H.; Ramachandran, A. Mechanisms and pathophysiological significance of sterile inflammation during acetaminophen hepatotoxicity. *Food Chem. Toxicol.* **2020**, *138*, 111240. [CrossRef] [PubMed]
27. Jaeschke, H.; Williams, C.D.; Ramachandran, A.; Bajt, M.L. Acetaminophen hepatotoxicity and repair: The role of sterile inflammation and innate immunity. *Liver Int.* **2012**, *32*, 8–20. [CrossRef]
28. Jungermann, K. Metabolic zonation of liver parenchyma. *Semin. Liver Dis.* **1988**, *8*, 329–341. [CrossRef]
29. Umbaugh, D.S.; Ramachandran, A.; Jaeschke, H. Spatial Reconstruction of the Early Hepatic Transcriptomic Landscape After an Acetaminophen Overdose Using Single-Cell RNA-Sequencing. *Toxicol. Sci.* **2021**, *182*, 327–345. [CrossRef]
30. Ben-Moshe, S.; Veg, T.; Manco, R.; Dan, S.; Papinutti, D.; Lifshitz, A.; Kolodziejczyk, A.A.; Bahar Halpern, K.; Elinav, E.; Itzkovitz, S. The spatiotemporal program of zonal liver regeneration following acute injury. *Cell Stem Cell* **2022**, *29*, 973–989. [CrossRef]
31. Jaeschke, H.; Adelusi, O.B.; Akakpo, J.Y.; Nguyen, N.T.; Sanchez-Guerrero, G.; Umbaugh, D.S.; Ding, W.X.; Ramachandran, A. Recommendations for the use of the acetaminophen hepatotoxicity model for mechanistic studies and how to avoid common pitfalls. *Acta Pharm. Sin. B* **2021**, *11*, 3740–3755. [CrossRef] [PubMed]

livers

MDPI

Review

Role of Pyroptosis in Acetaminophen-Induced Hepatotoxicity

Hartmut Jaeschke *, David S. Umbaugh and Anup Ramachandran

Department of Pharmacology, Toxicology and Therapeutics, University of Kansas Medical Center, Kansas City, KS 66160, USA
* Correspondence: hjaeschke@kumc.edu; Tel.: +1-913-588-7969

Abstract: Acetaminophen (APAP) is a widely used pain reliever that can cause liver injury or liver failure in response to an overdose. Understanding the mechanisms of APAP-induced cell death is critical for identifying new therapeutic targets. In this respect it was hypothesized that hepatocytes die by oncotic necrosis, apoptosis, necroptosis, ferroptosis and more recently pyroptosis. The latter cell death is characterized by caspase-dependent gasdermin cleavage into a C-terminal and an N-terminal fragment, which forms pores in the plasma membrane. The gasdermin pores can release potassium, interleukin-1β (IL-1β), IL-18, and other small molecules in a sublytic phase, which can be the main function of the pores in certain cell types such as inflammatory cells. Alternatively, the process can progress to full lysis of the cell (pyroptosis) with extensive cell contents release. This review discusses the experimental evidence for the involvement of pyroptosis in APAP hepatotoxicity as well as the arguments against pyroptosis as a relevant mechanism of APAP-induced cell death in hepatocytes. Based on the critical evaluation of the currently available literature and understanding of the pathophysiology, it can be concluded that pyroptotic cell death is unlikely to be a relevant contributor to APAP-induced liver injury.

Keywords: acetaminophen; hepatotoxicity; pyroptosis; gasdermin; inflammasome; caspases

1. Introduction

Acetaminophen (N-acetyl-p-aminophenol, APAP, paracetamol) is one of the most widely used pain reliever worldwide. At therapeutic doses, the drug is considered safe, but an overdose can induce liver injury and even acute liver failure [1,2]. Because of the wide-spread availability of APAP, intentional and accidental overdosing is relatively common, especially in western countries. Thus, APAP overdose is responsible for almost 50% and 70% of all acute liver failure cases in the US and the UK, respectively [3,4]. Because of the clinical significance, understanding the mechanisms of APAP-induced liver injury has been a priority for decades. Early investigations in mice showed that APAP is metabolized by cytochrome P450 enzymes to a reactive metabolite, now known as N-acetyl-p-benzoquinone imine (NAPQI), which can be detoxified by glutathione (GSH), and after hepatic GSH depletion, NAPQI binds to cellular proteins and initiates toxicity [5–7]. The identification of the critical role of GSH in protecting against APAP-induced cell death in preclinical models led to the development of the GSH precursor N-acetylcysteine (NAC) as clinical antidote against APAP poisoning [8]. More recently, the critical role of a mitochondrial oxidant stress and peroxynitrite formation was established in animals [9]. In addition, it was recognized that although the mitochondrial oxidant stress is initiated by protein adducts in mitochondria [10], activation of c-jun N-terminal kinase (JNK) in the cytosol and subsequent translocation of phospho-JNK to the mitochondria amplifies the formation of reactive oxygen and peroxynitrite in the mitochondrial matrix [11,12] leading to the opening of the mitochondrial membrane permeability transition pore (MPTP) and subsequent cell death [13]. This more detailed mechanistic insight resulted in the recognition of 4-methylpyrazole (Fomepizole), an effective inhibitor of cytochrome P450

2E1 (Cyp2E1) and JNK in mice, human hepatocytes and in patients [14–16], as a second possible clinical antidote against APAP poisoning [17,18].

Given that the mode of cell death is related to specific signaling events, substantial efforts were made to characterize the cell death after APAP overdose. Earlier studies in animals suggested necrosis or oncotic necrosis as the mode of cell death for drug- or chemical-induced liver injury due to cell and organelle swelling and release of cell contents [19]. It was thought that the cell death is caused by a catastrophic event, e.g., lipid peroxidation, calcium dysregulation, or protein adducts formation) [5–7,19,20]. However, over time more details emerged of the cellular signaling events resulting in APAP-induced necrosis [21–23], which led to the use of the term programmed necrosis [24,25]. During this time, it was also suggested that there might be substantial apoptotic cell death [26,27] but the lack of relevant caspase activation and cell shrinkage and absence of many other characteristics of apoptotic cell death did not support this hypothesis [28,29]. Necroptosis, a specific form of programmed necrosis, was also hypothesized to be involved in APAP-induced liver injury [30]. Although evidence for a role of receptor-interacting serine/threonine-protein 1 kinase (RIP1K) [30,31] and RIP3K [32,33] was provided, the fact that deficiency of mixed lineage kinase domain like pseudokinase (MLKL) did not protect against APAP hepatotoxicity [31], did not support necroptosis as a key cell death mode. In addition, ferroptosis, a cell death mechanism characterized by iron-dependent lipid peroxidation, was suggested to be involved in APAP-induced cell death [34]. However, under normal conditions, lipid peroxidation after APAP overdose is quantitatively insufficient to cause cell death and vitamin E does not protect [35]. Furthermore, lysosomal iron is taken up into mitochondria [36,37] and functions as a catalyst for peroxynitrite-mediated protein nitration critical for the mitochondrial MPTP opening, not lipid peroxidation [38]. This makes it unlikely that the key mode of cell death caused by APAP is ferroptosis [39]. More recently, it was suggested that the mode of cell death is actually pyroptosis [40–42], which raises the question whether there is any stronger evidence to support this newest idea for a mechanism of APAP hepatotoxicity than previously for apoptosis, necroptosis or ferroptosis.

2. Pyroptotic Cell Death Signaling

Pyroptosis is a necrotic programmed cell death mechanism that depends on gasdermin processing [43]. Although there are 6 known gasdermins, gasdermin D (GSDMD) is the prototypic gasdermin, which is present in most cell types including the liver [44]. GSDMD, as most other gasdermins, consists of a 31 kD N-terminal $GSDMD^{NT}$ fragment and a 22 kD C-terminal $GSDMD^{CT}$ fragment, which are connected through a linker region [44]. $GSDMD^{NT}$ forms pores in the cell membrane and $GSDMD^{CT}$ acts as a repressor of this pore formation [45–47]. The linker region contains caspase cleavage domains. Thus, based on the caspases involved, there is a canonical and a non-canonical inflammasome activation leading to pyroptosis [44] (Figure 1). In the canonical pathway, pathogen associated molecular patterns (PAMPs) or damage associated molecular patterns (DAMPs) activate cytosolic pattern recognition receptors including NOD-, LRR- and pyrin domain-containing protein 3 (NLRP3), which recruits the Apoptosis-associated speck-like protein containing a CARD (ASC) and pro-caspase-1. Caspase-1 is activated within the inflammasome and cleaves pro-IL-1β/pro-IL-18 to the active cytokine. In addition, caspase-1 also proteolytically releases $GSDMD^{NT}$ from GSDMD and the N-terminal fragment translocates to the plasma membrane and forms $GSDMD^{NT}$ pores [48]. These pores can trigger the release of IL-1β and IL-18 from the cell but eventually induce lytic cell death (pyroptosis) with extensive release of cellular contents through the ruptured cell membrane [44]. In contrast, the non-canonical inflammasome activation and pyroptosis is mediated by activation of caspase-11 (mice) or caspase 4 and 5 (humans) by lipopolysaccharide from Gram-negative bacteria. The active caspase-11 cleaves GSDMD, and the N-terminal fragments form a $GSDMD^{NT}$ pores. Cellular potassium release through the $GSDMD^{NT}$ pores triggers activation of the NLRP3 inflammasome with caspase 1 activation and pro-IL-1β/pro-IL-18 cleavage and release. In addition, GSDMD^{NT} pores induce the lytic cell death (pyroptosis) with cell swelling, plasma membrane rupture and extensive release of cellular contents [44].

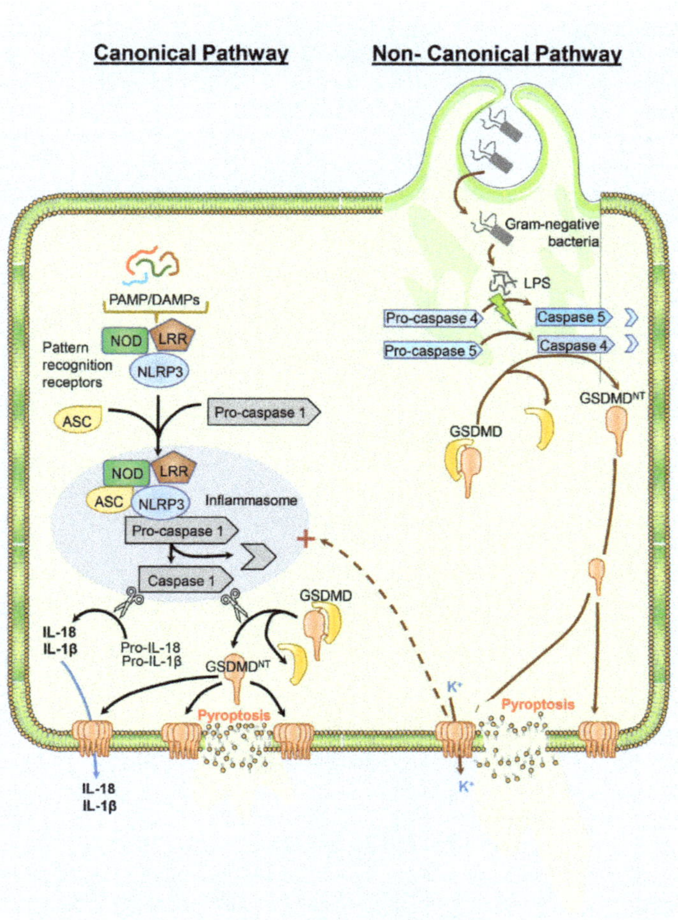

Figure 1. Pathways of pyroptosis. Gasdermin (GSDMD) cleavage and activation are central to pyroptotic cell death and can occur through a canonical or non-canonical pathway. The canonical pathway is initiated by recognition of pathogen associated molecular patterns (PAMPs) or damage associated molecular patterns (DAMPs) by cytosolic pattern recognition receptors such as NOD, LRR and NLRP3. These then recruit ASC and pro-caspase-1, which is activated to caspase-1 within the inflammasome. Caspase 1 cleaves pro-IL1β and pro-IL18 to the active cytokines, and also cleaves GSDMD to release the N-terminal domain (GSDMD^{NT}), which translocates to the plasma membrane to form pores. While the active cytokines can be released through the GSDMD^{NT} pores, these eventually cause lytic cell death with release of cellular contents through damaged cell membranes. In contrast to PAMPs and DAMPs, the non-canonical pyroptotic pathway is initiated by LPS from Gram-negative bacteria, which activates caspase 4 and 5 in humans. Activated caspase cleaves GSDMD as in the canonical pathway with formation of membrane pores, but cellular potassium release through the GSDMD^{NT} pores can induce activation of the NLRP3 inflammasome for IL-1β and IL-18 release. Ultimately, the pores again induce lytic cell death due to release of cell contents.

In addition to the classical cleavage of GSDMD by caspase-1, or -11 (mice) and -4, -5 (humans), there is evidence for some crosstalk between apoptotic and pyroptotic signaling [44]. For example, caspase-8 activated during apoptosis, can also cleave GSDMD and promote pore formation, although at a slower rate [49]. However, active caspase-3 can cleave and inactive the N-terminal fragment [50,51]. Thus, GSDMD can trigger pyroptosis during apoptotic cell death, however, the physiological function of GSDMD activation/inactivation during apoptosis remains to be determined [44].

Despite the well-described mechanism of pyroptosis, GSDMD cleavage may not always end up with cell lysis. In some cell types, especially monocytes and neutrophils, the main function of gasdermin pores may be just the release of mature IL-1β and IL-18 in the absence of cell death [52,53]. These sublytic gasdermin pores can not only release the cytokines IL-1β and IL-18 but also other small cytosolic proteins [53,54]. Importantly, the membrane channels can release ions such as potassium, which triggers activation of the NLRP3 inflammasome after initiation of the non-canonical pathway by lipopolysaccharide [55,56]. An interesting question is what determines sublytic versus lytic gasdermin pore formation. Although cell type-specific expression of gasdermins and activation of caspases may be important factors, it was also recognized that GSDMD pores can be removed by an endosomal sorting complex required for transport (ESCRT) [57]. The ESCRT is recruited to the plasma membrane by calcium influx through the GSDMD pore and promotes the budding and release of vesicles with the GSDMD pore-containing membrane parts [58]. This process can completely repair the membrane damage or at least limit the function of GSDMD pores to the sublytic phase. Together, the process of pyroptosis is well regulated by cell type-specific expression of gasdermins, the degree of caspase activation and gasdermin cleavage and pore formation and the counteracting repair processes.

3. Evidence for Pyroptosis in APAP Toxicity

Recently, pyroptosis has been suggested to be a relevant cell death pathway in the standard murine model of APAP hepatotoxicity, i.e., 12–24 h after a dose of 300 mg/kg APAP in fasted mice [40–42]. Wang et al. provided evidence for cleavage of gasdermin D and of caspase-1 along with a minor increase in IL-1β and IL-18 in plasma. These changes were observed in both Kupffer cells and in hepatocytes. In addition, knock-down of peroxiredoxin 3 (Prdx3) aggravated the injury and all pyroptosis parameters, and knock-down of NLRP3 reduced all pyroptosis parameters and the overall liver injury [40]. The authors concluded that Prdx3 inhibits APAP-induced pyroptosis by attenuating the mitochondrial oxidant stress and preventing NLRP3 inflammasome activation [40]. However, there are many concerns with the interpretation of these experiments. First, the mitochondria-specific peroxidase Prdx3 protects against mitochondrial dysfunction by removing hydrogen peroxide and especially peroxynitrite [59,60]. It is well documented that peroxynitrite is the most important mitochondrial oxidant generated during APAP overdose [61]. APAP toxicity was greatly diminished by facilitating the synthesis of GSH as scavenger of peroxynitrite [62], the deficiency of the mitochondrial SOD2 dramatically enhanced peroxynitrite formation and injury [63,64] and the mitochondria-specific SOD mimetic mito-tempo eliminated peroxynitrite formation and effectively protected [65]. Thus, it is not surprising that Prdx3, an effective peroxynitrite scavenger located in mitochondria, reduced APAP toxicity [40]. However, the mitochondrial stress and dysfunction after an APAP overdose causes the MPT pore opening and nuclear DNA fragmentation leading to programmed necrosis not pyroptosis [23,66]. Second, the overall changes in pyroptotic parameters such as cleavage of gasdermin D or caspase 1 is generally below 2–3-fold of baseline, which leads to very limited IL-1β and IL-18 formation [40]. In fact, the increase of plasma IL-1β levels from <10 pg/mL in controls to 20 pg/mL after APAP reported by the authors [40] is almost identical to levels published previously in a similar mouse model [67]. However, the minor changes in IL-1β were insufficient to impact the injury [67]. Moreover, a recent study did not observe protection against APAP or thioacetamide hepatotoxicity in gasdermin D- and E-knock-out mice [68]. Interestingly, this study also demonstrated that thioacetamide toxicity did not involve gasdermin D or E cleavage, but no data were provided on gasdermin cleavage after APAP [68]. In contrast, another report indicated increased APAP-induced liver injury in gasdermin D-deficient mice [69]. However, as discussed [25], this alleged protection by gasdermin D may have been the result of a substrain mismatch between the KO mice and the wildtype animals.

More recently, 2 additional manuscripts were published with the conclusion that pyroptosis may be a mode of cell death during APAP hepatotoxicity in mice [41,42]. The conclusion was based on only minor (<2-fold) increases in gasdermin-D, caspase-1 and NLRP3 protein expression at the whole liver level [41,42]. However, minor changes in protein expression are insufficient to explain extensive cellular necrosis and are certainly not specific for pyroptotic cell death. Furthermore, no specific intervention for pyroptosis was used to justify the conclusion that pyroptosis may be relevant for APAP-induced liver injury. Thus, most of the data and conclusions regarding the critical role of pyroptosis in APAP-induced liver injury are based on correlations and have to be questioned.

4. Evidence against Pyroptosis in Acetaminophen-Induced Liver Injury

As discussed above, key signaling events in pyroptotic cell death are the activation of the NLRP3 inflammasome with cleavage of pro-caspase 1. The active caspase cleaves gasdermin and the N-terminal fragments translocate to the cell membrane forming a pore to facilitate the release of IL-1β, and eventually cause cell death. A recent study showed that gasdermin D- and E-deficient mice are not protected against APAP hepatotoxicity [68]. Caspase 1 is one of many caspases that are all effectively inhibited by suicide substrates like Z-VAD-fmk. These caspase inhibitors bind irreversibly to the active caspase and block the enzyme activity [70]). Pancaspase inhibitors and inhibitors more specific for individual caspases, e.g., caspase 3 or -8, are highly effective in models of hepatocellular apoptosis such as galactosamine/endotoxin shock [71–73], or agonistic Fas antibody-induced liver injury [74–76] but fail to protect against APAP hepatotoxicity [28,67,77,78]. The few studies that claim a beneficial effect of pancaspase inhibitors in the APAP model [27,79] were later shown to be effects of the solvent dimethyl sulfoxide (DMSO) [78,80], which is an effective inhibitor of cytochrome P450 enzymes [81]. Nevertheless, when IL-1β formation was evaluated after an APAP overdose, there was a significant but moderate increase of IL-1β mRNA and mature IL-1β protein formation [67,82] suggesting activation of the inflammasome and caspase-1 in the mouse model. Indeed, a pancaspase inhibitor reduced IL-1β protein levels but did not affect IL-1β mRNA levels [67]. However, the IL-1β levels were far below concentrations that could have affected APAP-induced liver injury both in mice [67,83] and in human overdose patients [84], which is consistent with the fact that IL-1 receptor-deficient mice are not protected against APAP hepatotoxicity [67].

The sterile inflammatory response after an APAP overdose is initiated by the release of DAMPs from necrotic hepatocytes including mitochondrial DNA and nuclear DNA fragments [85], which bind to Toll-like receptors, e.g., TLR9, on Kupffer cells and trigger the transcriptional activation of pro-inflammatory cytokine genes [82,86]. Additional DAMPs like ATP activate the NLRP3 inflammasome by binding to the purine receptor P2X7 on Kupffer cells, which causes the activation of caspase-1 and processing of pro-IL-1β to the active cytokine [48]. In addition to the relatively moderate formation of these active cytokines, the fundamental issue is that the activation of the inflammasome and caspase-1 and IL-1β formation occurs mainly in Kupffer cells [83] whereas the main APAP-induced cell death occurs in hepatocytes. This would question the possibility that caspase-mediated pyroptosis could be responsible for APAP-induced hepatocyte necrosis. Consistent with these findings, analysis of time series single-cell RNA sequencing data during APAP hepatotoxicity reveals that Kupffer cells and infiltrating macrophages are the primary cells expressing the pyroptotic genes Casp1, IL-1β, Gsdmd and Nlrp3 while hepatocytes, regardless of spatial location within the liver lobule, maintain very low expression levels for these pyroptotic genes (Figure 2) [87–89]. A limitation of the single cell data is that it cannot distinguish between the original Kupffer cells and monocyte-derived macrophages that may have shifted their phenotype during the resolution phase of the injury. However, this does not affect our conclusion that genes related to pyroptosis are primarily located in macrophages and not in hepatocytes, which means that hepatocytes are unlikely to be able to die by pyroptosis. Collectively, these findings support a potential role of pyroptosis to resolve the sterile inflammatory response after an APAP overdose, however, pyroptosis as the primary mode of hepatocyte cell death is unlikely.

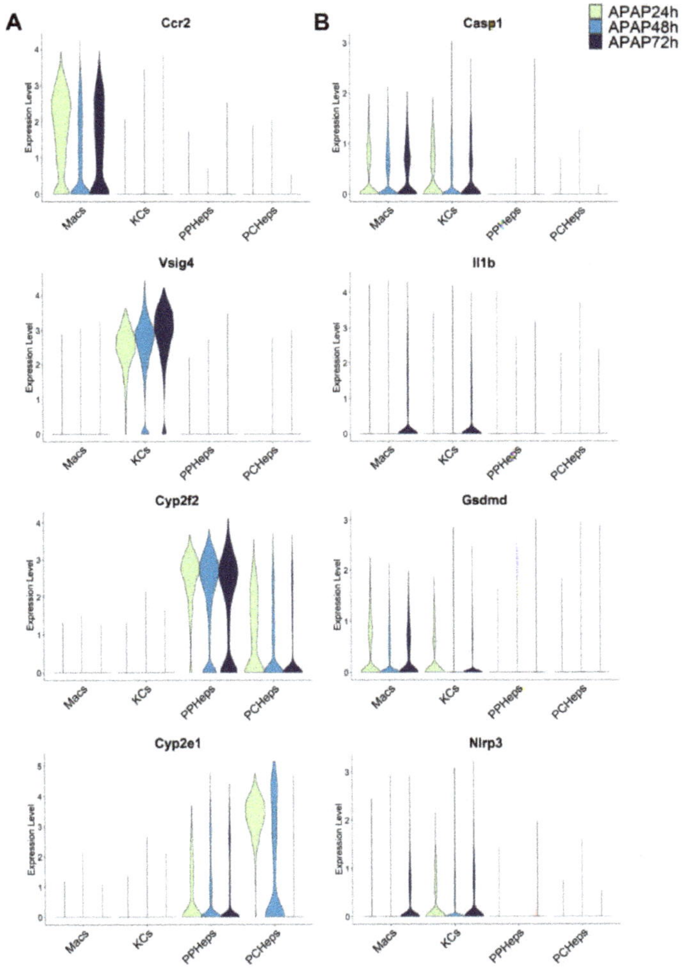

Figure 2. Single-cell RNA sequencing data reveal pyroptotic genes are expressed predominantly in infiltrating macrophages (Macs) or Kupffer cells (KCs) during the acetaminophen time course (24, 48, 72 h) in mice. Data in the left column (**A**) show representative cell type markers for infiltrating macrophages (Ccr2), KCs (Vsig4), periportal hepatocytes (cyp2f2) and pericentral hepatocytes (cyp2e1). Data in the right column (**B**) show canonical genes of pyroptosis (Casp1, IL-1β, Gsdmd, and Nlrp3). Single-cell RNA seq data were aggregated from publicly available datasets (GSE136679, GSE200771, zenodo.6035873).

5. Summary and Conclusions

The mode of cell death after an APAP overdose has been extensively investigated and discussed [24,25]. Besides oncotic necrosis, other forms of cell death including apoptosis, necroptosis, ferroptosis and most recently pyroptosis have been implicated in APAP-induced liver injury. However, one glaring weakness of many studies claiming one of these cell death pathways as central to the toxicity is the lack of discussion of other cell death pathways and the fact that others have come to fundamentally different conclusions. A problem in this respect is that there are overlap in signaling pathways between different modes of cell death (discussed in detail: [25,90]), which can lead to misinterpretations. For example, the translocation of Bax to the mitochondria and formation of pores in the outer mitochondrial membrane, which can induce release of cytochrome c and other intermembrane proteins, is generally considered a pro-apoptotic signaling event [91]. However, mitochondrial Bax translocation is an early event in APAP hepatotoxicity that facilitates the release of endonuclease G and apoptosis-inducing factor (AIF) from mitochondria and promotes nuclear DNA fragmentation [92]. Thus, Bax pores amplify caspase activation through mitochondrial cytochrome c release during apoptosis but promote nuclear DNA degradation through mitochondrial endonuclease G release and its translocation to the nucleus during APAP-induced necrosis. Importantly, these events do not require transcriptional activation of Bax. It is therefore important to not just associate the increased expression of mRNAs or proteins of certain genes presumably associated with a cell death pathway but fully understand the functional importance of the genes in the signaling events of cell death. For pyroptosis, this means that neither increased protein expression of inflammasome components, caspase-1 nor gasdermins are evidence for pyroptotic cell death. In contrast, activation of caspase-1, cleavage of gasdermins and translocation of the N-terminal fragment to the cell membrane and pore formation are the critical events [44]. Although evidence was provided for modest caspase-1 and gasdermin D cleavage and limited formation of IL-1β and IL-18 in both hepatocytes and Kupffer cells after APAP overdose [40], gasdermin D gene knockout mice were not protected against APAP toxicity [68,69] suggesting no relevant pyroptosis in APAP-induced liver injury. However, based on the experience with apoptosis [29,93] and ferroptosis [39] in APAP hepatotoxicity, questionable evidence (minor increases of mRNAs or protein expression of genes presumably related to pyroptosis) can be expected to be used by other authors in the future as evidence for pyroptosis. Unfortunately, this will only add to the confusion but not advance our understanding of the pathophysiology of APAP or the mechanism of protection with various interventions. We hope that our discussion can limit the casual use of cell death modes like pyroptosis based on gene expression data and encourage proper investigations into this cell death pathway using specific interventions, e.g., gasdermin D gene knockout mice, and documentation of quantitively relevant inflammasome activation and gasdermin pore formation in specific cell types of the liver. Furthermore, authors should integrate their new findings with earlier available information on necrotic cell signaling after an APAP overdose in order to make progress in understanding the nuances of APAP pathophysiology.

Author Contributions: H.J. conceived the manuscript and wrote the first draft. A.R. edited the manuscript and generated the graphic. D.S.U. edited the manuscript and performed the bioinformatic analysis of scRNA seq data and generated the figure. All authors have read and agreed to the published version of the manuscript.

Funding: The work discussed was supported in part by the U.S. National Institutes of Health grants R01 DK102142 (H.J.) and R01 DK125465 (A.R).

Data Availability Statement: Single-cell RNA seq data were aggregated from publicly available datasets (GSE136679, GSE200771, zenodo.6035873).

Conflicts of Interest: The authors declare no conflict of interest.

References

1. Jaeschke, H. Acetaminophen: Dose-Dependent Drug Hepatotoxicity and Acute Liver Failure in Patients. *Dig. Dis.* **2015**, *33*, 464–471. [CrossRef] [PubMed]
2. Larson, A.M. Acetaminophen hepatotoxicity. *Clin. Liver Dis.* **2007**, *11*, 525–548. [CrossRef] [PubMed]
3. Bernal, W.; Wendon, J. Acute liver failure. *N. Engl. J. Med.* **2013**, *369*, 2525–2534. [CrossRef] [PubMed]

4. Stravitz, R.T.; Lee, W.M. Acute liver failure. *Lancet* **2019**, *394*, 869–881. [CrossRef] [PubMed]
5. Mitchell, J.R.; Jollow, D.J.; Potter, W.Z.; Davis, D.C.; Gillette, J.R.; Brodie, B.B. Acetaminophen-induced hepatic necrosis. I. Role of drug metabolism. *J. Pharmacol. Exp. Ther.* **1973**, *187*, 185–194.
6. Jollow, D.J.; Mitchell, J.R.; Potter, W.Z.; Davis, D.C.; Gillette, J.R.; Brodie, B.B. Acetaminophen-induced hepatic necrosis. II. Role of covalent binding in vivo. *J. Pharmacol. Exp. Ther.* **1973**, *187*, 195–202.
7. Mitchell, J.R.; Jollow, D.J.; Potter, W.Z.; Gillette, J.R.; Brodie, B.B. Acetaminophen-induced hepatic necrosis. IV. Protective role of glutathione. *J. Pharmacol. Exp. Ther.* **1973**, *187*, 211–217.
8. Rumack, B.H.; Bateman, D.N. Acetaminophen and acetylcysteine dose and duration: Past, present and future. *Clin. Toxicol.* **2012**, *50*, 91–98. [CrossRef]
9. Du, K.; Ramachandran, A.; Jaeschke, H. Oxidative stress during acetaminophen hepatotoxicity: Sources, pathophysiological role and therapeutic potential. *Redox Biol.* **2016**, *10*, 148–156. [CrossRef]
10. Nguyen, N.T.; Du, K.; Akakpo, J.Y.; Umbaugh, D.S.; Jaeschke, H.; Ramachandran, A. Mitochondrial protein adduct and superoxide generation are prerequisites for early activation of c-jun N-terminal kinase within the cytosol after an acetaminophen overdose in mice. *Toxicol. Lett.* **2021**, *338*, 21–31. [CrossRef]
11. Hanawa, N.; Shinohara, M.; Saberi, B.; Gaarde, W.A.; Han, D.; Kaplowitz, N. Role of JNK translocation to mitochondria leading to inhibition of mitochondria bioenergetics in acetaminophen-induced liver injury. *J. Biol. Chem.* **2008**, *283*, 13565–13577. [CrossRef] [PubMed]
12. Saito, C.; Lemasters, J.J.; Jaeschke, H. c-Jun N-terminal kinase modulates oxidant stress and peroxynitrite formation independent of inducible nitric oxide synthase in acetaminophen hepatotoxicity. *Toxicol. Appl. Pharmacol.* **2010**, *246*, 8–17. [CrossRef] [PubMed]
13. Kon, K.; Kim, J.S.; Jaeschke, H.; Lemasters, J.J. Mitochondrial permeability transition in acetaminophen-induced necrosis and apoptosis of cultured mouse hepatocytes. *Hepatology* **2004**, *40*, 1170–1179. [CrossRef] [PubMed]
14. Akakpo, J.Y.; Ramachandran, A.; Kandel, S.E.; Ni, H.M.; Kumer, S.C.; Rumack, B.H.; Jaeschke, H. 4-Methylpyrazole protects against acetaminophen hepatotoxicity in mice and in primary human hepatocytes. *Hum. Exp. Toxicol.* **2018**, *37*, 1310–1322. [CrossRef] [PubMed]
15. Kang, A.M.; Padilla-Jones, A.; Fisher, E.S.; Akakpo, J.Y.; Jaeschke, H.; Rumack, B.H.; Gerkin, R.D.; Curry, S.C. The Effect of 4-Methylpyrazole on Oxidative Metabolism of Acetaminophen in Human Volunteers. *J. Med. Toxicol.* **2020**, *16*, 169–176. [CrossRef]
16. Akakpo, J.Y.; Ramachandran, A.; Duan, L.; Schaich, M.A.; Jaeschke, M.W.; Freudenthal, B.D.; Ding, W.X.; Rumack, B.H.; Jaeschke, H. Delayed Treatment With 4-Methylpyrazole Protects Against Acetaminophen Hepatotoxicity in Mice by Inhibition of c-Jun n-Terminal Kinase. *Toxicol. Sci.* **2019**, *170*, 57–68. [CrossRef]
17. Akakpo, J.Y.; Ramachandran, A.; Curry, S.C.; Rumack, B.H.; Jaeschke, H. Comparing N-acetylcysteine and 4-methylpyrazole as antidotes for acetaminophen overdose. *Arch. Toxicol.* **2022**, *96*, 453–465. [CrossRef]
18. Kaiser, S.K.; Dart, R.C. The roles of antidotes in emergency situations. *Emerg. Med. Clin. N. Am.* **2022**, *40*, 381–394. [CrossRef]
19. Farber, J.L. The biochemical pathology of toxic cell death. *Monogr. Pathol.* **1985**, *26*, 19–31.
20. Poli, G.; Albano, E.; Dianzani, M.U. The role of lipid peroxidation in liver damage. *Chem. Phys. Lipids* **1987**, *45*, 117–142. [CrossRef]
21. Jaeschke, H.; Bajt, M.L. Intracellular signaling mechanisms of acetaminophen-induced liver cell death. *Toxicol. Sci.* **2006**, *89*, 31–41. [CrossRef] [PubMed]
22. Jaeschke, H.; McGill, M.R.; Ramachandran, A. Oxidant stress, mitochondria, and cell death mechanisms in drug-induced liver injury: Lessons learned from acetaminophen hepatotoxicity. *Drug Metab. Rev.* **2012**, *44*, 88–106. [CrossRef] [PubMed]
23. Ramachandran, A.; Jaeschke, H. Acetaminophen hepatotoxicity. *Semin. Liver Dis.* **2019**, *39*, 221–234. [CrossRef] [PubMed]
24. Jaeschke, H.; Ramachandran, A.; Chao, X.; Ding, W.X. Emerging and established modes of cell death during acetaminophen-induced liver injury. *Arch. Toxicol.* **2019**, *93*, 3491–3502. [CrossRef]
25. Iorga, A.; Dara, L. Cell death in drug-induced liver injury. *Adv. Pharmacol.* **2019**, *85*, 31–74.
26. Ray, S.D.; Mumaw, V.R.; Raje, R.R.; Fariss, M.W. Protection of acetaminophen-induced hepatocellular apoptosis and necrosis by cholesteryl hemisuccinate pretreatment. *J. Pharmacol. Exp. Ther.* **1996**, *279*, 1470–1483.
27. El-Hassan, H.; Anwar, K.; Macanas-Pirard, P.; Crabtree, M.; Chow, S.C.; Johnson, V.L.; Lee, P.C.; Hinton, R.H.; Price, S.C.; Kass, G.E. Involvement of mitochondria in acetaminophen-induced apoptosis and hepatic injury: Roles of cytochrome c, Bax, Bid, and caspases. *Toxicol. Appl. Pharmacol.* **2003**, *191*, 118–129. [CrossRef]
28. Gujral, J.S.; Knight, T.R.; Farhood, A.; Bajt, M.L.; Jaeschke, H. Mode of cell death after acetaminophen overdose in mice: Apoptosis or oncotic necrosis? *Toxicol. Sci.* **2002**, *67*, 322–328. [CrossRef]
29. Jaeschke, H.; Duan, L.; Akakpo, J.Y.; Farhood, A.; Ramachandran, A. The role of apoptosis in acetaminophen hepatotoxicity. *Food Chem. Toxicol.* **2018**, *118*, 709–718. [CrossRef]
30. Zhang, Y.F.; He, W.; Zhang, C.; Liu, X.J.; Lu, Y.; Wang, H.; Zhang, Z.H.; Chen, X.; Xu, D.X. Role of receptor interacting protein (RIP)1 on apoptosis-inducing factor-mediated necroptosis during acetaminophen-evoked acute liver failure in mice. *Toxicol. Lett.* **2014**, *225*, 445–453. [CrossRef]
31. Dara, L.; Johnson, H.; Suda, J.; Win, S.; Gaarde, W.; Han, D.; Kaplowitz, N. Receptor interacting protein kinase 1 mediates murine acetaminophen toxicity independent of the necrosome and not through necroptosis. *Hepatology* **2015**, *62*, 1847–1857. [CrossRef]
32. Ramachandran, A.; McGill, M.R.; Xie, Y.; Ni, H.M.; Ding, W.X.; Jaeschke, H. Receptor interacting protein kinase 3 is a critical early mediator of acetaminophen-induced hepatocyte necrosis in mice. *Hepatology* **2013**, *58*, 2099–2108. [CrossRef] [PubMed]

33. Deutsch, M.; Graffeo, C.S.; Rokosh, R.; Pansari, M.; Ochi, A.; Levie, E.M.; Van Heerden, E.; Tippens, D.M.; Greco, S.; Barilla, R.; et al. Divergent effects of RIP1 or RIP3 blockade in murine models of acute liver injury. *Cell Death Dis.* **2015**, *6*, e1759. [CrossRef]
34. Yamada, N.; Karasawa, T.; Kimura, H.; Watanabe, S.; Komada, T.; Kamata, R.; Sampilvanjil, A.; Ito, J.; Nakagawa, K.; Kuwata, H.; et al. Ferroptosis driven by radical oxidation of n-6 polyunsaturated fatty acids mediates acetaminophen-induced acute liver failure. *Cell Death Dis.* **2020**, *11*, 144. [CrossRef] [PubMed]
35. Knight, T.R.; Fariss, M.W.; Farhood, A.; Jaeschke, H. Role of lipid peroxidation as a mechanism of liver injury after acetaminophen overdose in mice. *Toxicol. Sci.* **2003**, *76*, 229–236. [CrossRef] [PubMed]
36. Kon, K.; Kim, J.S.; Uchiyama, A.; Jaeschke, H.; Lemasters, J.J. Lysosomal iron mobilization and induction of the mitochondrial permeability transition in acetaminophen-induced toxicity to mouse hepatocytes. *Toxicol. Sci.* **2010**, *117*, 101–108. [CrossRef] [PubMed]
37. Hu, J.; Kholmukhamedov, A.; Lindsey, C.C.; Beeson, C.C.; Jaeschke, H.; Lemasters, J.J. Translocation of iron from lysosomes to mitochondria during acetaminophen-induced hepatocellular injury: Protection by starch-desferal and minocycline. *Free Radic. Biol. Med.* **2016**, *97*, 418–426. [CrossRef]
38. Adelusi, O.B.; Ramachandran, A.; Lemasters, J.J.; Jaeschke, H. The role of iron in lipid peroxidation and protein nitration during acetaminophen-induced liver injury in mice. *Toxicol. Appl. Pharmacol.* **2022**, *445*, 116043. [CrossRef]
39. Jaeschke, H.; Adelusi, O.B.; Ramachandran, A. Ferroptosis and Acetaminophen Hepatotoxicity: Are We Going Down Another Rabbit Hole? *Gene Expr.* **2021**, *20*, 169–178. [CrossRef]
40. Wang, Y.; Zhao, Y.; Wang, Z.; Sun, R.; Zou, B.; Li, R.; Liu, D.; Lin, M.; Zhou, J.; Ning, S.; et al. Peroxiredoxin 3 Inhibits Acetaminophen-Induced Liver Pyroptosis Through the Regulation of Mitochondrial ROS. *Front. Immunol.* **2021**, *12*, 652782. [CrossRef]
41. Liu, T.; Yang, L.; Gao, H.; Zhuo, Y.; Tu, Z.; Wang, Y.; Xun, J.; Zhang, Q.; Zhang, L.; Wang, X. 3,4-dihydroxyphenylethyl alcohol glycoside reduces acetaminophen-induced acute liver failure in mice by inhibiting hepatocyte ferroptosis and pyroptosis. *PeerJ* **2022**, *10*, e13082. [CrossRef] [PubMed]
42. Rousta, A.M.; Mirahmadi, S.M.; Shahmohammadi, A.; Mehrabi, Z.; Fallah, S.; Baluchnejadmojarad, T.; Roghani, M. Therapeutic Potential of Isorhamnetin following Acetaminophen-Induced Hepatotoxicity through Targeting NLRP3/NF-κB/Nrf2. *Drug Res.* **2022**, *72*, 245–254. [CrossRef] [PubMed]
43. Shi, J.; Gao, W.; Shao, F. Pyroptosis: Gasdermin-Mediated Programmed Necrotic Cell Death. *Trends Biochem. Sci.* **2017**, *42*, 245–254. [CrossRef] [PubMed]
44. Broz, P.; Pelegrín, P.; Shao, F. The gasdermins, a protein family executing cell death and inflammation. *Nat. Rev. Immunol.* **2020**, *20*, 143–157. [CrossRef] [PubMed]
45. Kayagaki, N.; Stowe, I.B.; Lee, B.L.; O'Rourke, K.; Anderson, K.; Warming, S.; Cuellar, T.; Haley, B.; Roose-Girma, M.; Phung, Q.T.; et al. Caspase-11 cleaves gasdermin D for non-canonical inflammasome signalling. *Nature* **2015**, *526*, 666–671. [CrossRef] [PubMed]
46. Shi, J.; Zhao, Y.; Wang, K.; Shi, X.; Wang, Y.; Huang, H.; Zhuang, Y.; Cai, T.; Wang, F.; Shao, F. Cleavage of GSDMD by inflammatory caspases determines pyroptotic cell death. *Nature* **2015**, *526*, 660–665. [CrossRef]
47. He, W.T.; Wan, H.; Hu, L.; Chen, P.; Wang, X.; Huang, Z.; Yang, Z.H.; Zhong, C.Q.; Han, J. Gasdermin D is an executor of pyroptosis and required for interleukin-1β secretion. *Cell Res.* **2015**, *25*, 1285–1298. [CrossRef]
48. Woolbright, B.L.; Jaeschke, H. Role of the inflammasome in acetaminophen-induced liver injury and acute liver failure. *J. Hepatol.* **2017**, *66*, 836–848. [CrossRef]
49. Orning, P.; Weng, D.; Starheim, K.; Ratner, D.; Best, Z.; Lee, B.; Brooks, A.; Xia, S.; Wu, H.; Kelliher, M.A.; et al. Pathogen blockade of TAK1 triggers caspase-8-dependent cleavage of gasdermin D and cell death. *Science* **2018**, *362*, 1064–1069. [CrossRef]
50. Rogers, C.; Fernandes-Alnemri, T.; Mayes, L.; Alnemri, D.; Cingolani, G.; Alnemri, E.S. Cleavage of DFNA5 by caspase-3 during apoptosis mediates progression to secondary necrotic/pyroptotic cell death. *Nat. Commun.* **2017**, *8*, 14128. [CrossRef]
51. Taabazuing, C.Y.; Okondo, M.C.; Bachovchin, D.A. Pyroptosis and Apoptosis Pathways Engage in Bidirectional Crosstalk in Monocytes and Macrophages. *Cell Chem. Biol.* **2017**, *24*, 507–514. [CrossRef] [PubMed]
52. Evavold, C.L.; Ruan, J.; Tan, Y.; Xia, S.; Wu, H.; Kagan, J.C. The Pore-Forming Protein Gasdermin D Regulates Interleukin-1 Secretion from Living Macrophages. *Immunity* **2018**, *48*, 35–44.e6. [CrossRef] [PubMed]
53. Heilig, R.; Dick, M.S.; Sborgi, L.; Meunier, E.; Hiller, S.; Broz, P. The Gasdermin-D pore acts as a conduit for IL-1β secretion in mice. *Eur. J. Immunol.* **2018**, *48*, 584–592. [CrossRef] [PubMed]
54. de Torre-Minguela, C.; Barberà-Cremades, M.; Gómez, A.I.; Martín-Sánchez, F.; Pelegrín, P. Macrophage activation and polarization modify P2X7 receptor secretome influencing the inflammatory process. *Sci. Rep.* **2016**, *6*, 22586. [CrossRef] [PubMed]
55. Kayagaki, N.; Warming, S.; Lamkanfi, M.; Vande Walle, L.; Louie, S.; Dong, J.; Newton, K.; Qu, Y.; Liu, J.; Heldens, S.; et al. Non-canonical inflammasome activation targets caspase-11. *Nature* **2011**, *479*, 117–121. [CrossRef] [PubMed]
56. Rühl, S.; Broz, P. Caspase-11 activates a canonical NLRP3 inflammasome by promoting K(+) efflux. *Eur. J. Immunol.* **2015**, *45*, 2927–2936. [CrossRef] [PubMed]
57. Cooper, S.T.; McNeil, P.L. Membrane Repair: Mechanisms and Pathophysiology. *Physiol. Rev.* **2015**, *95*, 1205–1240. [CrossRef] [PubMed]
58. Rühl, S.; Shkarina, K.; Demarco, B.; Heilig, R.; Santos, J.C.; Broz, P. ESCRT-dependent membrane repair negatively regulates pyroptosis downstream of GSDMD activation. *Science* **2018**, *362*, 956–960. [CrossRef] [PubMed]

59. Trujillo, M.; Ferrer-Sueta, G.; Radi, R. Kinetic studies on peroxynitrite reduction by peroxiredoxins. *Methods Enzymol.* **2008**, *441*, 173–196.
60. Trujillo, M.; Ferrer-Sueta, G.; Thomson, L.; Flohé, L.; Radi, R. Kinetics of peroxiredoxins and their role in the decomposition of peroxynitrite. *Subcell. Biochem.* **2007**, *44*, 83–113.
61. Cover, C.; Mansouri, A.; Knight, T.R.; Bajt, M.L.; Lemasters, J.J.; Pessayre, D.; Jaeschke, H. Peroxynitrite-induced mitochondrial and endonuclease-mediated nuclear DNA damage in acetaminophen hepatotoxicity. *J. Pharmacol. Exp. Ther.* **2005**, *315*, 879–887. [CrossRef] [PubMed]
62. Knight, T.R.; Ho, Y.S.; Farhood, A.; Jaeschke, H. Peroxynitrite is a critical mediator of acetaminophen hepatotoxicity in murine livers: Protection by glutathione. *J. Pharmacol. Exp. Ther.* **2002**, *303*, 468–475. [CrossRef] [PubMed]
63. Fujimoto, K.; Kumagai, K.; Ito, K.; Arakawa, S.; Ando, Y.; Oda, S.; Yamoto, T.; Manabe, S. Sensitivity of liver injury in heterozygous Sod2 knockout mice treated with troglitazone or acetaminophen. *Toxicol. Pathol.* **2009**, *37*, 193–200. [CrossRef] [PubMed]
64. Ramachandran, A.; Lebofsky, M.; Weinman, S.A.; Jaeschke, H. The impact of partial manganese superoxide dismutase (SOD2)-deficiency on mitochondrial oxidant stress, DNA fragmentation and liver injury during acetaminophen hepatotoxicity. *Toxicol. Appl. Pharmacol.* **2011**, *251*, 226–233. [CrossRef] [PubMed]
65. Du, K.; Farhood, A.; Jaeschke, H. Mitochondria-targeted antioxidant Mito-Tempo protects against acetaminophen hepatotoxicity. *Arch. Toxicol.* **2017**, *91*, 761–773. [CrossRef] [PubMed]
66. Ramachandran, A.; Jaeschke, H. Acetaminophen Toxicity: Novel Insights into Mechanisms and Future Perspectives. *Gene Expr.* **2018**, *18*, 19–30. [CrossRef] [PubMed]
67. Williams, C.D.; Farhood, A.; Jaeschke, H. Role of caspase-1 and interleukin-1beta in acetaminophen-induced hepatic inflammation and liver injury. *Toxicol. Appl. Pharmacol.* **2010**, *247*, 169–178. [CrossRef]
68. Li, Z.; Wang, H.; Zhu, J.; Nan, N.; Lin, Y.; Zhuang, X.; Li, L.; Zhang, Y.; Huang, P. Inhibition of TWEAK/Tnfrsf12a axis protects against acute liver failure by suppressing RIPK1-dependent apoptosis. *Cell Death Discov.* **2022**, *8*, 328. [CrossRef]
69. Yang, C.; Sun, P.; Deng, M.; Loughran, P.; Li, W.; Yi, Z.; Li, S.; Zhang, X.; Fan, J.; Billiar, T.R.; et al. Gasdermin D protects against noninfectious liver injury by regulating apoptosis and necroptosis. *Cell Death Dis.* **2019**, *10*, 481. [CrossRef]
70. Concha, N.O.; Abdel-Meguid, S.S. Controlling apoptosis by inhibition of caspases. *Curr. Med. Chem.* **2002**, *9*, 713–726. [CrossRef]
71. Jaeschke, H.; Fisher, M.; Lawson, J.A.; Simmons, C.A.; Farhood, A.; Jones, D.A. Activation of caspase 3 (CPP32)-like proteases is essential for TNF-alpha-induced hepatic parenchymal cell apoptosis and neutrophil-mediated necrosis in a murine endotoxin shock model. *J. Immunol.* **1998**, *160*, 3480–3486. [PubMed]
72. Jaeschke, H.; Farhood, A.; Cai, S.X.; Tseng, B.Y.; Bajt, M.L. Protection against TNF-induced liver parenchymal cell apoptosis during endotoxemia by a novel caspase inhibitor in mice. *Toxicol. Appl. Pharmacol.* **2000**, *169*, 77–83. [CrossRef] [PubMed]
73. Bajt, M.L.; Vonderfecht, S.L.; Jaeschke, H. Differential protection with inhibitors of caspase-8 and caspase-3 in murine models of tumor necrosis factor and Fas receptor-mediated hepatocellular apoptosis. *Toxicol. Appl. Pharmacol.* **2001**, *175*, 243–252. [CrossRef]
74. Rodriguez, I.; Matsuura, K.; Ody, C.; Nagata, S.; Vassalli, P. Systemic injection of a tripeptide inhibits the intracellular activation of CPP32-like proteases in vivo and fully protects mice against Fas-mediated fulminant liver destruction and death. *J. Exp. Med.* **1996**, *184*, 2067–2072. [CrossRef] [PubMed]
75. Künstle, G.; Leist, M.; Uhlig, S.; Revesz, L.; Feifel, R.; MacKenzie, A.; Wendel, A. ICE-protease inhibitors block murine liver injury and apoptosis caused by CD95 or by TNF-alpha. *Immunol. Lett.* **1997**, *55*, 5–10. [CrossRef] [PubMed]
76. Bajt, M.L.; Lawson, J.A.; Vonderfecht, S.L.; Gujral, J.S.; Jaeschke, H. Protection against Fas receptor-mediated apoptosis in hepatocytes and nonparenchymal cells by a caspase-8 inhibitor in vivo: Evidence for a postmitochondrial processing of caspase-8. *Toxicol. Sci.* **2000**, *58*, 109–117. [CrossRef] [PubMed]
77. Lawson, J.A.; Fisher, M.A.; Simmons, C.A.; Farhood, A.; Jaeschke, H. Inhibition of Fas receptor (CD95)-induced hepatic caspase activation and apoptosis by acetaminophen in mice. *Toxicol. Appl. Pharmacol.* **1999**, *156*, 179–186. [CrossRef]
78. Jaeschke, H.; Cover, C.; Bajt, M.L. Role of caspases in acetaminophen-induced liver injury. *Life Sci.* **2006**, *78*, 1670–1676. [CrossRef]
79. Hu, B.; Colletti, L.M. CXC receptor-2 knockout genotype increases X-linked inhibitor of apoptosis protein and protects mice from acetaminophen hepatotoxicity. *Hepatology* **2010**, *52*, 691–702. [CrossRef]
80. Jaeschke, H.; Williams, C.D.; Farhood, A. No evidence for caspase-dependent apoptosis in acetaminophen hepatotoxicity. *Hepatology* **2011**, *53*, 718–719. [CrossRef]
81. Kelava, T.; Cavar, I.; Culo, F. Influence of small doses of various drug vehicles on acetaminophen-induced liver injury. *Can. J. Physiol. Pharmacol.* **2010**, *88*, 960–967. [CrossRef] [PubMed]
82. Imaeda, A.B.; Watanabe, A.; Sohail, M.A.; Mahmood, S.; Mohamadnejad, M.; Sutterwala, F.S.; Flavell, R.A.; Mehal, W.Z. Acetaminophen-induced hepatotoxicity in mice is dependent on Tlr9 and the Nalp3 inflammasome. *J. Clin. Investig.* **2009**, *119*, 305–314. [CrossRef] [PubMed]
83. Zhang, C.; Feng, J.; Du, J.; Zhuo, Z.; Yang, S.; Zhang, W.; Wang, W.; Zhang, S.; Iwakura, Y.; Meng, G.; et al. Macrophage-derived IL-1α promotes sterile inflammation in a mouse model of acetaminophen hepatotoxicity. *Cell. Mol. Immunol.* **2018**, *15*, 973–982. [CrossRef] [PubMed]
84. Woolbright, B.L.; Nguyen, N.T.; McGill, M.R.; Sharpe, M.R.; Curry, S.C.; Jaeschke, H. Generation of pro-and anti-inflammatory mediators after acetaminophen overdose in surviving and non-surviving patients. *Toxicol. Lett.* **2022**, *367*, 59–66. [CrossRef]

85. McGill, M.R.; Sharpe, M.R.; Williams, C.D.; Taha, M.; Curry, S.C.; Jaeschke, H. The mechanism underlying acetaminophen-induced hepatotoxicity in humans and mice involves mitochondrial damage and nuclear DNA fragmentation. *J. Clin. Investig.* **2012**, *122*, 1574–1583. [CrossRef] [PubMed]
86. Marques, P.E.; Oliveira, A.G.; Pereira, R.V.; David, B.A.; Gomides, L.F.; Saraiva, A.M.; Pires, D.A.; Novaes, J.T.; Patricio, D.O.; Cisalpino, D.; et al. Hepatic DNA deposition drives drug-induced liver injury and inflammation in mice. *Hepatology* **2015**, *61*, 348–360. [CrossRef] [PubMed]
87. Umbaugh, D.S.; Ramachandran, A.; Jaeschke, H. Spatial Reconstruction of the Early Hepatic Transcriptomic Landscape After an Acetaminophen Overdose Using Single-Cell RNA-Sequencing. *Toxicol. Sci.* **2021**, *182*, 327–345. [CrossRef]
88. Walesky, C.M.; Kolb, K.E.; Winston, C.L.; Henderson, J.; Kruft, B.; Fleming, I.; Ko, S.; Monga, S.P.; Mueller, F.; Apte, U.; et al. Functional compensation precedes recovery of tissue mass following acute liver injury. *Nat. Commun.* **2020**, *11*, 5785. [CrossRef]
89. Ben-Moshe, S.; Veg, T.; Manco, R.; Dan, S.; Papinutti, D.; Lifshitz, A.; Kolodziejczyk, A.A.; Bahar Halpern, K.; Elinav, E.; Itzkovitz, S. The spatiotemporal program of zonal liver regeneration following acute injury. *Cell Stem Cell* **2022**, *29*, 973–989.e10. [CrossRef]
90. Iorga, A.; Dara, L.; Kaplowitz, N. Drug-Induced Liver Injury: Cascade of Events Leading to Cell Death, Apoptosis or Necrosis. *Int. J. Mol. Sci.* **2017**, *18*, 1018. [CrossRef]
91. Renault, T.T.; Floros, K.V.; Elkholi, R.; Corrigan, K.A.; Kushnareva, Y.; Wieder, S.Y.; Lindtner, C.; Serasinghe, M.N.; Asciolla, J.J.; Buettner, C.; et al. Mitochondrial shape governs BAX-induced membrane permeabilization and apoptosis. *Mol. Cell* **2015**, *57*, 69–82. [CrossRef] [PubMed]
92. Bajt, M.L.; Farhood, A.; Lemasters, J.J.; Jaeschke, H. Mitochondrial bax translocation accelerates DNA fragmentation and cell necrosis in a murine model of acetaminophen hepatotoxicity. *J. Pharmacol. Exp. Ther.* **2008**, *324*, 8–14. [CrossRef] [PubMed]
93. Jaeschke, H.; Ramachandran, A. Acetaminophen-induced apoptosis: Facts versus fiction. *J. Clin. Transl. Res.* **2020**, *6*, 36–47. [PubMed]

livers

MDPI

Review

Acetaminophen-Induced Hepatotoxicity in Obesity and Nonalcoholic Fatty Liver Disease: A Critical Review

Karima Begriche, Clémence Penhoat, Pénélope Bernabeu-Gentey, Julie Massart and Bernard Fromenty *

INSERM, Univ Rennes, INRAE, Institut NUMECAN (Nutrition Metabolisms and Cancer) UMR_A 1341, UMR_S 1241, F-35000 Rennes, France
* Correspondence: bernard.fromenty@inserm.fr; Tel.: +33-2-23-23-30-44

Abstract: The epidemic of obesity, type 2 diabetes and nonalcoholic liver disease (NAFLD) favors drug consumption, which augments the risk of adverse events including liver injury. For more than 30 years, a series of experimental and clinical investigations reported or suggested that the common pain reliever acetaminophen (APAP) could be more hepatotoxic in obesity and related metabolic diseases, at least after an overdose. Nonetheless, several investigations did not reproduce these data. This discrepancy might come from the extent of obesity and steatosis, accumulation of specific lipid species, mitochondrial dysfunction and diabetes-related parameters such as ketonemia and hyperglycemia. Among these factors, some of them seem pivotal for the induction of cytochrome P450 2E1 (CYP2E1), which favors the conversion of APAP to the toxic metabolite N-acetyl-*p*-benzoquinone imine (NAPQI). In contrast, other factors might explain why obesity and NAFLD are not always associated with more frequent or more severe APAP-induced acute hepatotoxicity, such as increased volume of distribution in the body, higher hepatic glucuronidation and reduced CYP3A4 activity. Accordingly, the occurrence and outcome of APAP-induced liver injury in an obese individual with NAFLD would depend on a delicate balance between metabolic factors that augment the generation of NAPQI and others that can mitigate hepatotoxicity.

Keywords: acetaminophen; drug-induced liver injury; obesity; nonalcoholic fatty liver disease; steatosis; nonalcoholic steatohepatitis; diabetes; cytochrome P450 2E1; fatty acids; mitochondria

1. Introduction

The epidemic of obesity is associated with a steady rise in drug consumption in order to treat several associated diseases such as type 2 diabetes mellitus (T2DM), hypertension, atherosclerosis, dyslipidemia and osteoarthritis [1,2]. In addition, numerous drugs are currently being developed in order to specifically treat nonalcoholic fatty liver disease (NAFLD), which is frequently associated with obesity and overweight [3,4]. This implies increased polypharmacy among obese patients, which can augment the risk of adverse events including drug-induced liver injury (DILI) [5,6]. In line with this, recent investigations reported a higher frequency of DILI in patients with NAFLD [7,8]. More specifically, the common pain reliever acetaminophen (APAP) is one of the identified drugs that could be more hepatotoxic in obesity and NAFLD, at least after an overdose [9]. The present article reviews the clinical and experimental investigations published on APAP-induced liver injury in the context of these metabolic diseases and also discusses the possible reasons that might explain why some studies are discrepant from others. Because our previous review on this matter was published in 2014 [9], many recent investigations are now discussed in this updated review.

2. APAP Hepatotoxicity

2.1. General Overview

APAP, also referred to as paracetamol, is one of the most widely prescribed drugs for the management of pain and hyperthermia. The current maximum recommended dosage of APAP is 4 g/day in adults even though the Food and Drug Administration (FDA) advises doses below 3.25 g/day for chronic use [10]. Although therapeutic doses of APAP can induce hepatic cytolysis in some patients [11,12], most cases of severe APAP-induced acute liver injury occur after accidental or intentional overdoses [13,14]. Actually, APAP is deemed to have a narrow therapeutic margin since as little as 7.5 g/day might be hazardous [15]. Currently, administration of N-acetylcysteine (NAC) is the only approved therapy to treat APAP overdose-induced liver injury in patients [10,14]. The rationale of NAC administration is to restore hepatic levels of glutathione (GSH), a major endogenous antioxidant limiting the noxious effects of the APAP toxic metabolite N-acetyl-*p*-benzoquinone imine (NAPQI) (Figure 1) [16,17]. Notably, repeated or long-term intake of APAP at therapeutic doses can occasionally cause acute hepatic cytolysis of different severities [11,12] but also chronic liver injury such as granulomatous hepatitis and cirrhosis [18–20].

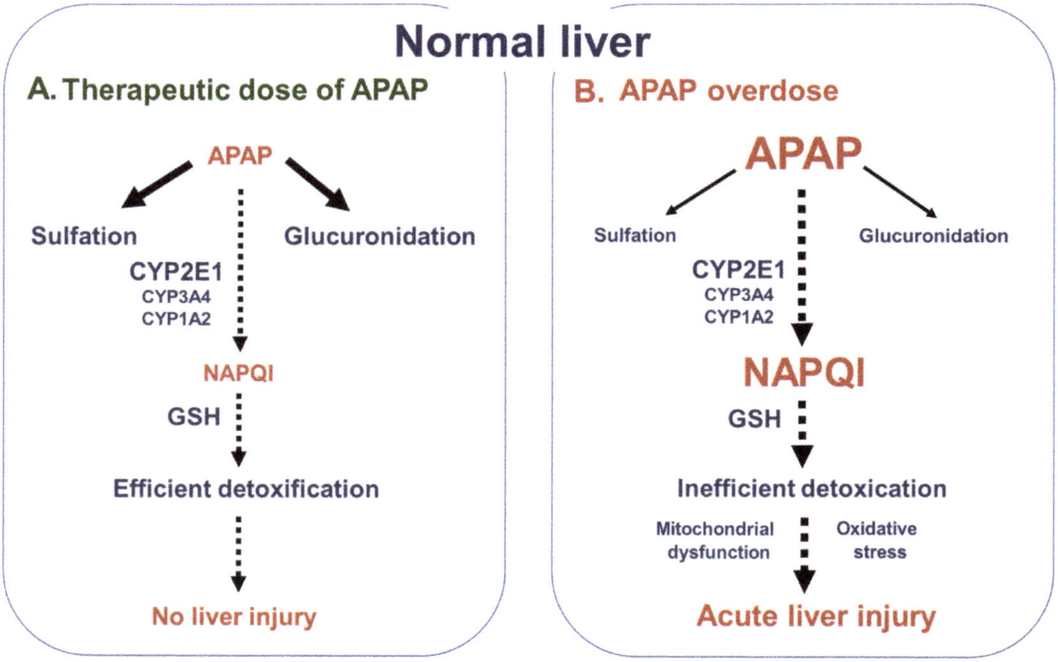

Figure 1. Biotransformation and toxicity of APAP in normal liver. (**A**). For therapeutic dose, APAP is mainly detoxified through sulfation and glucuronidation, while a small proportion is metabolized to N-acetyl-*p*-benzoquinone imine (NAPQI) via the cytochrome P450 2E1 (CYP2E1) and to a lesser extent CYP3A4 and CYP1A2. In normal liver, the low amounts of NAPQI are efficiently detoxified by glutathione (GSH), a major antioxidant molecule present in different cellular compartments including mitochondria. (**B**). After APAP overdoses, the sulfation and glucuronidation pathways are overwhelmed and more APAP undergoes CYP-dependent oxidation to NAPQI. However, GSH concentrations in hepatocytes are not sufficient to allow the efficient detoxification of NAPQI, which then induces major mitochondrial dysfunction, oxidative stress and acute liver injury. More information is provided in the text.

A key player in APAP liver injury is cytochrome P450 2E1 (CYP2E1), an enzyme that catalyzes the oxidation of APAP to NAPQI (Figure 1) [10,21,22]. Indeed, NAPQI is a highly reactive metabolite inducing severe mitochondrial dysfunction, overproduction of reactive oxygen species (ROS), and c-jun N-terminal kinase (JNK) activation, eventually leading to ATP depletion and massive hepatocellular necrosis [17,22,23]. Importantly, mitochondrial CYP2E1 could play a major role in APAP-induced cytotoxicity [24,25]. Finally, CYP3A4 (referred to as CYP3A2 in rats and CYP3A11 in mice) and CYP1A2 might also play a role in the conversion of APAP to NAPQI (Figure 1), although to a lesser extent than CYP2E1 in normal physiological conditions [26,27].

2.2. Predisposing Factors

Except for APAP ingested dose, APAP-induced hepatotoxicity could be favored by different factors such as chronic alcohol abuse, severe or chronic liver diseases, prolonged fasting and malnutrition, older age, and some comedications such as antituberculosis and antiepileptic drugs [12,16,28,29]. Importantly, increased activity of hepatic CYP2E1 (and possibly other CYPs) seems to be a common mechanism whereby chronic alcohol abuse, prolonged fasting and some comedications favor APAP-induced liver injury [16,30]. As discussed in this review, obesity, NAFLD and both types 1 and 2 diabetes could also predispose to APAP liver injury, at least in part, due to higher hepatic CYP2E1 activity [9,10,13]. Finally, the risk of APAP hepatotoxicity could be modulated by polymorphisms in different genes [16], such as *UGT1A* encoding UDP-glucuronosyltransferase (UGT) 1A, which plays a pivotal role in APAP glucuronidation and detoxification (Figure 1) [28,31].

3. APAP Hepatotoxicity in NAFLD

3.1. Main Features of NAFLD

Because of the epidemic of obesity and T2DM, NAFLD is now the most frequent chronic liver disease worldwide with a global prevalence of 25% [32]. NAFLD comprises a large spectrum of histologic changes including simple fatty liver, nonalcoholic steatohepatitis (NASH), advanced fibrosis and cirrhosis [33], which can evolve into hepatocellular carcinoma (HCC) [34]. It is estimated that simple fatty liver progresses to NASH in about 10 to 20% of the patients [35]. NASH itself is defined by the presence of steatosis (mostly macrovacuolar), some necrosis and apoptosis, hepatocellular ballooning and lobular inflammation [33]. Of note, the presence of microvesicular steatosis has been associated with histological markers of NASH severity [36]. Although the mechanisms of progression of fatty liver to NASH in some patients are not fully understood, mitochondrial dysfunction, oxidative stress and lipid peroxidation are deemed to play a primary role in the occurrence of cell death and inflammation [37–39].

3.2. Clinical Investigations on Acute APAP Hepatotoxicity in Obesity and NAFLD

There is some clinical evidence that obesity and NAFLD can predispose to APAP hepatotoxicity in the setting of APAP overdose (Table 1). Two large retrospective studies reported that APAP-induced acute liver injury was more frequent in NAFLD patients [40,41]. In these studies, patients with pre-existing NAFLD hospitalized for APAP overdose had a four- to sevenfold higher prevalence of acute liver injury as compared to those without NAFLD [40,41]. In another study, APAP-induced acute liver injury was more frequent in overweight or obese patients, but NAFLD presence was not investigated [42]. Obesity might also favor APAP hepatotoxicity when this analgesic and antipyretic drug is taken at therapeutic doses. Indeed, mild to moderate hepatic cytolysis, as evidenced by increased plasma transaminases (ALT and AST), was reported in some morbidly obese patients but not in nonobese individuals after receiving 4–5 g of intravenous APAP [43].

In contrast to these studies, the occurrence of APAP-induced acute liver injury was reported to be similar, or even lower, in obese patients compared to nonobese individuals (Table 1) [44,45]. However, one of these studies showed that obese patients had significantly poorer clinical outcomes after acute liver failure [44]. The discrepancies between the aforementioned studies might arise from several factors including the degree of obesity, the existence of NASH and advanced fibrosis and the presence of insulin resistance and T2DM. Indeed, these factors could alter APAP absorption, distribution, metabolism and excretion (ADME) but also basal antioxidant defenses and mitochondrial function, as discussed in Section 4.

Table 1. Summary of the clinical studies (ordered by increasing year) carried out on APAP-induced acute liver injury in obesity and NAFLD.

Authors, Year [References]	Design of the Study	Presence of NAFLD	Hepatic CYP2E1 Activity	APAP Overdose	APAP-Induced Acute Liver Injury
Rutherford et al., 2006 [44]	Prospective	Not reported in this study [1]	Not reported in this study	Yes	Lower incidence (but poorer outcomes) in obese patients
Nguyen et al., 2008 [40]	Retrospective	Yes	Not reported in this study	Yes	Higher prevalence in patients with NAFLD
Myers and Shaheen, 2009 [41]	Retrospective	Yes	Not reported in this study	Yes	Higher prevalence in patients with NAFLD
Radosevich et al., 2016 [45]	Retrospective	Not reported in this study [1]	Not reported in this study	Yes	Equal prevalence between obese and nonobese patients
Van Rongen et al., 2016 [43]	Prospective	Not reported in this study [1]	Increased	No (4 to 5 g)	Increased plasma ALT and AST in morbidly obese patients but not in nonobese individuals
Chomchai and Chomchai, 2018 [42]	Retrospective	Not reported in this study [1]	Not reported in this study	Yes	Higher prevalence in overweight and obese patients

[1] There is now ample evidence that obesity is strongly associated with NAFLD (reviewed in [32,35]).

3.3. Rodent Studies on Acute APAP Hepatotoxicity in Obesity and NAFLD

APAP-induced acute hepatotoxicity has also been investigated in different rodent models of obesity and NAFLD (Table 2). However, while several investigations reported greater APAP hepatotoxicity in obese rodents [9,46–53], others showed no difference or even lower APAP-induced liver injury compared to lean rodents [9,46,54–57]. In addition to some factors mentioned in the previous section, discrepancies between these experimental investigations might be due to differences in the rodent model (rats vs. mice), the origin of obesity (genetic vs. diet-induced) and the composition of the hypercaloric diet, as discussed in Section 4.

In some aforementioned investigations, APAP not only caused more severe hepatic cytolysis in obese mice (as evidenced by increased ALT and AST) but also worsened liver fat accumulation through a mechanism that might involve inhibition of autophagy and exacerbation of oxidative stress [52,53]. Interestingly, aggravation of steatosis was also observed in ob/ob mice acutely intoxicated with APAP although this was not associated with higher plasma transaminases and more severe hepatic necrosis [49]. In NAFLD, distinct mechanisms might thus be involved in APAP-induced hepatic cytolysis and worsening of steatosis, respectively.

Table 2. Summary of the rodent studies (ordered by increasing year) carried out on APAP-induced hepatotoxicity in obesity and NAFLD.

Authors, Year [References]	Rodent Models of Obesity and NAFLD	Presence of NAFLD	Hepatic CYP2E1 Activity	Dose of APAP	APAP-Induced Hepatotoxicity
Corcoran and Wong, 1987 [47]	Male Sprague–Dawley rats fed a high-fat diet for 24 weeks	Not reported in this study [1]	Not reported in this study	710 mg/kg (i.p.)	Higher hepatotoxicity after 48 h, compared to rats fed a standard diet
Blouin et al., 1987 [58]	Male obese Zucker fa/fa rats	Not reported in this study [2]	Not reported in this study [2]	1300 mg (p.o.)	Similar hepatotoxicity after 48 h, compared to lean rats

Table 2. *Cont.*

Authors, Year [References]	Rodent Models of Obesity and NAFLD	Presence of NAFLD	Hepatic CYP2E1 Activity	Dose of APAP	APAP-Induced Hepatotoxicity
Tuntaterdtum et al., 1993 [54].	Male obese Zucker fa/fa rats	Not reported in this study [2]	Not reported in this study [2]	3000 mg/kg (p.o)	Lower hepatotoxicity after 48 h, compared to lean rats
Ito et al., 2006 [55]	Male C57Bl/6 mice fed a Western-style diet for 16 weeks	Yes	Not reported in this study	300 mg/kg (p.o.)	Lower hepatotoxicity after 6 h, compared to mice fed a standard diet
	Male ob/ob mice	Not reported in this study [3]	Not reported in this study [3]	300 mg/kg (p.o.)	Lower hepatotoxicity after 6 h, compared to wild-type mice
Donthamsetty et al., 2008 [59]	Male Swiss Webster mice fed a MCD diet for 1 month [4]	Yes	Unchanged	360 mg/kg (i.p.)	Higher hepatotoxicity from 6 to 48 h after overdose, compared to mice fed a standard diet
Kon et al., 2010 [48]	Male KK-A^y mice	Yes	Not reported in this study [5]	300 or 600 mg/kg (p.o.)	Higher hepatotoxicity after 6 h, compared to wild-type mice
Kucera et al., 2012 [50]	Male Sprague-Dawley rats fed a high-fat diet for 6 weeks	Yes	Not reported in this study	1 g/kg (p.o)	Higher hepatotoxicity after 24 and 48 h, compared to rats fed a standard diet
Aubert et al., 2012 [49]	Female db/db mice	Yes	Increased	500 mg/kg (p.o.)	Higher hepatotoxicity after 8 h, compared to wild-type mice
	Female ob/ob mice	Yes	Unchanged	500 mg/kg (p.o.)	Similar hepatotoxicity after 8 h, compared to wild-type mice
Kim et al., 2017 [56]	Male C57Bl/6 mice fed a fast food diet for 14 weeks	Yes	Not reported in this study (but higher CYP2E1 protein levels)	200 mg/kg (i.p.)	Lower hepatotoxicity compared to wild-type mice (timing not specified)
Piccinin et al., 2019 [51]	Male FVB/N mice fed a high-fat diet for 1 month	Yes	Not reported in this study	300 mg/kg (i.p.)	Higher hepatotoxicity after 6 h, compared to wild-type mice
Shi et al., 2019 [52]	Male C57Bl/6 mice fed a high-fat diet for 8 weeks	Yes	Not reported in this study	50, 100 or 200 mg/kg (p.o.)	Significant hepatotoxicity after 24 h but no comparison with wild-type mice
Wang et al., 2021 [53]	Male C57Bl/6J mice fed a high-fat diet for 8 weeks	Yes	Not reported in this study	100 mg/kg (p.o.)	Significant hepatotoxicity after 24 h but no comparison with wild-type mice
Ghallab et al., 2021 [57]	Male C57Bl/6N mice fed a Western diet for 48 to 50 weeks	Yes	Not reported in this study (but lower CYP2E1 immunostaining)	300 mg/kg (i.p.)	Lower hepatotoxicity compared to wild-type mice (timing not specified)

[1] Numerous investigations in rodents including rats showed that long-term feeding of high-fat diets consistently induces NAFLD (reviewed in [60–62]). [2] Other studies showed that male obese and insulin resistant Zucker fa/fa rats present moderate fatty liver [63,64] but reduced CYP2E1 activity [63,65]. [3] Other investigations showed that male obese and diabetic ob/ob mice present major fatty liver [66,67], with unchanged [49] or reduced [68] CYP2E1 activity. [4] Methionine and choline-deficient (MCD) diet is known to induce NASH, which is however associated with reduced body weight and blood glycemia [9,60]. [5] Previous studies showed that hepatic CYP2E1 mRNA expression [69] and activity [70] are unchanged in KK-A^y mice.

3.4. *In Vitro Studies on Acute APAP Hepatotoxicity in Models of Fatty Acid Exposure and NAFLD*

Several in vitro studies investigated APAP acute cytotoxicity in different models of fatty acid exposure and NAFLD. Two studies were carried out in hepatocytes isolated from rats fed different types of lipids. The first study reported that liver slices from rats fed a diet rich in butter (which mainly contains saturated fatty acids) were significantly more sensitive to APAP cytotoxicity than those from rats fed a diet enriched in polyunsaturated fatty acids (PUFAs) [71]. Unfortunately, lipid accumulation was not evaluated in this study nor were included liver slices from rats fed a standard diet. Nevertheless, this study suggests that exposure to long-chain saturated fatty acids could be more detrimental than to polyunsaturated linoleic acid (C18:2) and arachidonic acid (C20:4) [71]. In the second study, steatotic primary hepatocytes isolated from rats fed a diet enriched in corn oil (which mainly contains PUFAs) were more sensitive to APAP cytotoxicity than those from rats fed a standard diet [72]. The role of n-3 PUFAs (also referred to as ω-3 PUFAs) in APAP hepatotoxicity is discussed in Section 4.2.5.

Two other studies were performed in hepatocyte cell lines incubated with different fatty acids. In the first study, carried out in L02 liver cells, the investigations showed that a 24 h exposure to the monounsaturated oleic acid (C18:1) exacerbated APAP cytotoxicity whereas different medium chain fatty acids did not cause this effect [73]. Unfortunately, this study did not determine whether these different fatty acids induced steatosis in L02 liver cells. Other investigations performed in differentiated HepaRG cells incubated 7 days with stearic acid (C18:0) or oleic acid (which both induced steatosis) showed that only stearate supplementation induced greater APAP-induced cytotoxicity, which was blunted by the CYP2E1 inhibitor chlormethiazole [74]. The apparent discrepancy between these two studies could be due to the cell lines and the duration of oleic acid exposure. Nonetheless, these in vitro investigations clearly indicate that exposure to some fatty acids could favor APAP hepatotoxicity. Although this might be due to their propensity to induce CYP2E1, other possible mechanisms cannot be excluded, as briefly discussed in Section 4.1.3.

Finally, in vitro investigations also reported that APAP worsened lipid deposition in steatotic L02 cells [52,53], thus confirming in vivo results in diet-induced and genetically obese mice [49,52,53]. However, steatosis in L02 cells was induced by cotreating the cells with oleic acid and ethanol, which does not reflect pure NAFLD. Nevertheless, these investigations suggest that acute APAP could aggravate steatosis through a direct effect on hepatocytes and not via extrahepatic pathways such as fat mobilization from adipose tissue [75,76].

3.5. *Investigations on Chronic APAP Hepatotoxicity in Obesity and NAFLD*

Repeated or chronic intake of therapeutic doses of APAP can sporadically cause different types of liver injury, as previously mentioned [18–20]. Unfortunately, there are no clinical studies investigating the occurrence of repeated or chronic APAP hepatotoxicity in obesity and NAFLD. In rodents, a 13-week treatment with APAP was less hepatotoxic in leptin receptor-deficient obese (fa/fa) Zucker rats than in lean rats [77]. According to the authors, this might be explained by lower hepatic CYP2E1 expression in obese Zucker rats [77]. This is in line with previous studies showing downregulation of hepatic CYP2E1 in obese Zucker rats [63,68] and lower acute APAP hepatotoxicity in obese Zucker rats compared with their lean littermates [54]. The role of the adipokine leptin in CYP2E1 expression is briefly discussed in Section 4.2.2. In another study, a 35-day treatment with APAP caused more severe hepatic cytolysis in spontaneously diabetic torii (SDT) rats as compared to nondiabetic rats [78]. While SDT rats are not obese, this study did not investigate fatty liver [78]. APAP hepatotoxicity in type 1 diabetes is discussed in Section 6.

4. Factors Modulating APAP Hepatotoxicity in Obesity and NAFLD

From the abovementioned studies carried out in humans and rodents, it appears that obesity and NAFLD do not always increase the risk or the severity of APAP-induced liver injury. Hence, while several factors would favor APAP hepatotoxicity in these metabolic diseases, others might limit APAP toxicity.

4.1. Factors That Could Favor APAP Hepatotoxicity in Obesity and NAFLD

4.1.1. CYP2E1 Induction

Hepatic CYP2E1 induction could be a major mechanism associated with greater APAP hepatotoxicity observed in most clinical and experimental studies (Figure 2A), although other explanations can be considered as discussed below. Indeed, higher CYP2E1 activity is expected to cause an overproduction of NAPQI and deeper GSH depletion, thus leading to more severe mitochondrial dysfunction and oxidative stress [9,13,79]. In line with this hypothesis, the study by van Rongen et al. reported higher CYP2E1 activity in morbidly obese patients, which was associated with mild to moderate hepatic cytolysis after administration of 4–5 g of APAP [43]. However, CYP2E1 activity was not determined in the other investigations reporting a higher risk of APAP-induced liver injury in patients with obesity and NAFLD [40–42]. Experimentally, investigations in ob/ob and db/db obese mice showed that APAP hepatotoxicity correlated with hepatic CYP2E1 activity but not with liver fat accumulation [49]. Unfortunately, most other rodent studies showing higher APAP hepatotoxicity in obese animals did not investigate CYP2E1 expression, or activity [47,48,50–53].

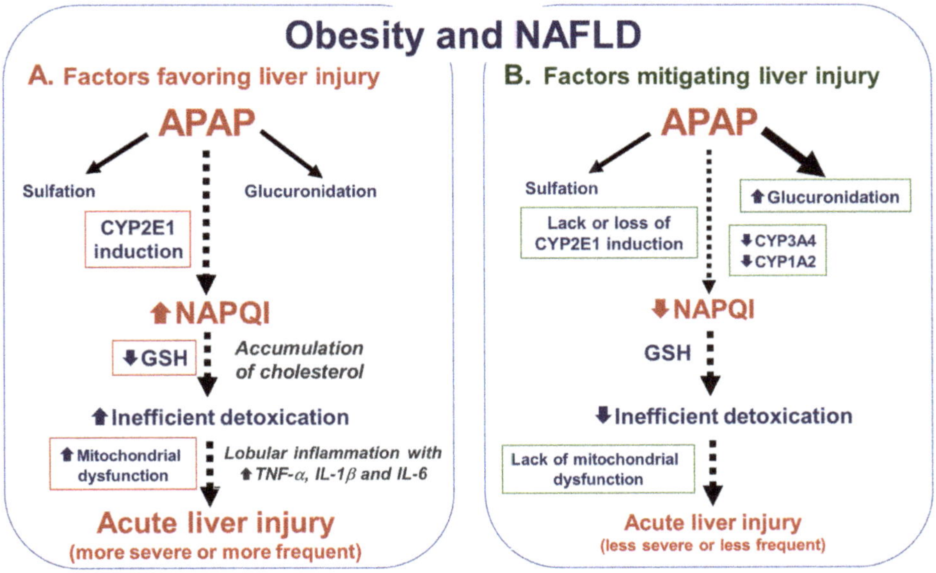

Figure 2. Hepatotoxicity of APAP in obesity and NAFLD. (**A**). Different factors in obesity and NAFLD could favor liver injury induced by APAP overdose, for instance by increasing cytochrome P450 2E1 (CYP2E1) activity, reducing basal concentrations of glutathione (GSH) and promoting preexisting mitochondrial dysfunction. In addition, the accumulation of cholesterol could sensitize the liver to APAP-induced hepatotoxicity by favoring mitochondrial GSH depletion. Lobular inflammation might also favor APAP hepatotoxicity via several cytokines such as tumor necrosis factor-α (TNF-α), interleukin-1β (IL-1β) and IL-6. (**B**). On the contrary, some factors in obesity and NAFLD could mitigate APAP-induced liver injury, for instance by increasing APAP glucuronidation and reducing CYP3A4 and CYP1A2 activity. Moreover, CYP2E1 induction could be absent or lost in some metabolic and pathological conditions. The absence of preexisting mitochondrial dysfunction in some patients might also mitigate APAP-induced hepatotoxicity. Consequently, obese people with one or several of these mitigating factors might not have a higher risk of severe APAP-induced liver injury. More information is provided in the text.

In a study carried out in mice fed a fast food diet enriched in saturated fatty acids, cholesterol and fructose, less severe APAP liver injury was observed despite enhanced hepatic CYP2E1 protein expression but CYP2E1 activity was not measured [56]. Adaptive responses in different antioxidant and anti-inflammatory pathways might explain this protective effect in this mouse model of obesity [56]. Conversely, higher APAP hepatotoxicity was observed in a mouse model of NASH despite unchanged CYP2E1 activity [59]. Although the reasons for the lack of CYP2E1 induction are unclear, it should be underlined that NASH was induced in this work with a methionine and choline-deficient (MCD) diet [59], which significantly reduces body weight and blood glycemia and does not cause systemic insulin resistance [9,60]. Hence, this peculiar metabolic profile might have removed some cues that otherwise might have led to CYP2E1 induction, as discussed in Section 4.2.2.

Hepatic CYP2E1 induction is a salient feature of obesity and NAFLD. Indeed, many clinical investigations consistently reported higher hepatic CYP2E1 expression and activity in patients with these metabolic diseases [9,43,80–85]. Hepatic CYP2E1 induction has also been found in many studies performed in different rodent models of obesity and NAFLD [49,57,82,86–91], although there are some exceptions as mentioned in Section 4.2.2.

Hepatic CYP2E1 induction in obese patients would not only cause more frequent or more severe APAP hepatotoxicity but may also favor the transition of fatty liver to NASH [82,89,92–94]. In steatotic hepatocytes, ROS overproduction secondary to CYP2E1 induction is indeed deemed to cause lipid peroxidation and the generation of noxious reactive aldehydes such as malondialdehyde (MDA) and 4-hydroxynonenal (4-HNE), which then promote necroinflammation and fibrosis [82,92–95]. Accordingly, the key role of CYP2E1 in NASH pathophysiology makes CYP2E1 inhibition or downregulation a promising therapeutic strategy in NAFLD [92,96,97].

The mechanisms of CYP2E1 induction in NAFLD are poorly understood. Accumulation of some fatty acids such as palmitic acid (C16:0) and stearic acid (C18:0) might play a role [74,98,99]. In keeping with the role of some fatty acids or lipids, a recent interventional study in healthy individuals showed that a short-term regular diet supplemented with whipped cream induced hepatic steatosis and significantly enhanced CYP2E1 activity [100]. Other mechanisms might involve hyperleptinemia, hyperglucagonemia and insulin resistance [10,25,82]. The exact downstream signaling pathways involved in CYP2E1 induction in NAFLD are still unknown.

4.1.2. Low Basal Levels of GSH

Low basal levels of liver GSH might also favor APAP hepatotoxicity in NAFLD as this is expected to hasten and even promote the profound GSH depletion taking place after APAP overdose (Figure 2A). Consequently, less NAPQI can be detoxified by hepatic GSH thus allowing the APAP reactive metabolite to covalently bind to different proteins and other cellular components, especially in mitochondria [16,17,23]. Significant reduction of basal levels of liver GSH has been reported in NAFLD, either in patients [101,102] or in some rodent models [103,104]. However, other animal investigations did not find any significant decrease in hepatic GSH content [49,50,105,106], although this was sometimes associated with higher levels of oxidized GSH (GSSG) [105].

The mechanisms that can cause low basal levels of liver GSH in NAFLD might be complex. Several factors might be involved including the extent of ROS overproduction via mitochondrial dysfunction, reduced synthesis of GSH and impairment of other antioxidant defenses, which can occur during the progression of NAFLD [37,105,107,108].

4.1.3. Extent of Steatosis and Accumulation of Deleterious Fatty Acids and Lipid Species

Investigations in genetically obese mice intoxicated with APAP showed that higher basal levels of hepatic triglycerides did not cause more severe APAP-induced hepatic cytolysis [49]. Hence, the extent of steatosis per se does not seem to favor APAP hepatotoxicity in NAFLD. In contrast, the accumulation of some fatty acids might specifically favor liver injury. For instance, palmitic and stearic acids could be particularly harmful by promoting hepatic CYP2E1 induction [74,98,99], as previously mentioned. Furthermore, studies carried out in transgenic fat-1 mice, which endogenously convert n-6 PUFAs to n-3 PUFAs, showed that male animals were more susceptible to APAP-induced acute liver injury, possibly via a JNK-dependent mechanism and downregulation of signal transducer and activator of transcription 3 (STAT3) [109,110].

Cholesterol accumulation might also favor APAP hepatotoxicity in NAFLD (Figure 2A). Indeed, investigations in mice fed a high-cholesterol diet for 4 weeks showed more severe APAP-induced acute liver injury, possibly through the Toll-like receptor 9 (TLR9)/inflammasome pathway [111]. Interestingly, mitochondrial free cholesterol loading leads to mitochondrial GSH depletion in hepatocytes [112], which could promote mitochondrial dysfunction and cell death [113]. In contrast, CYP2E1 might not be involved because hepatic CYP2E1 expression and activity were reduced in rats fed a high-cholesterol diet for 11 weeks [114].

4.1.4. Mitochondrial Dysfunction

NAFLD is associated with complex mitochondrial alterations. In simple fatty liver, mitochondrial oxidative metabolism is stimulated, most probably as an adaptation to the increased levels of different substrates including fatty acids [37,38,108,115]. However, this adaptation can be lost in NASH, which is associated with reduced expression and activity of different mitochondrial respiratory complexes [37,38,108,115–117]. Accordingly, NASH-associated mitochondrial dysfunction might favor APAP hepatotoxicity (Figure 2A) since respiratory chain impairment is pivotal in APAP-induced liver injury [118–120]. However, there are currently no available data to confirm this hypothesis but different rodent models reproducing NAFLD progression can be useful for this [60,61,121].

4.1.5. Presence of Lobular Inflammation

Simple fatty liver can progress in some patients to NASH which is characterized by lobular inflammation, hepatocellular ballooning and the presence of some necrotic hepatocytes and apoptotic bodies, as previously mentioned. These pathological lesions are due at least in part to the overproduction of several proinflammatory cytokines such as tumor necrosis factor-α (TNF-α), interleukin-1β (IL-1β) and IL-6 [122,123], which could sensitize the liver to APAP-induced hepatotoxicity (Figure 2A). Interestingly, APAP-induced acute liver injury is exacerbated in Nlrp6$^{-/-}$ mice [124], a well-established mouse model of intestinal dysbiosis associated with enhanced gut–liver inflammatory responses [125]. However, it remains to be determined whether obesity- and NAFLD-associated gut dysbiosis [126,127] could play a role in higher APAP hepatotoxicity in these metabolic diseases. Other investigations showed that hepatic inflammation favors liver injury induced by different drugs and chemicals [128–130].

4.2. Factors That Could Mitigate APAP Hepatotoxicity in Obesity and NAFLD

4.2.1. Alteration in APAP Absorption and Distribution

Only a few clinical studies dealt with the impact of obesity on gastrointestinal absorption of APAP and its whole-body distribution. To our knowledge, only one study reported a lower absorption rate of APAP in obese subjects, which was associated with a decrease in the maximum plasma concentrations of the pain reliever [131]. Regarding whole-body distribution, two studies reported higher APAP volume of distribution (Vd) in obese subjects [43,132]. However, all these investigations were carried out in morbidly obese persons and further investigations would be needed to confirm these data for body mass index (BMI) below 40 kg/m^2. Nevertheless, decreased APAP gastrointestinal absorption and higher Vd could favor lower APAP plasma and liver concentrations, at least in some obese patients [9].

4.2.2. Lack of CYP2E1 Induction or CYP2E1 Downregulation

Although hepatic CYP2E1 activity is frequently increased in NAFLD (see Section 4.1.1), some investigations reported a lack of CYP2E1 induction, which might not allow NAPQI overproduction (Figure 2B). Indeed, several clinical studies showed that some obese patients had CYP2E1 activity in the range of nonobese individuals [43,46,85,133]. Experimentally, hepatic CYP2E1 expression and activity are not increased in obese leptin-deficient ob/ob mice and leptin receptor-deficient fa/fa Zucker rats [49,68,134]. Although this might suggest that the leptin signaling pathway is needed for CYP2E1 induction in obesity and NAFLD, hepatic CYP2E1 activity is enhanced in leptin receptor-deficient db/db mice, especially in females [49]. The very high glycemia and ketonemia in these mice [49,66] might play a role in CYP2E1 induction in this context of severe diabetes [10]. Because many endogenous molecules, hormones and cytokines are deemed to regulate hepatic CYP2E1 expression and activity, sometimes with opposite effects [10,82,135–137], it is possible that CYP2E1 induction might not always occur in obesity and NAFLD.

Another possibility could be the loss of CYP2E1 induction during NAFLD progression (Figure 2B). Indeed, recent investigations suggested that CYP2E1 induction seems to wane when NASH progresses toward advanced fibrosis [57], in line with clinical data reporting a significant reduction of CYP2E1 expression with the progression of liver fibrosis [138,139]. Increased production of proinflammatory cytokines including TNF-α might play a role in this progressive decline of CYP2E1 expression [135,139]. In contrast, the profibrotic cytokine transforming growth factor-beta (TGF-β) does not seem to be involved in fibrosis-associated CYP2E1 downregulation [140,141].

4.2.3. Reduced CYP3A4 and CYP1A2 Activity

CYP3A4 (also referred to as CYP3A) and CYP1A2 are also involved in APAP biotransformation to NAPQI, although to a lesser extent than CYP2E1 [26,27]. Many clinical and experimental studies consistently reported lower hepatic expression and activity of CYP3A4 in obesity and NAFLD [83,142–150]. Hence, lower CYP3A4 activity in obesity and NAFLD might reduce the generation of NAPQI after an APAP overdose (Figure 2B).

Several clinical studies on CYP1A2 activity reported little or no change in obesity [83,147,149]. Interestingly, investigations in patients with NAFLD reported that CYP1A2 expression and activity were unaltered in fatty liver but significantly reduced in NASH [151,152]. These data seem to be in line with the investigations carried out in obese patients since NASH occurs only in a minority of those people [35]. In rodent models of NAFLD, CYP1A2 expression and activity were significantly decreased in most investigations [153–158], but increased or unchanged in some others [143,159]. Like CYP3A4, lower CYP1A2 activity in NAFLD might also reduce the generation of NAPQI after an APAP overdose (Figure 2B).

4.2.4. Increased APAP Glucuronidation

Clinical and experimental investigations consistently reported increased APAP glucuronidation in obesity and NAFLD [9,43,49,83,160,161], which is expected to reduce the extent of APAP bioactivation to NAPQI (Figure 2B). Of note, UGT1A6 and UGT1A9 are the main UGT isoforms involved in APAP glucuronidation in humans [162] but only UGT1A9 protein expression tended to be increased in patients with obesity-related fatty liver [163].

4.2.5. Exposure and Accumulation of Protective Fatty Acids

Two studies carried out in female transgenic fat-1 mice (which endogenously convert n-6 PUFAs to n-3 PUFAs) showed significant protection against APAP-induced acute liver injury [109,164]. In the study by Liu et al., the opposite effect was observed in male mice and this gender difference was attributed to estrogens [109]. Of note, the expression of hepatic CYP2E1 in female mice was unchanged in one study [164], whereas CYP2E1 was not investigated in the second one [109]. Other investigations in rats showed that dietary supplementation with the n-3 polyunsaturated eicosapentaenoic and docosahexaenoic acids (EPA and DHA) protected against acute APAP liver injury [165]. According to the authors, the hepatoprotective effect of n-3 PUFAs against APAP liver injury might be mediated via their anti-inflammatory and antioxidant properties [164,165]. Another study in rats fed a diet with 20% fish oil (i.e., rich in n-3 PUFAs) also reported protection against APAP-induced acute liver injury, which was deemed to be related to higher APAP glucuronidation [166]. Interestingly, n-3 PUFAs reduced hepatic CYP2E1 activity in insulinopenic diabetic rats [167] but their protective effect against APAP hepatotoxicity was not investigated in this study.

5. APAP-Induced Liver Injury after Bariatric Surgery

Roux-en-Y gastric bypass and sleeve gastrectomy are surgical procedures increasingly used for the treatment of morbid obesity and comorbidities including NAFLD [168,169]. A retrospective study suggested that weight loss surgery may predispose to acute liver failure after APAP overdose and this was independent of alcohol abuse and the use of APAP–narcotic combination drugs [170]. More recently, a case of fulminant hepatitis was observed after laparoscopic sleeve gastrectomy in a young woman who received therapeutic doses of APAP [171]. In addition to malnutrition and vitamin deficiency, the authors pointed to other possible risk factors including rapid weight loss, which might have aggravated preexisting fatty liver [171]. Notably, although CYP2E1 activity in obese patients decreases after bariatric surgery it remains higher than in healthy volunteers [133,172]. Thus, increased CYP2E1 activity might favor APAP-induced liver injury in obese patients even after such surgery. However, beyond CYP2E1 activity, other metabolic parameters most probably explain the profound alterations of APAP bioavailability observed after weight loss surgery [173,174]. Hence, further investigations would be needed to determine the mechanisms whereby bariatric surgery might predispose to APAP hepatotoxicity.

6. APAP-Hepatotoxicity in Type 1 Diabetes Mellitus

Type 1 diabetes mellitus (T1DM) is a chronic autoimmune disease caused by insulin deficiency and leading to severe hyperglycemia [175]. Importantly, the pathogenesis of T1DM significantly differs from that of obesity-related T2DM [176,177]. Nonetheless, T1DM seems to be frequently associated with fatty liver, which can progress to steatohepatitis and cirrhosis in some patients [178,179]. Some clinical investigations disclosed that diabetes increases the risk and the severity of DILI but these studies did not specify whether there was a difference between T1DM and T2DM [180–182]. Moreover, these investigations did not provide specific information on APAP.

T1DM can be induced in rats and mice by single or repeated injections of streptozotocin, a pancreatic β-cell poison [10,183]. Using this experimental model, a recent study reported that APAP-induced acute liver injury was exacerbated in diabetic mice possibly via a hyperglycemia-induced proinflammatory response in liver Kupffer cells [184]. Although not investigated in this study, it is possible that CYP2E1 induction might also have played a role in liver injury aggravation [10]. Indeed, numerous studies (but not all—see below) showed that streptozotocin-induced diabetes is associated with higher hepatic CYP2E1 protein expression and activity [10,167,185–188].

Contrasting with the study by Wang et al. [184], several investigations in streptozotocin-treated rodents showed that T1DM protected against APAP-induced acute hepatotoxicity [189–191]. The exact reasons for these discrepancies are unknown although higher APAP glucuronidation and improved liver repair in diabetic animals might play a role [189–191]. However, it is worth mentioning that hepatic CYP2E1 activity was not increased in these studies, thus contrasting with many other investigations reporting CYP2E1 induction in streptozotocin-treated rodents [10,167,185–188]. Further studies would be needed in order to determine why hepatic CYP2E1 induction is not always observed in streptozotocin-induced experimental diabetes. The extent of insulinopenia, ketonemia and hyperglycemia might be pivotal [10], in addition to other metabolic factors already discussed in this review.

7. Conclusions

Although obesity and NAFLD appear to increase the risk or the severity of APAP-induced acute liver injury, this relationship has not always been reported. As discussed in previous reviews [9,13,46] and this one, we propose that the occurrence and outcome of APAP-induced liver injury in these metabolic diseases might depend on a subtle balance between metabolic factors that can be protective for the liver and others that favor the generation of NAPQI (Figure 2). Hence, further investigations are needed in order to understand why some obese individuals could be at risk for APAP-induced hepatotoxicity and why some others are not. Although the absence of hepatic CYP2E1 induction might explain the lack of increased risk, other mechanisms might be involved including reduced APAP gastrointestinal absorption, enhanced Vd, higher hepatic glucuronidation and lower hepatic CYP3A4 activity (Figure 2B). In contrast, robust CYP2E1 induction, lobular inflammation, low basal concentrations of hepatic GSH and NASH-associated mitochondrial dysfunction might favor APAP hepatotoxicity in obesity and NAFLD (Figure 2A). While some of these factors are difficult to investigate in patients, many rodent models can be useful for mechanistic purposes [60,61,121]. Of note, these rodent models of obesity and NAFLD could also be valuable in order to determine whether repeated or chronic administration of APAP at therapeutic doses can cause more severe liver injury.

From a clinical viewpoint, physicians are encouraged to carry out regular monitoring of liver function in obese patients treated with chronic APAP administration, in particular in patients with pre-existing NAFLD. Finally, it should be underlined that chronic ethanol consumption constantly causes hepatic CYP2E1 induction while recent investigations reported that alcohol consumption and obesity (or metabolic syndrome) can synergistically augment the risk and severity of steatohepatitis, cirrhosis and HCC [192–194]. Hence, further investigations would be required to determine whether obese people who regularly consume alcohol have an even higher risk of APAP-induced hepatotoxicity.

Finally, a major issue for the future is to better prevent liver failure and mortality after APAP overdose, irrespective of the patient's body weight. Although NAC is the only approved antidote to treat APAP-induced liver injury [10,14], other therapeutic compounds are currently being developed to inhibit CYP2E1 activity (fomepizole), or to prevent mitochondrial oxidative stress (MitoTEMPO) and peroxynitrite formation (calmangafodipir) [195]. Numerous phytochemicals with efficient antioxidant properties might also be promising antidotes [196]. As for NAC, these compounds might be able to protect against APAP-induced necrosis [17,197] and other possible types of cell death including necroptosis and apoptosis [198,199]. Furthermore, targeting autophagy, mitophagy and mitochondrial biogenesis could also be promising therapeutic strategies [22,195,200].

Author Contributions: Conceptualization, K.B., J.M. and B.F.; writing—original draft preparation, B.F.; writing—review and editing, K.B., C.P., P.B.-G. and J.M.; visualization, K.B., J.M. and B.F.; supervision, B.F.; project administration, B.F. All authors have read and agreed to the published version of the manuscript.

Funding: This research received no external funding.

Institutional Review Board Statement: Not applicable.

Informed Consent Statement: Not applicable.

Data Availability Statement: Not applicable.

Acknowledgments: We are grateful to the Institut National de la Santé et de la Recherche Médicale (INSERM) for its constant support.

Conflicts of Interest: The authors declare no conflict of interest.

References

1. Barrett, L.A.; Xing, A.; Sheffler, J.; Steidley, E.; Adam, T.J.; Zhang, R.; He, Z. Assessing the Use of Prescription Drugs and Dietary Supplements in Obese Respondents in the National Health and Nutrition Examination Survey. *PLoS ONE* **2022**, *17*, e0269241. [CrossRef] [PubMed]
2. Pulipati, V.P.; Pannain, S. Pharmacotherapy of Obesity in Complex Diseases. *Clin. Obes.* **2022**, *12*, e12497. [CrossRef] [PubMed]
3. Chew, N.W.S.; Ng, C.H.; Truong, E.; Noureddin, M.; Kowdley, K.V. Nonalcoholic Steatohepatitis Drug Development Pipeline: An Update. *Semin. Liver Dis.* **2022**, *42*, 379–400. [CrossRef]
4. Negi, C.K.; Babica, P.; Bajard, L.; Bienertova-Vasku, J.; Tarantino, G. Insights into the Molecular Targets and Emerging Pharmacotherapeutic Interventions for Nonalcoholic Fatty Liver Disease. *Metabolism* **2022**, *126*, 154925. [CrossRef] [PubMed]
5. Scott, I.A.; Hilmer, S.N.; Reeve, E.; Potter, K.; Le Couteur, D.; Rigby, D.; Gnjidic, D.; Del Mar, C.B.; Roughead, E.E.; Page, A.; et al. Reducing Inappropriate Polypharmacy: The Process of Deprescribing. *JAMA Intern. Med.* **2015**, *175*, 827–834. [CrossRef]
6. Suzuki, A.; Yuen, N.A.; Ilic, K.; Miller, R.T.; Reese, M.J.; Brown, H.R.; Ambroso, J.I.; Falls, J.G.; Hunt, C.M. Comedications Alter Drug-Induced Liver Injury Reporting Frequency: Data Mining in the WHO VigiBase^{TM}. *Regul. Toxicol. Pharm.* **2015**, *72*, 481–490. [CrossRef]
7. Lammert, C.; Imler, T.; Teal, E.; Chalasani, N. Patients With Chronic Liver Disease Suggestive of Nonalcoholic Fatty Liver Disease May Be at Higher Risk for Drug-Induced Liver Injury. *Clin. Gastroenterol. Hepatol.* **2019**, *17*, 2814–2815. [CrossRef]
8. Hwang, S.; Won, S.; Lee, S. Nonalcoholic Fatty Liver Disease for the Incidence of Drug-Induced Liver Injury. *Clin. Gastroenterol. Hepatol.* **2022**, *20*, 964–965. [CrossRef]
9. Michaut, A.; Moreau, C.; Robin, M.-A.; Fromenty, B. Acetaminophen-Induced Liver Injury in Obesity and Nonalcoholic Fatty Liver Disease. *Liver Int.* **2014**, *34*, e171–e179. [CrossRef]
10. Massart, J.; Begriche, K.; Fromenty, B. Cytochrome P450 2E1 Should Not Be Neglected for Acetaminophen-Induced Liver Injury in Metabolic Diseases with Altered Insulin Levels or Glucose Homeostasis. *Clin. Res. Hepatol. Gastroenterol.* **2021**, *45*, 101470. [CrossRef]
11. Borlak, J.; Chatterji, B.; Londhe, K.B.; Watkins, P.B. Serum Acute Phase Reactants Hallmark Healthy Individuals at Risk for Acetaminophen-Induced Liver Injury. *Genome Med.* **2013**, *5*, 86. [CrossRef] [PubMed]
12. Louvet, A.; Ntandja Wandji, L.C.; Lemaître, E.; Khaldi, M.; Lafforgue, C.; Artru, F.; Quesnel, B.; Lassailly, G.; Dharancy, S.; Mathurin, P. Acute Liver Injury With Therapeutic Doses of Acetaminophen: A Prospective Study. *Hepatology* **2021**, *73*, 1945–1955. [CrossRef] [PubMed]
13. Massart, J.; Begriche, K.; Moreau, C.; Fromenty, B. Role of Nonalcoholic Fatty Liver Disease as Risk Factor for Drug-Induced Hepatotoxicity. *J. Clin. Transl. Res.* **2017**, *3*, 212–232. [CrossRef] [PubMed]
14. Licata, M.; Minisalle, M.G.; Stankeviciute, S.; Sanabria-Cabrera, J.; Lucena, M.M.; Andrade, R.J.; Almasio, P.L. N-Acetylcysteine for Preventing Acetaminophen-Induced Liver Injury: A Comprehensive Review. *Front. Pharm.* **2022**, *13*, 828565. [CrossRef] [PubMed]
15. Larson, A.M.; Polson, J.; Fontana, R.J.; Davern, T.J.; Lalani, E.; Hynan, L.S.; Reisch, J.S.; Schiodt, F.V.; Ostapowicz, G.; Shakil, A.O.; et al. Acetaminophen-Induced Acute Liver Failure: Results of a United States Multicenter, Prospective Study. *Hepatology* **2005**, *42*, 1364–1372. [CrossRef]
16. Yoon, E.; Babar, A.; Choudhary, M.; Kutner, M.; Pyrsopoulos, N. Acetaminophen-Induced Hepatotoxicity: A Comprehensive Update. *J. Clin. Transl. Hepatol.* **2016**, *4*, 131–142. [CrossRef]
17. Ramachandran, A.; Jaeschke, H. A Mitochondrial Journey through Acetaminophen Hepatotoxicity. *Food Chem. Toxicol.* **2020**, *140*, 111282. [CrossRef]
18. Biour, M.; Ben Salem, C.; Chazouillères, O.; Grangé, J.-D.; Serfaty, L.; Poupon, R. Drug-induced liver injury; fourteenth updated edition of the bibliographic database of liver injuries and related drugs. *Gastroenterol. Clin. Biol.* **2004**, *28*, 720–759. [CrossRef]
19. Watelet, J.; Laurent, V.; Bressenot, A.; Bronowicki, J.-P.; Larrey, D.; Peyrin-Biroulet, L. Toxicity of Chronic Paracetamol Ingestion. *Aliment. Pharm.* **2007**, *26*, 1543–1544. [CrossRef]
20. Yaghi, C.; Assaf, A. Acetaminophen Toxicity at Therapeutic Doses. *Intern. Med. Rev.* **2017**, *3*, 1–13.
21. McGill, M.R.; Hinson, J.A. The Development and Hepatotoxicity of Acetaminophen: Reviewing over a Century of Progress. *Drug Metab. Rev.* **2020**, *52*, 472–500. [CrossRef] [PubMed]
22. Jaeschke, H. Acetaminophen Hepatotoxicity: Not as Simple as One Might Think! Introductory Comments on the Special Issue-Recent Advances in Acetaminophen Hepatotoxicity. *Livers* **2022**, *2*, 105–107. [CrossRef] [PubMed]
23. Fernandez-Checa, J.C.; Bagnaninchi, P.; Ye, H.; Sancho-Bru, P.; Falcon-Perez, J.M.; Royo, F.; Garcia-Ruiz, C.; Konu, O.; Miranda, J.; Lunov, O.; et al. Advanced Preclinical Models for Evaluation of Drug-Induced Liver Injury–Consensus Statement by the European Drug-Induced Liver Injury Network [PRO-EURO-DILI-NET]. *J. Hepatol.* **2021**, *75*, 935–959. [CrossRef] [PubMed]
24. Knockaert, L.; Descatoire, V.; Vadrot, N.; Fromenty, B.; Robin, M.-A. Mitochondrial CYP2E1 Is Sufficient to Mediate Oxidative Stress and Cytotoxicity Induced by Ethanol and Acetaminophen. *Toxicol. Vitr.* **2011**, *25*, 475–484. [CrossRef] [PubMed]
25. Massart, J.; Begriche, K.; Hartman, J.H.; Fromenty, B. Role of Mitochondrial Cytochrome P450 2E1 in Healthy and Diseased Liver. *Cells* **2022**, *11*, 288. [CrossRef]

26. Brackett, C.C.; Bloch, J.D. Phenytoin as a Possible Cause of Acetaminophen Hepatotoxicity: Case Report and Review of the Literature. *Pharmacotherapy* **2000**, *20*, 229–233. [CrossRef]
27. McGill, M.R.; Jaeschke, H. Metabolism and Disposition of Acetaminophen: Recent Advances in Relation to Hepatotoxicity and Diagnosis. *Pharm. Res.* **2013**, *30*, 2174–2187. [CrossRef]
28. Caparrotta, T.M.; Antoine, D.J.; Dear, J.W. Are Some People at Increased Risk of Paracetamol-Induced Liver Injury? A Critical Review of the Literature. *Eur. J. Clin. Pharm.* **2018**, *74*, 147–160. [CrossRef]
29. Hidaka, N.; Kaji, Y.; Takatori, S.; Tanaka, A.; Matsuoka, I.; Tanaka, M. Risk Factors for Acetaminophen-Induced Liver Injury: A Single-Center Study from Japan. *Clin. Ther.* **2020**, *42*, 704–710. [CrossRef]
30. Tsuchiya, Y.; Sakai, H.; Hirata, A.; Yanai, T. Effects of Food Restriction on the Expression of Genes Related to Acetaminophen-Induced Liver Toxicity in Rats. *J. Toxicol. Pathol.* **2018**, *31*, 267–274. [CrossRef]
31. Court, M.H.; Freytsis, M.; Wang, X.; Peter, I.; Guillemette, C.; Hazarika, S.; Duan, S.X.; Greenblatt, D.J.; Lee, W.M. Acute Liver Failure Study Group The UDP-Glucuronosyltransferase (UGT) 1A Polymorphism c.2042C>G (Rs8330) Is Associated with Increased Human Liver Acetaminophen Glucuronidation, Increased UGT1A Exon 5a/5b Splice Variant MRNA Ratio, and Decreased Risk of Unintentional Acetaminophen-Induced Acute Liver Failure. *J. Pharm. Exp.* **2013**, *345*, 297–307. [CrossRef]
32. Henry, L.; Paik, J.; Younossi, Z.M. Review Article: The Epidemiologic Burden of Non-Alcoholic Fatty Liver Disease across the World. *Aliment. Pharm.* **2022**, *56*, 942–956. [CrossRef] [PubMed]
33. Brunt, E.M.; Kleiner, D.E.; Carpenter, D.H.; Rinella, M.; Harrison, S.A.; Loomba, R.; Younossi, Z.; Neuschwander-Tetri, B.A.; Sanyal, A.J. American Association for the Study of Liver Diseases NASH Task Force NAFLD: Reporting Histologic Findings in Clinical Practice. *Hepatology* **2021**, *73*, 2028–2038. [CrossRef] [PubMed]
34. Ahmad, M.I.; Khan, M.U.; Kodali, S.; Shetty, A.; Bell, S.M.; Victor, D. Hepatocellular Carcinoma Due to Nonalcoholic Fatty Liver Disease: Current Concepts and Future Challenges. *J. Hepatocell. Carcinoma* **2022**, *9*, 477–496. [CrossRef]
35. Koch, L.K.; Yeh, M.M. Nonalcoholic Fatty Liver Disease (NAFLD): Diagnosis, Pitfalls, and Staging. *Ann. Diagn. Pathol.* **2018**, *37*, 83–90. [CrossRef] [PubMed]
36. Tandra, S.; Yeh, M.M.; Brunt, E.M.; Vuppalanchi, R.; Cummings, O.W.; Ünalp-Arida, A.; Wilson, L.A.; Chalasani, N. Presence and Significance of Microvesicular Steatosis in Nonalcoholic Fatty Liver Disease. *J. Hepatol.* **2011**, *55*, 654–659. [CrossRef] [PubMed]
37. Begriche, K.; Massart, J.; Robin, M.-A.; Bonnet, F.; Fromenty, B. Mitochondrial Adaptations and Dysfunctions in Nonalcoholic Fatty Liver Disease. *Hepatology* **2013**, *58*, 1497–1507. [CrossRef]
38. Sunny, N.E.; Bril, F.; Cusi, K. Mitochondrial Adaptation in Nonalcoholic Fatty Liver Disease: Novel Mechanisms and Treatment Strategies. *Trends Endocrinol. Metab.* **2017**, *28*, 250–260. [CrossRef]
39. Pafili, K.; Roden, M. Nonalcoholic Fatty Liver Disease (NAFLD) from Pathogenesis to Treatment Concepts in Humans. *Mol. Metab.* **2021**, *50*, 101122. [CrossRef]
40. Nguyen, G.C.; Sam, J.; Thuluvath, P.J. Hepatitis C Is a Predictor of Acute Liver Injury among Hospitalizations for Acetaminophen Overdose in the United States: A Nationwide Analysis. *Hepatology* **2008**, *48*, 1336–1341. [CrossRef]
41. Myers, R.P.; Shaheen, A.A.M. Hepatitis C, Alcohol Abuse, and Unintentional Overdoses Are Risk Factors for Acetaminophen-Related Hepatotoxicity. *Hepatology* **2009**, *49*, 1399–1400. [CrossRef] [PubMed]
42. Chomchai, S.; Chomchai, C. Being Overweight or Obese as a Risk Factor for Acute Liver Injury Secondary to Acute Acetaminophen Overdose. *Pharm. Drug Saf.* **2018**, *27*, 19–24. [CrossRef] [PubMed]
43. van Rongen, A.; Välitalo, P.A.J.; Peeters, M.Y.M.; Boerma, D.; Huisman, F.W.; van Ramshorst, B.; van Dongen, E.P.A.; van den Anker, J.N.; Knibbe, C.A.J. Morbidly Obese Patients Exhibit Increased CYP2E1-Mediated Oxidation of Acetaminophen. *Clin. Pharm.* **2016**, *55*, 833–847. [CrossRef]
44. Rutherford, A.; Davern, T.; Hay, J.E.; Murray, N.G.; Hassanein, T.; Lee, W.M.; Chung, R.T. Acute Liver Failure Study Group Influence of High Body Mass Index on Outcome in Acute Liver Failure. *Clin. Gastroenterol. Hepatol.* **2006**, *4*, 1544–1549. [CrossRef] [PubMed]
45. Radosevich, J.J.; Patanwala, A.E.; Erstad, B.L. Hepatotoxicity in Obese Versus Nonobese Patients With Acetaminophen Poisoning Who Are Treated With Intravenous N-Acetylcysteine. *Am. J. Ther.* **2016**, *23*, e714–e719. [CrossRef]
46. Allard, J.; Le Guillou, D.; Begriche, K.; Fromenty, B. Drug-Induced Liver Injury in Obesity and Nonalcoholic Fatty Liver Disease. *Adv. Pharm.* **2019**, *85*, 75–107. [CrossRef]
47. Corcoran, G.B.; Wong, B.K. Obesity as a Risk Factor in Drug-Induced Organ Injury: Increased Liver and Kidney Damage by Acetaminophen in the Obese Overfed Rat. *J. Pharm. Exp. Ther.* **1987**, *241*, 921–927.
48. Kon, K.; Ikejima, K.; Okumura, K.; Arai, K.; Aoyama, T.; Watanabe, S. Diabetic KK-A(y) Mice Are Highly Susceptible to Oxidative Hepatocellular Damage Induced by Acetaminophen. *Am. J. Physiol. Gastrointest. Liver Physiol.* **2010**, *299*, G329–G337. [CrossRef] [PubMed]
49. Aubert, J.; Begriche, K.; Delannoy, M.; Morel, I.; Pajaud, J.; Ribault, C.; Lepage, S.; McGill, M.R.; Lucas-Clerc, C.; Turlin, B.; et al. Differences in Early Acetaminophen Hepatotoxicity between Obese Ob/Ob and Db/Db Mice. *J. Pharm. Exp. Ther.* **2012**, *342*, 676–687. [CrossRef]
50. Kučera, O.; Roušar, T.; Staňková, P.; Haňáčková, L.; Lotková, H.; Podhola, M.; Cervinková, Z. Susceptibility of Rat Non-Alcoholic Fatty Liver to the Acute Toxic Effect of Acetaminophen. *J. Gastroenterol. Hepatol.* **2012**, *27*, 323–330. [CrossRef]

51. Piccinin, E.; Ducheix, S.; Peres, C.; Arconzo, M.; Vegliante, M.C.; Ferretta, A.; Bellafante, E.; Villani, G.; Moschetta, A. PGC-1β Induces Susceptibility To Acetaminophen-Driven Acute Liver Failure. *Sci. Rep.* **2019**, *9*, 16821. [CrossRef]
52. Shi, C.; Xue, W.; Han, B.; Yang, F.; Yin, Y.; Hu, C. Acetaminophen Aggravates Fat Accumulation in NAFLD by Inhibiting Autophagy via the AMPK/MTOR Pathway. *Eur. J. Pharm.* **2019**, *850*, 15–22. [CrossRef]
53. Wang, J.; Jiang, W.; Xin, J.; Xue, W.; Shi, C.; Wen, J.; Huang, Y.; Hu, C. Caveolin-1 Alleviates Acetaminophen-Induced Fat Accumulation in Non-Alcoholic Fatty Liver Disease by Enhancing Hepatic Antioxidant Ability via Activating AMPK Pathway. *Front. Pharm.* **2021**, *12*, 717276. [CrossRef]
54. Tuntaterdtum, S.; Chaudhary, I.P.; Cibull, M.; Robertson, L.W.; Blouin, R.A. Acetaminophen Hepatotoxicity: Influence of Phenobarbital and Beta-Naphthoflavone Treatment in Obese and Lean Zucker Rats. *Toxicol. Appl. Pharm.* **1993**, *123*, 219–225. [CrossRef]
55. Ito, Y.; Abril, E.R.; Bethea, N.W.; McCuskey, M.K.; McCuskey, R.S. Dietary Steatotic Liver Attenuates Acetaminophen Hepatotoxicity in Mice. *Microcirculation* **2006**, *13*, 19–27. [CrossRef]
56. Kim, T.H.; Choi, D.; Kim, J.Y.; Lee, J.H.; Koo, S.-H. Fast Food Diet-Induced Non-Alcoholic Fatty Liver Disease Exerts Early Protective Effect against Acetaminophen Intoxication in Mice. *BMC Gastroenterol.* **2017**, *17*, 124. [CrossRef]
57. Ghallab, A.; Myllys, M.; Friebel, A.; Duda, J.; Edlund, K.; Halilbasic, E.; Vucur, M.; Hobloss, Z.; Brackhagen, L.; Begher-Tibbe, B.; et al. Spatio-Temporal Multiscale Analysis of Western Diet-Fed Mice Reveals a Translationally Relevant Sequence of Events during NAFLD Progression. *Cells* **2021**, *10*, 2516. [CrossRef]
58. Blouin, R.A.; Dickson, P.; McNamara, P.J.; Cibull, M.; McClain, C. Phenobarbital induction and acetaminophen hepatotoxi-city: Resistance in the obese Zucker rodent. *J. Pharm. Exp. Ther.* **1987**, *243*, 270–565.
59. Donthamsetty, S.; Bhave, V.S.; Mitra, M.S.; Latendresse, J.R.; Mehendale, H.M. Nonalcoholic Steatohepatitic (NASH) Mice Are Protected from Higher Hepatotoxicity of Acetaminophen upon Induction of PPARalpha with Clofibrate. *Toxicol. Appl. Pharm.* **2008**, *230*, 327–337. [CrossRef]
60. Jahn, D.; Kircher, S.; Hermanns, H.M.; Geier, A. Animal Models of NAFLD from a Hepatologist's Point of View. *Biochim. Biophys. Acta Mol. Basis Dis.* **2019**, *1865*, 943–953. [CrossRef]
61. Radhakrishnan, S.; Yeung, S.F.; Ke, J.-Y.; Antunes, M.M.; Pellizzon, M.A. Considerations When Choosing High-Fat, High-Fructose, and High-Cholesterol Diets to Induce Experimental Nonalcoholic Fatty Liver Disease in Laboratory Animal Models. *Curr. Dev. Nutr.* **2021**, *5*, nzab138. [CrossRef]
62. Carreres, L.; Jilkova, Z.M.; Vial, G.; Marche, P.N.; Decaens, T.; Lerat, H. Modeling Diet-Induced NAFLD and NASH in Rats: A Comprehensive Review. *Biomedicines* **2021**, *9*, 378. [CrossRef]
63. Carmiel-Haggai, M.; Cederbaum, A.I.; Nieto, N. Binge Ethanol Exposure Increases Liver Injury in Obese Rats. *Gastroenterology* **2003**, *125*, 1818–1833. [CrossRef]
64. Cipriani, S.; Mencarelli, A.; Palladino, G.; Fiorucci, S. FXR activation reverses insulin resistance and lipid abnormalities and protects against liver steatosis in Zucker (fa/fa) obese rats. *J. Lipid Res.* **2010**, *51*, 771–784. [CrossRef]
65. Zaluzny, L.; Farrell, G.C.; Murray, M. Effect of genetic obesity and experimental diabetes on hepatic microsomal mixed function oxidase activities. *J. Gastroenterol. Hepatol.* **1990**, *5*, 256–263. [CrossRef]
66. Trak-Smayra, V.; Paradis, V.; Massart, J.; Nasser, S.; Jebara, V.; Fromenty, B. Pathology of the Liver in Obese and Diabetic Ob/Ob and Db/Db Mice Fed a Standard or High-Calorie Diet. *Int. J. Exp. Pathol.* **2011**, *92*, 413–421. [CrossRef]
67. Robin, M.A.; Demeilliers, C.; Sutton, A.; Paradis, V.; Maisonneuve, C.; Dubois, S.; Poirel, O.; Lettéron, P.; Pessayre, D.; Fromenty, B. Alcohol increases tumor necrosis factor alpha and decreases nuclear factor-kB to activate hepatic apoptosis in genetically obese mice. *Hepatology* **2005**, *42*, 1280–1290. [CrossRef]
68. Enriquez, A.; Leclercq, I.; Farrell, G.C.; Robertson, G. Altered Expression of Hepatic CYP2E1 and CYP4A in Obese, Diabetic Ob/Ob Mice, and Fa/Fa Zucker Rats. *Biochem. Biophys. Res. Commun.* **1999**, *255*, 300–306. [CrossRef]
69. Okumura, K.; Ikejima, K.; Kon, K.; Abe, W.; Yamashina, S.; Enomoto, N.; Takei, Y.; Sato, N. Exacerbation of dietary steatohepatitis and fibrosis in obese, diabetic KK-A(y) mice. *Hepatol. Res.* **2006**, *36*, 217–228. [CrossRef]
70. Teraoka, N.; Mutoh, M.; Takasu, S.; Ueno, T.; Nakano, K.; Takahashi, M.; Imai, T.; Masuda, S.; Sugimura, T.; Wakabayashi, K. High susceptibility to azoxymethane-induced colorectal carcinogenesis in obese KK-Ay mice. *Int. J. Cancer* **2011**, *129*, 528–535. [CrossRef]
71. McDanell, R.E.; Beales, D.; Henderson, L.; Sethi, J.K. Effect of Dietary Fat on the in Vitro Hepatotoxicity of Paracetamol. *Biochem. Pharm.* **1992**, *44*, 1303–1306. [CrossRef]
72. Kučera, O.; Al-Dury, S.; Lotková, H.; Roušar, T.; Rychtrmoc, D.; Červinková, Z. Steatotic Rat Hepatocytes in Primary Culture Are More Susceptible to the Acute Toxic Effect of Acetaminophen. *Physiol. Res.* **2012**, *61*, S93–S101. [CrossRef]
73. Yang, J.; Peng, T.; Huang, J.; Zhang, G.; Xia, J.; Ma, M.; Deng, D.; Gong, D.; Zeng, Z. Effects of Medium- and Long-Chain Fatty Acids on Acetaminophen- or Rifampicin-Induced Hepatocellular Injury. *Food Sci. Nutr.* **2020**, *8*, 3590–3601. [CrossRef]
74. Michaut, A.; Le Guillou, D.; Moreau, C.; Bucher, S.; McGill, M.R.; Martinais, S.; Gicquel, T.; Morel, I.; Robin, M.-A.; Jaeschke, H.; et al. A Cellular Model to Study Drug-Induced Liver Injury in Nonalcoholic Fatty Liver Disease: Application to Acetaminophen. *Toxicol. Appl. Pharm.* **2016**, *292*, 40–55. [CrossRef]
75. Hubel, E.; Fishman, S.; Holopainen, M.; Käkelä, R.; Shaffer, O; Houri, I.; Zvibel, I.; Shibolet, O. Repetitive Amiodarone Administration Causes Liver Damage via Adipose Tissue ER Stress-Dependent Lipolysis, Leading to Hepatotoxic Free Fatty Acid Accumulation. *Am. J. Physiol. Gastrointest. Liver Physiol.* **2021**, *321*, G298–G307. [CrossRef]

76. Mathur, M.; Yeh, Y.-T.; Arya, R.K.; Jiang, L.; Pornour, M.; Chen, W.; Ma, Y.; Gao, B.; He, L.; Ying, Z.; et al. Adipose Lipolysis Is Important for Ethanol to Induce Fatty Liver in the National Institute on Alcohol Abuse and Alcoholism Murine Model of Chronic and Binge Ethanol Feeding. *Hepatology* **2022**. [CrossRef]
77. Toyoda, T.; Cho, Y.-M.; Akagi, J.-I.; Mizuta, Y.; Matsushita, K.; Nishikawa, A.; Imaida, K.; Ogawa, K. A 13-Week Subchronic Toxicity Study of Acetaminophen Using an Obese Rat Model. *J. Toxicol. Sci.* **2018**, *43*, 423–433. [CrossRef]
78. Kondo, K.; Yamada, N.; Suzuki, Y.; Hashimoto, T.; Toyoda, K.; Takahashi, T.; Kobayashi, A.; Sugai, S.; Yoshinari, K. Enhancement of Acetaminophen-Induced Chronic Hepatotoxicity in Spontaneously Diabetic Torii (SDT) Rats. *J. Toxicol. Sci.* **2020**, *45*, 245–260. [CrossRef]
79. Arconzo, M.; Piccinin, E.; Moschetta, A. Increased Risk of Acute Liver Failure by Pain Killer Drugs in NAFLD: Focus on Nuclear Receptors and Their Coactivators. *Dig. Liver Dis.* **2021**, *53*, 26–34. [CrossRef]
80. Chalasani, N.; Gorski, J.C.; Asghar, M.S.; Asghar, A.; Foresman, B.; Hall, S.D.; Crabb, D.W. Hepatic Cytochrome P450 2E1 Activity in Nondiabetic Patients with Nonalcoholic Steatohepatitis. *Hepatology* **2003**, *37*, 544–550. [CrossRef]
81. Chtioui, H.; Semela, D.; Ledermann, M.; Zimmermann, A.; Dufour, J.-F. Expression and Activity of the Cytochrome P450 2E1 in Patients with Nonalcoholic Steatosis and Steatohepatitis. *Liver Int.* **2007**, *27*, 764–771. [CrossRef]
82. Aubert, J.; Begriche, K.; Knockaert, L.; Robin, M.A.; Fromenty, B. Increased Expression of Cytochrome P450 2E1 in Nonalcoholic Fatty Liver Disease: Mechanisms and Pathophysiological Role. *Clin. Res. Hepatol. Gastroenterol.* **2011**, *35*, 630–637. [CrossRef]
83. Brill, M.J.E.; Diepstraten, J.; van Rongen, A.; van Kralingen, S.; van den Anker, J.N.; Knibbe, C.A.J. Impact of Obesity on Drug Metabolism and Elimination in Adults and Children. *Clin. Pharm.* **2012**, *51*, 277–304. [CrossRef]
84. Aljomah, G.; Baker, S.S.; Liu, W.; Kozielski, R.; Oluwole, J.; Lupu, B.; Baker, R.D.; Zhu, L. Induction of CYP2E1 in Non-Alcoholic Fatty Liver Diseases. *Exp. Mol. Pathol.* **2015**, *99*, 677–681. [CrossRef]
85. Gade, C.; Dalhoff, K.; Petersen, T.S.; Riis, T.; Schmeltz, C.; Chabanova, E.; Christensen, H.R.; Mikus, G.; Burhenne, J.; Holm, J.C.; et al. Higher Chlorzoxazone Clearance in Obese Children Compared with Nonobese Peers. *Br. J. Clin. Pharm.* **2018**, *84*, 1738–1747. [CrossRef]
86. Raucy, J.L.; Lasker, J.M.; Kraner, J.C.; Salazar, D.E.; Lieber, C.S.; Corcoran, G.B. Induction of Cytochrome P450IIE1 in the Obese Overfed Rat. *Mol. Pharm.* **1991**, *39*, 275–280.
87. Baumgardner, J.N.; Shankar, K.; Hennings, L.; Badger, T.M.; Ronis, M.J.J. A New Model for Nonalcoholic Steatohepatitis in the Rat Utilizing Total Enteral Nutrition to Overfeed a High-Polyunsaturated Fat Diet. *Am. J. Physiol. Gastrointest. Liver Physiol.* **2008**, *294*, G27–G38. [CrossRef]
88. Begriche, K.; Lettéron, P.; Abbey-Toby, A.; Vadrot, N.; Robin, M.-A.; Bado, A.; Pessayre, D.; Fromenty, B. Partial Leptin Deficiency Favors Diet-Induced Obesity and Related Metabolic Disorders in Mice. *Am. J. Physiol. Endocrinol. Metab.* **2008**, *294*, E939–E951. [CrossRef]
89. Abdelmegeed, M.A.; Banerjee, A.; Yoo, S.-H.; Jang, S.; Gonzalez, F.J.; Song, B.-J. Critical Role of Cytochrome P450 2E1 (CYP2E1) in the Development of High Fat-Induced Non-Alcoholic Steatohepatitis. *J. Hepatol.* **2012**, *57*, 860–866. [CrossRef]
90. Lai, Y.-S.; Lee, W.-C.; Lin, Y.-E.; Ho, C.-T.; Lu, K.-H.; Lin, S.-H.; Panyod, S.; Chu, Y.-L.; Sheen, L.-Y. Ginger Essential Oil Ameliorates Hepatic Injury and Lipid Accumulation in High Fat Diet-Induced Nonalcoholic Fatty Liver Disease. *J. Agric. Food Chem.* **2016**, *64*, 2062–2071. [CrossRef]
91. Liu, W.; Shang, J.; Deng, Y.; Han, X.; Chen, Y.; Wang, S.; Yang, R.; Dong, F.; Shang, H. Network Pharmacology Analysis on Mechanism of Jian Pi Qing Gan Yin Decoction Ameliorating High Fat Diet-Induced Non-Alcoholic Fatty Liver Disease and Validated in Vivo. *J. Ethnopharmacol.* **2022**, *295*, 115382. [CrossRef]
92. Seth, R.K.; Das, S.; Pourhoseini, S.; Dattaroy, D.; Igwe, S.; Ray, J.B.; Fan, D.; Michelotti, G.A.; Diehl, A.M.; Chatterjee, S. M1 Polarization Bias and Subsequent Nonalcoholic Steatohepatitis Progression Is Attenuated by Nitric Oxide Donor DETA NONOate via Inhibition of CYP2E1-Induced Oxidative Stress in Obese Mice. *J. Pharm. Exp. Ther.* **2015**, *352*, 77–89. [CrossRef]
93. Correia, M.A.; Kwon, D. Why Hepatic CYP2E1-Elevation by Itself Is Insufficient for Inciting NAFLD/NASH: Inferences from Two Genetic Knockout Mouse Models. *Biology* **2020**, *9*, 419. [CrossRef]
94. Leclercq, I.A.; Farrell, G.C.; Field, J.; Bell, D.R.; Gonzalez, F.J.; Robertson, G.R. CYP2E1 and CYP4A as Microsomal Catalysts of Lipid Peroxides in Murine Nonalcoholic Steatohepatitis. *J. Clin. Investig.* **2000**, *105*, 1067–1075. [CrossRef]
95. Abdelmegeed, M.A.; Choi, Y.; Godlewski, G.; Ha, S.-K.; Banerjee, A.; Jang, S.; Song, B.-J. Cytochrome P450-2E1 Promotes Fast Food-Mediated Hepatic Fibrosis. *Sci. Rep.* **2017**, *7*, 39764. [CrossRef]
96. Leung, T.-M.; Nieto, N. CYP2E1 and Oxidant Stress in Alcoholic and Non-Alcoholic Fatty Liver Disease. *J. Hepatol.* **2013**, *58*, 395–398. [CrossRef]
97. Wang, K.; Tan, W.; Liu, X.; Deng, L.; Huang, L.; Wang, X.; Gao, X. New Insight and Potential Therapy for NAFLD: CYP2E1 and Flavonoids. *Biomed. Pharm.* **2021**, *137*, 111326. [CrossRef]
98. Raucy, J.L.; Lasker, J.; Ozaki, K.; Zoleta, V. Regulation of CYP2E1 by Ethanol and Palmitic Acid and CYP4A11 by Clofibrate in Primary Cultures of Human Hepatocytes. *Toxicol. Sci.* **2004**, *79*, 233–241. [CrossRef]
99. Zhou, Z.; Qi, J.; Lim, C.W.; Kim, J.-W.; Kim, B. Dual TBK1/IKKε Inhibitor Amlexanox Mitigates Palmitic Acid-Induced Hepatotoxicity and Lipoapoptosis in Vitro. *Toxicology* **2020**, *444*, 152579. [CrossRef]

100. Achterbergh, R.; Lammers, L.A.; Klümpen, H.-J.; Mathôt, R.A.A.; Romijn, J.A. Short-Term High-Fat Diet Alters Acetaminophen Metabolism in Healthy Individuals. *Ther. Drug Monit.* **2022**, *44*, 797–804. [CrossRef]
101. Videla, L.A.; Rodrigo, R.; Orellana, M.; Fernandez, V.; Tapia, G.; Quiñones, L.; Varela, N.; Contreras, J.; Lazarte, R.; Csendes, A.; et al. Oxidative Stress-Related Parameters in the Liver of Non-Alcoholic Fatty Liver Disease Patients. *Clin. Sci.* **2004**, *106*, 261–268. [CrossRef]
102. Hardwick, R.N.; Fisher, C.D.; Canet, M.J.; Lake, A.D.; Cherrington, N.J. Diversity in Antioxidant Response Enzymes in Progressive Stages of Human Nonalcoholic Fatty Liver Disease. *Drug Metab. Dispos.* **2010**, *38*, 2293–2301. [CrossRef]
103. Lin, Z.; Cai, F.; Lin, N.; Ye, J.; Zheng, Q.; Ding, G. Effects of Glutamine on Oxidative Stress and Nuclear Factor-KB Expression in the Livers of Rats with Nonalcoholic Fatty Liver Disease. *Exp. Ther. Med.* **2014**, *7*, 365–370. [CrossRef]
104. Wang, G.; Wu, B.; Zhang, L.; Jin, X.; Wang, K.; Xu, W.; Zhang, B.; Wang, H. The Protective Effects of Trelagliptin on High-Fat Diet-Induced Nonalcoholic Fatty Liver Disease in Mice. *J. Biochem. Mol. Toxicol.* **2021**, *35*, e22696. [CrossRef]
105. Li, L.; Zhang, G.-F.; Lee, K.; Lopez, R.; Previs, S.F.; Willard, B.; McCullough, A.; Kasumov, T. A Western Diet Induced NAFLD in LDLR(-/)(-) Mice Is Associated with Reduced Hepatic Glutathione Synthesis. *Free Radic. Biol. Med.* **2016**, *96*, 13–21. [CrossRef]
106. Staňková, P.; Kučera, O.; Peterová, E.; Lotková, H.; Maseko, T.E.; Nožičková, K.; Červinková, Z. Adaptation of Mitochondrial Substrate Flux in a Mouse Model of Nonalcoholic Fatty Liver Disease. *Int. J. Mol. Sci.* **2020**, *21*, 1101. [CrossRef]
107. Smirne, C.; Croce, E.; Di Benedetto, D.; Cantaluppi, V.; Comi, C.; Sainaghi, P.P.; Minisini, R.; Grossini, E.; Pirisi, M. Oxidative Stress in Non-Alcoholic Fatty Liver Disease. *Livers* **2022**, *2*, 30–76. [CrossRef]
108. Fromenty, B.; Roden, M. Mitochondrial Alterations in Fatty Liver Diseases. *J. Hepatol.* **2022**, *Oct 7. 22*, S0168–S8278. [CrossRef]
109. Liu, Y.; Chen, Y.; Xie, X.; Yin, A.; Yin, Y.; Liu, Y.; Dong, L.; Zhu, Z.; Zhou, J.; Zeng, Q.; et al. Gender Difference on the Effect of Omega-3 Polyunsaturated Fatty Acids on Acetaminophen-Induced Acute Liver Failure. *Oxid. Med. Cell Longev.* **2020**, *2020*, 8096847. [CrossRef]
110. Liu, Y.; Lin, J.; Chen, Y.; Li, Z.; Zhou, J.; Lu, X.; Chen, Z.; Zuo, D. Omega-3 Polyunsaturated Fatty Acids Inhibit IL-11/STAT3 Signaling in Hepatocytes during Acetaminophen Hepatotoxicity. *Int. J. Mol. Med.* **2021**, *48*, 190. [CrossRef]
111. Teratani, T.; Tomita, K.; Suzuki, T.; Furuhashi, H.; Irie, R.; Hida, S.; Okada, Y.; Kurihara, C.; Ebinuma, H.; Nakamoto, N.; et al. Free Cholesterol Accumulation in Liver Sinusoidal Endothelial Cells Exacerbates Acetaminophen Hepatotoxicity via TLR9 Signaling. *J. Hepatol.* **2017**, *67*, 780–790. [CrossRef]
112. Marí, M.; Caballero, F.; Colell, A.; Morales, A.; Caballeria, J.; Fernandez, A.; Enrich, C.; Fernandez-Checa, J.C.; García-Ruiz, C. Mitochondrial Free Cholesterol Loading Sensitizes to TNF- and Fas-Mediated Steatohepatitis. *Cell Metab.* **2006**, *4*, 185–198. [CrossRef]
113. Ribas, V.; García-Ruiz, C.; Fernández-Checa, J.C. Glutathione and Mitochondria. *Front Pharm.* **2014**, *5*, 151. [CrossRef]
114. Xu, Y.; Lu, J.; Guo, Y.; Zhang, Y.; Liu, J.; Huang, S.; Zhang, Y.; Gao, L.; Wang, X. Hypercholesterolemia Reduces the Expression and Function of Hepatic Drug Metabolizing Enzymes and Transporters in Rats. *Toxicol. Lett.* **2022**, *364*, 1–11. [CrossRef]
115. Karkucinska-Wieckowska, A.; Simoes, I.C.M.; Kalinowski, P.; Lebiedzinska-Arciszewska, M.; Zieniewicz, K.; Milkiewicz, P.; Górska-Ponikowska, M.; Pinton, P.; Malik, A.N.; Krawczyk, M.; et al. Mitochondria, Oxidative Stress and Nonalcoholic Fatty Liver Disease: A Complex Relationship. *Eur. J. Clin. Investig.* **2022**, *52*, e13622. [CrossRef]
116. Pérez-Carreras, M.; Del Hoyo, P.; Martín, M.A.; Rubio, J.C.; Martín, A.; Castellano, G.; Colina, F.; Arenas, J.; Solis-Herruzo, J.A. Defective Hepatic Mitochondrial Respiratory Chain in Patients with Nonalcoholic Steatohepatitis. *Hepatology* **2003**, *38*, 999–1007. [CrossRef]
117. Koliaki, C.; Szendroedi, J.; Kaul, K.; Jelenik, T.; Nowotny, P.; Jankowiak, F.; Herder, C.; Carstensen, M.; Krausch, M.; Knoefel, W.T.; et al. Adaptation of Hepatic Mitochondrial Function in Humans with Non-Alcoholic Fatty Liver Is Lost in Steatohepatitis. *Cell Metab.* **2015**, *21*, 739–746. [CrossRef]
118. Ramsay, R.R.; Rashed, M.S.; Nelson, S.D. In Vitro Effects of Acetaminophen Metabolites and Analogs on the Respiration of Mouse Liver Mitochondria. *Arch. Biochem. Biophys.* **1989**, *273*, 449–457. [CrossRef]
119. Chrøis, K.M.; Larsen, S.; Pedersen, J.S.; Rygg, M.O.; Boilsen, A.E.B.; Bendtsen, F.; Dela, F. Acetaminophen Toxicity Induces Mitochondrial Complex I Inhibition in Human Liver Tissue. *Basic Clin. Pharm. Toxicol.* **2020**, *126*, 86–91. [CrossRef]
120. Fromenty, B. Alteration of Mitochondrial DNA Homeostasis in Drug-Induced Liver Injury. *Food Chem. Toxicol.* **2020**, *135*, 110916. [CrossRef]
121. Farrell, G.; Schattenberg, J.M.; Leclercq, I.; Yeh, M.M.; Goldin, R.; Teoh, N.; Schuppan, D. Mouse Models of Nonalcoholic Steatohepatitis: Toward Optimization of Their Relevance to Human Nonalcoholic Steatohepatitis. *Hepatology* **2019**, *69*, 2241–2257. [CrossRef]
122. Schuster, S.; Cabrera, D.; Arrese, M.; Feldstein, A.E. Triggering and Resolution of Inflammation in NASH. *Nat. Rev. Gastroenterol. Hepatol.* **2018**, *15*, 349–364. [CrossRef]
123. Kazankov, K.; Jørgensen, S.M.D.; Thomsen, K.L.; Møller, H.J.; Vilstrup, H.; George, J.; Schuppan, D.; Grønbæk, H. The Role of Macrophages in Nonalcoholic Fatty Liver Disease and Nonalcoholic Steatohepatitis. *Nat. Rev. Gastroenterol. Hepatol.* **2019**, *16*, 145–159. [CrossRef]
124. Schneider, K.M.; Elfers, C.; Ghallab, A.; Schneider, C.V.; Galvez, E.J.C.; Mohs, A.; Gui, W.; Candels, L.S.; Wirtz, T.H.; Zuehlke, S.; et al. Intestinal Dysbiosis Amplifies Acetaminophen-Induced Acute Liver Injury. *Cell Mol. Gastroenterol. Hepatol.* **2021**, *11*, 909–933. [CrossRef]

125. Levy, M.; Shapiro, H.; Thaiss, C.A.; Elinav, E. NLRP6: A Multifaceted Innate Immune Sensor. *Trends Immunol.* **2017**, *38*, 248–260. [CrossRef]
126. Aron-Wisnewsky, J.; Vigliotti, C.; Witjes, J.; Le, P.; Holleboom, A.G.; Verheij, J.; Nieuwdorp, M.; Clément, K. Gut Microbiota and Human NAFLD: Disentangling Microbial Signatures from Metabolic Disorders. *Nat. Rev. Gastroenterol. Hepatol.* **2020**, *17*, 279–297. [CrossRef]
127. Breton, J.; Galmiche, M.; Déchelotte, P. Dysbiotic Gut Bacteria in Obesity: An Overview of the Metabolic Mechanisms and Therapeutic Perspectives of Next-Generation Probiotics. *Microorganisms* **2022**, *10*, 452. [CrossRef]
128. Sneed, R.A.; Grimes, S.D.; Schultze, A.E.; Brown, A.P.; Ganey, P.E. Bacterial Endotoxin Enhances the Hepatotoxicity of Allyl Alcohol. *Toxicol. Appl. Pharm.* **1997**, *144*, 77–87. [CrossRef]
129. Shaw, P.J.; Ganey, P.E.; Roth, R.A. Idiosyncratic Drug-Induced Liver Injury and the Role of Inflammatory Stress with an Emphasis on an Animal Model of Trovafloxacin Hepatotoxicity. *Toxicol. Sci.* **2010**, *118*, 7–18. [CrossRef]
130. Wu, W.; Zhao, L.; Yang, P.; Zhou, W.; Li, B.; Moorhead, J.F.; Varghese, Z.; Ruan, X.Z.; Chen, Y. Inflammatory Stress Sensitizes the Liver to Atorvastatin-Induced Injury in ApoE-/- Mice. *PLoS ONE* **2016**, *11*, e0159512. [CrossRef]
131. Lee, W.H.; Kramer, W.G.; Granville, G.E. The Effect of Obesity on Acetaminophen Pharmacokinetics in Man. *J. Clin. Pharm.* **1981**, *21*, 284–287. [CrossRef]
132. Abernethy, D.R.; Divoll, M.; Greenblatt, D.J.; Ameer, B. Obesity, Sex, and Acetaminophen Disposition. *Clin. Pharm. Ther.* **1982**, *31*, 783–790. [CrossRef]
133. Emery, M.G.; Fisher, J.M.; Chien, J.Y.; Kharasch, E.D.; Dellinger, E.P.; Kowdley, K.V.; Thummel, K.E. CYP2E1 Activity before and after Weight Loss in Morbidly Obese Subjects with Nonalcoholic Fatty Liver Disease. *Hepatology* **2003**, *38*, 428–435. [CrossRef]
134. Leclercq, I.A.; Field, J.; Enriquez, A.; Farrell, G.C.; Robertson, G.R. Constitutive and Inducible Expression of Hepatic CYP2E1 in Leptin-Deficient Ob/Ob Mice. *Biochem. Biophys. Res. Commun.* **2000**, *268*, 337–344. [CrossRef]
135. Abdel-Razzak, Z.; Loyer, P.; Fautrel, A.; Gautier, J.C.; Corcos, L.; Turlin, B.; Beaune, P.; Guillouzo, A. Cytokines Down-Regulate Expression of Major Cytochrome P-450 Enzymes in Adult Human Hepatocytes in Primary Culture. *Mol. Pharm.* **1993**, *44*, 707–715.
136. Wang, J.; Hu, Y.; Nekvindova, J.; Ingelman-Sundberg, M.; Neve, E.P.A. IL-4-Mediated Transcriptional Regulation of Human CYP2E1 by Two Independent Signaling Pathways. *Biochem. Pharm.* **2010**, *80*, 1592–1600. [CrossRef]
137. Lin, Q.; Kang, X.; Li, X.; Wang, T.; Liu, F.; Jia, J.; Jin, Z.; Xue, Y. NF-KB-Mediated Regulation of Rat CYP2E1 by Two Independent Signaling Pathways. *PLoS ONE* **2019**, *14*, e0225531. [CrossRef]
138. Drozdzik, M.; Lapczuk-Romanska, J.; Wenzel, C.; Szelag-Pieniek, S.; Post, M.; Skalski, Ł.; Kurzawski, M.; Oswald, S. Gene Expression and Protein Abundance of Hepatic Drug Metabolizing Enzymes in Liver Pathology. *Pharmaceutics* **2021**, *13*, 1334. [CrossRef]
139. Nakai, K.; Tanaka, H.; Hanada, K.; Ogata, H.; Suzuki, F.; Kumada, H.; Miyajima, A.; Ishida, S.; Sunouchi, M.; Habano, W.; et al. Decreased Expression of Cytochromes P450 1A2, 2E1, and 3A4 and Drug Transporters Na+-Taurocholate-Cotransporting Polypeptide, Organic Cation Transporter 1, and Organic Anion-Transporting Peptide-C Correlates with the Progression of Liver Fibrosis in Chronic Hepatitis C Patients. *Drug Metab. Dispos.* **2008**, *36*, 1786–1793. [CrossRef]
140. Müller, G.F.; Döhr, O.; El-Bahay, C.; Kahl, R.; Abel, J. Effect of Transforming Growth Factor-Beta1 on Cytochrome P450 Expression: Inhibition of CYP1 MRNA and Protein Expression in Primary Rat Hepatocytes. *Arch. Toxicol.* **2000**, *74*, 145–152. [CrossRef]
141. Ciuclan, L.; Ehnert, S.; Ilkavets, I.; Weng, H.-L.; Gaitantzi, H.; Tsukamoto, H.; Ueberham, E.; Meindl-Beinker, N.M.; Singer, M.V.; Breitkopf, K.; et al. TGF-Beta Enhances Alcohol Dependent Hepatocyte Damage via down-Regulation of Alcohol Dehydrogenase I. *J. Hepatol.* **2010**, *52*, 407–416. [CrossRef]
142. Kolwankar, D.; Vuppalanchi, R.; Ethell, B.; Jones, D.R.; Wrighton, S.A.; Hall, S.D.; Chalasani, N. Association between Nonalcoholic Hepatic Steatosis and Hepatic Cytochrome P-450 3A Activity. *Clin. Gastroenterol. Hepatol.* **2007**, *5*, 388–393. [CrossRef]
143. Chiba, T.; Noji, K.; Shinozaki, S.; Suzuki, S.; Umegaki, K.; Shimokado, K. Diet-Induced Non-Alcoholic Fatty Liver Disease Affects Expression of Major Cytochrome P450 Genes in a Mouse Model. *J. Pharm. Pharm.* **2016**, *68*, 1567–1576. [CrossRef]
144. Woolsey, S.J.; Mansell, S.E.; Kim, R.B.; Tirona, R.G.; Beaton, M.D. CYP3A Activity and Expression in Nonalcoholic Fatty Liver Disease. *Drug Metab. Dispos.* **2015**, *43*, 1484–1490. [CrossRef]
145. Cobbina, E.; Akhlaghi, F. Non-Alcoholic Fatty Liver Disease (NAFLD)—Pathogenesis, Classification, and Effect on Drug Metabolizing Enzymes and Transporters. *Drug Metab. Rev.* **2017**, *49*, 197–211. [CrossRef]
146. Jamwal, R.; de la Monte, S.M.; Ogasawara, K.; Adusumalli, S.; Barlock, B.B.; Akhlaghi, F. Nonalcoholic Fatty Liver Disease and Diabetes Are Associated with Decreased CYP3A4 Protein Expression and Activity in Human Liver. *Mol. Pharm.* **2018**, *15*, 2621–2632. [CrossRef]
147. Smit, C.; De Hoogd, S.; Brüggemann, R.J.M.; Knibbe, C.A.J. Obesity and Drug Pharmacology: A Review of the Influence of Obesity on Pharmacokinetic and Pharmacodynamic Parameters. *Expert. Opin. Drug Metab. Toxicol.* **2018**, *14*, 275–285. [CrossRef]
148. Zeng, H.; Lin, Y.; Gong, J.; Lin, S.; Gao, J.; Li, C.; Feng, Z.; Zhang, H.; Zhang, J.; Li, Y.; et al. CYP3A Suppression during Diet-Induced Nonalcoholic Fatty Liver Disease Is Independent of PXR Regulation. *Chem. Biol. Interact.* **2019**, *308*, 185–193. [CrossRef]
149. Krogstad, V.; Peric, A.; Robertsen, I.; Kringen, M.K.; Vistnes, M.; Hjelmesæth, J.; Sandbu, R.; Johnson, L.K.; Angeles, P.C.; Jansson-Löfmark, R.; et al. Correlation of Body Weight and Composition With Hepatic Activities of Cytochrome P450 Enzymes. *J. Pharm. Sci.* **2021**, *110*, 432–437. [CrossRef]

150. Wiese, M.D.; Meakin, A.S.; Varcoe, T.J.; Darby, J.R.T.; Sarr, O.; Kiser, P.; Bradshaw, E.L.; Regnault, T.R.H.; Morrison, J.L. Hepatic Cytochrome P450 Function Is Reduced by Life-Long Western Diet Consumption in Guinea Pig Independent of Birth Weight. *Life Sci.* **2021**, *287*, 120133. [CrossRef]
151. Fisher, C.D.; Lickteig, A.J.; Augustine, L.M.; Ranger-Moore, J.; Jackson, J.P.; Ferguson, S.S.; Cherrington, N.J. Hepatic Cytochrome P450 Enzyme Alterations in Humans with Progressive Stages of Nonalcoholic Fatty Liver Disease. *Drug Metab. Dispos.* **2009**, *37*, 2087–2094. [CrossRef]
152. Lake, A.D.; Novak, P.; Fisher, C.D.; Jackson, J.P.; Hardwick, R.N.; Billheimer, D.D.; Klimecki, W.T.; Cherrington, N.J. Analysis of Global and Absorption, Distribution, Metabolism, and Elimination Gene Expression in the Progressive Stages of Human Nonalcoholic Fatty Liver Disease. *Drug Metab. Dispos.* **2011**, *39*, 1954–1960. [CrossRef]
153. Li, H.; Clarke, J.D.; Dzierlenga, A.L.; Bear, J.; Goedken, M.J.; Cherrington, N.J. In Vivo Cytochrome P450 Activity Alterations in Diabetic Nonalcoholic Steatohepatitis Mice. *J. Biochem. Mol. Toxicol.* **2017**, *31*, e21840. [CrossRef]
154. Hou, C.; Feng, W.; Wei, S.; Wang, Y.; Xu, X.; Wei, J.; Ma, Z.; Du, Y.; Guo, J.; He, Y.; et al. Bioinformatics Analysis of Key Differentially Expressed Genes in Nonalcoholic Fatty Liver Disease Mice Models. *Gene Expr.* **2018**, *19*, 25–35. [CrossRef]
155. Gabbia, D.; Roverso, M.; Guido, M.; Sacchi, D.; Scaffidi, M.; Carrara, M.; Orso, G.; Russo, F.P.; Floreani, A.; Bogialli, S.; et al. Western Diet-Induced Metabolic Alterations Affect Circulating Markers of Liver Function before the Development of Steatosis. *Nutrients* **2019**, *11*, 1602. [CrossRef]
156. Al Nebaihi, H.M.; Al Batran, R.; Ussher, J.R.; Maayah, Z.H.; El-Kadi, A.O.S.; Brocks, D.R. Dietary-Induced Obesity, Hepatic Cytochrome P450, and Lidocaine Metabolism: Comparative Effects of High-Fat Diets in Mice and Rats and Reversibility of Effects With Normalization of Diet. *J. Pharm. Sci.* **2020**, *109*, 1199–1210. [CrossRef]
157. Wu, J.; Lou, Y.-G.; Yang, X.; Wang, R.; Zhang, R.; Aa, J.-Y.; Wang, G.-J.; Xie, Y. Silybin Regulates P450s Activity by Attenuating Endoplasmic Reticulum Stress in Mouse Nonalcoholic Fatty Liver Disease. *Acta Pharm. Sin.* **2022**, *44*, 133–144. [CrossRef]
158. Xiang, L.; Jiao, Y.; Qian, Y.; Li, Y.; Mao, F.; Lu, Y. Comparison of Hepatic Gene Expression Profiles between Three Mouse Models of Nonalcoholic Fatty Liver Disease. *Genes Dis.* **2022**, *9*, 201–215. [CrossRef]
159. Wahlang, B.; Song, M.; Beier, J.I.; Cameron Falkner, K.; Al-Eryani, L.; Clair, H.B.; Prough, R.A.; Osborne, T.S.; Malarkey, D.E.; States, J.C.; et al. Evaluation of Aroclor 1260 Exposure in a Mouse Model of Diet-Induced Obesity and Non-Alcoholic Fatty Liver Disease. *Toxicol. Appl. Pharm.* **2014**, *279*, 380–390. [CrossRef]
160. Abernethy, D.R.; Greenblatt, D.J.; Divoll, M.; Shader, R.I. Enhanced Glucuronide Conjugation of Drugs in Obesity: Studies of Lorazepam, Oxazepam, and Acetaminophen. *J. Lab. Clin. Med.* **1983**, *101*, 873–880.
161. Barshop, N.J.; Capparelli, E.V.; Sirlin, C.B.; Schwimmer, J.B.; Lavine, J.E. Acetaminophen Pharmacokinetics in Children with Nonalcoholic Fatty Liver Disease. *J. Pediatr. Gastroenterol. Nutr.* **2011**, *52*, 198–202. [CrossRef]
162. Mazaleuskaya, L.L.; Sangkuhl, K.; Thorn, C.F.; FitzGerald, G.A.; Altman, R.B.; Klein, T.E. PharmGKB Summary: Pathways of Acetaminophen Metabolism at the Therapeutic versus Toxic Doses. *Pharm. Genom.* **2015**, *25*, 416–426. [CrossRef]
163. Hardwick, R.N.; Ferreira, D.W.; More, V.R.; Lake, A.D.; Lu, Z.; Manautou, J.E.; Slitt, A.L.; Cherrington, N.J. Altered UDP-Glucuronosyltransferase and Sulfotransferase Expression and Function during Progressive Stages of Human Nonalcoholic Fatty Liver Disease. *Drug Metab. Dispos.* **2013**, *41*, 554–561. [CrossRef]
164. Feng, R.; Wang, Y.; Liu, C.; Yan, C.; Zhang, H.; Su, H.; Kang, J.X.; Shang, C.-Z.; Wan, J.-B. Acetaminophen-Induced Liver Injury Is Attenuated in Transgenic Fat-1 Mice Endogenously Synthesizing Long-Chain n-3 Fatty Acids. *Biochem. Pharm.* **2018**, *154*, 75–88. [CrossRef]
165. Eraky, S.M.; Abo El-Magd, N.F. Omega-3 Fatty Acids Protect against Acetaminophen-Induced Hepatic and Renal Toxicity in Rats through HO-1-Nrf2-BACH1 Pathway. *Arch. Biochem. Biophys.* **2020**, *687*, 108387. [CrossRef]
166. Speck, R.F.; Lauterburg, B.H. Fish Oil Protects Mice against Acetaminophen Hepatotoxicity in Vivo. *Hepatology* **1991**, *13*, 557–561. [CrossRef]
167. Maksymchuk, O.; Shysh, A.; Stroy, D. Treatment with Omega-3 PUFAs Does Not Increase the Risk of CYP2E1-Dependent Oxidative Stress and Diabetic Liver Pathology. *Front. Endocrinol.* **2022**, *13*, 1004564. [CrossRef]
168. Jain, P.; Hejjaji, V.; Thomas, M.B.; Garcia, R.A.; Kennedy, K.F.; Goyal, A.; Sperling, L.; Das, S.R.; Hafida, S.; Enriquez, J.R.; et al. Use of Primary Bariatric Surgery among Patients with Obesity and Diabetes. Insights from the Diabetes Collaborative Registry. *Int. J. Obes.* **2022**, *46*, 2163–2167. [CrossRef]
169. Zhou, H.; Luo, P.; Li, P.; Wang, G.; Yi, X.; Fu, Z.; Sun, X.; Cui, B.; Zhu, L.; Zhu, S. Bariatric Surgery Improves Nonalcoholic Fatty Liver Disease: Systematic Review and Meta-Analysis. *Obes. Surg.* **2022**, *32*, 1872–1883. [CrossRef]
170. Holt, E.W.; DeMartini, S.; Davern, T.J. Acute Liver Failure Due to Acetaminophen Poisoning in Patients With Prior Weight Loss Surgery: A Case Series. *J. Clin. Gastroenterol.* **2015**, *49*, 790–793. [CrossRef]
171. Abusabeib, A.; El Ansari, W.; Alobaidan, J.; Elhag, W. First Case Report of Fulminant Hepatitis After Laparoscopic Sleeve Gastrectomy Associated with Concomitant Maximal Therapeutic Dose of Acetaminophen Use, Protein Calorie Malnutrition, and Vitamins A and D, Selenium, and Glutathione Deficiencies. *Obes. Surg.* **2021**, *31*, 899–903. [CrossRef]
172. Puris, E.; Pasanen, M.; Ranta, V.-P.; Gynther, M.; Petsalo, A.; Käkelä, P.; Männistö, V.; Pihlajamäki, J. Laparoscopic Roux-En-Y Gastric Bypass Surgery Influenced Pharmacokinetics of Several Drugs given as a Cocktail with the Highest Impact Observed for CYP1A2, CYP2C8 and CYP2E1 Substrates. *Basic. Clin. Pharm. Toxicol.* **2019**, *125*, 123–132. [CrossRef]

173. Porat, D.; Markovic, M.; Zur, M.; Fine-Shamir, N.; Azran, C.; Shaked, G.; Czeiger, D.; Vaynshtein, J.; Replyanski, I.; Sebbag, G.; et al. Increased Paracetamol Bioavailability after Sleeve Gastrectomy: A Crossover Pre- vs. Post-Operative Clinical Trial. *J. Clin. Med.* **2019**, *8*, 1949. [CrossRef]
174. Chen, K.-F.; Chan, L.-N.; Senn, T.D.; Oelschlager, B.K.; Flum, D.R.; Shen, D.D.; Horn, J.R.; Lin, Y.S. The Impact of Proximal Roux-En-Y Gastric Bypass Surgery on Acetaminophen Absorption and Metabolism. *Pharmacotherapy* **2020**, *40*, 191–203. [CrossRef]
175. Katsarou, A.; Gudbjörnsdottir, S.; Rawshani, A.; Dabelea, D.; Bonifacio, E.; Anderson, B.J.; Jacobsen, L.M.; Schatz, D.A.; Lernmark, Å. Type 1 Diabetes Mellitus. *Nat. Rev. Dis. Prim.* **2017**, *3*, 17016. [CrossRef]
176. Zaccardi, F.; Webb, D.R.; Yates, T.; Davies, M.J. Pathophysiology of Type 1 and Type 2 Diabetes Mellitus: A 90-Year Perspective. *Postgrad. Med. J.* **2016**, *92*, 63–69. [CrossRef]
177. Eizirik, D.L.; Pasquali, L.; Cnop, M. Pancreatic β-Cells in Type 1 and Type 2 Diabetes Mellitus: Different Pathways to Failure. *Nat. Rev. Endocrinol.* **2020**, *16*, 349–362. [CrossRef]
178. de Vries, M.; Westerink, J.; Kaasjager, K.H.A.H.; de Valk, H.W. Prevalence of Nonalcoholic Fatty Liver Disease (NAFLD) in Patients With Type 1 Diabetes Mellitus: A Systematic Review and Meta-Analysis. *J. Clin. Endocrinol. Metab.* **2020**, *105*, 3842–3853. [CrossRef]
179. Mertens, J.; De Block, C.; Spinhoven, M.; Driessen, A.; Francque, S.M.; Kwanten, W.J. Hepatopathy Associated With Type 1 Diabetes: Distinguishing Non-Alcoholic Fatty Liver Disease From Glycogenic Hepatopathy. *Front. Pharm.* **2021**, *12*, 768576. [CrossRef]
180. El-Serag, H.B.; Everhart, J.E. Diabetes Increases the Risk of Acute Hepatic Failure. *Gastroenterology* **2002**, *122*, 1822–1828. [CrossRef]
181. Chalasani, N.; Fontana, R.J.; Bonkovsky, H.L.; Watkins, P.B.; Davern, T.; Serrano, J.; Yang, H.; Rochon, J. Drug Induced Liver Injury Network (DILIN) Causes, Clinical Features, and Outcomes from a Prospective Study of Drug-Induced Liver Injury in the United States. *Gastroenterology* **2008**, *135*, 1924–1934, 1934.e1-4. [CrossRef]
182. Lu, R.-J.; Zhang, Y.; Tang, F.-L.; Zheng, Z.-W.; Fan, Z.-D.; Zhu, S.-M.; Qian, X.-F.; Liu, N.-N. Clinical Characteristics of Drug-Induced Liver Injury and Related Risk Factors. *Exp. Ther. Med.* **2016**, *12*, 2606–2616. [CrossRef]
183. Deeds, M.C.; Anderson, J.M.; Armstrong, A.S.; Gastineau, D.A.; Hiddinga, H.J.; Jahangir, A.; Eberhardt, N.L.; Kudva, Y.C. Single Dose Streptozotocin-Induced Diabetes: Considerations for Study Design in Islet Transplantation Models. *Lab. Anim.* **2011**, *45*, 131–140. [CrossRef]
184. Wang, Q.; Wei, S.; Zhou, H.; Shen, G.; Gan, X.; Zhou, S.; Qiu, J.; Shi, C.; Lu, L. Hyperglycemia Exacerbates Acetaminophen-Induced Acute Liver Injury by Promoting Liver-Resident Macrophage Proinflammatory Response via AMPK/PI3K/AKT-Mediated Oxidative Stress. *Cell Death Discov.* **2019**, *5*, 119. [CrossRef]
185. Wu, D.; Cederbaum, A.I. Combined Effects of Streptozotocin-Induced Diabetes plus 4-Methylpyrazole Treatment on Rat Liver Cytochrome P4502E1. *Arch. Biochem. Biophys.* **1993**, *302*, 175–182. [CrossRef]
186. Raza, H.; Prabu, S.K.; Robin, M.-A.; Avadhani, N.G. Elevated Mitochondrial Cytochrome P450 2E1 and Glutathione S-Transferase A4-4 in Streptozotocin-Induced Diabetic Rats: Tissue-Specific Variations and Roles in Oxidative Stress. *Diabetes* **2004**, *53*, 185–194. [CrossRef]
187. Sindhu, R.K.; Koo, J.R.; Sindhu, K.K.; Ehdaie, A.; Farmand, F.; Roberts, C.K. Differential Regulation of Hepatic Cytochrome P450 Monooxygenases in Streptozotocin-Induced Diabetic Rats. *Free Radic. Res.* **2006**, *40*, 921–928. [CrossRef]
188. Maksymchuk, O.; Shysh, A.; Rosohatska, I.; Chashchyn, M. Quercetin Prevents Type 1 Diabetic Liver Damage through Inhibition of CYP2E1. *Pharmacol. Rep.* **2017**, *69*, 1386–1392. [CrossRef]
189. Price, V.F.; Jollow, D.J. Increased Resistance of Diabetic Rats to Acetaminophen-Induced Hepatotoxicity. *J. Pharm. Exp. Ther.* **1982**, *220*, 504–513.
190. Shankar, K.; Vaidya, V.S.; Apte, U.M.; Manautou, J.E.; Ronis, M.J.J.; Bucci, T.J.; Mehendale, H.M. Type 1 Diabetic Mice Are Protected from Acetaminophen Hepatotoxicity. *Toxicol. Sci.* **2003**, *73*, 220–234. [CrossRef]
191. Shankar, K.; Vaidya, V.S.; Corton, J.C.; Bucci, T.J.; Liu, J.; Waalkes, M.P.; Mehendale, H.M. Activation of PPAR-Alpha in Streptozotocin-Induced Diabetes Is Essential for Resistance against Acetaminophen Toxicity. *FASEB J.* **2003**, *17*, 1748–1750. [CrossRef]
192. Boyle, M.; Masson, S.; Anstee, Q.M. The Bidirectional Impacts of Alcohol Consumption and the Metabolic Syndrome: Cofactors for Progressive Fatty Liver Disease. *J. Hepatol.* **2018**, *68*, 251–267. [CrossRef]
193. Di Ciaula, A.; Bonfrate, L.; Krawczyk, M.; Frühbeck, G.; Portincasa, P. Synergistic and Detrimental Effects of Alcohol Intake on Progression of Liver Steatosis. *Int. J. Mol. Sci.* **2022**, *23*, 2636. [CrossRef]
194. Massart, J.; Begriche, K.; Corlu, A.; Fromenty, B. Xenobiotic-Induced Aggravation of Metabolic-Associated Fatty Liver Disease. *Int. J. Mol. Sci.* **2022**, *23*, 1062. [CrossRef]
195. Akakpo, J.Y.; Ramachandran, A.; Jaeschke, H. Novel strategies for the treatment of acetaminophen hepatotoxicity. *Expert. Opin. Drug Metab. Toxicol.* **2020**, *16*, 1039–1050. [CrossRef]
196. Subramanya, S.B.; Venkataraman, B.; Meeran, M.F.N.; Goyal, S.N.; Patil, C.R.; Ojha, S. Therapeutic Potential of Plants and Plant Derived Phytochemicals against Acetaminophen-Induced Liver Injury. *Int. J. Mol. Sci.* **2018**, *19*, 3776. [CrossRef]
197. Jaeschke, H.; Adelusi, O.B.; Ramachandran, A. Ferroptosis and Acetaminophen Hepatotoxicity: Are We Going Down Another Rabbit Hole? *Gene Expr.* **2021**, *20*, 169–178. [CrossRef]
198. Liao, Y.; Yang, Y.; Wang, X.; Wei, M.; Guo, Q.; Zhao, L. Oroxyloside ameliorates acetaminophen-induced hepatotoxicity by inhibiting JNK related apoptosis and necroptosis. *J. Ethnopharmacol.* **2020**, *258*, 112917. [CrossRef]

199. Hwang, K.A.; Hwang, Y.; Hwang, H.J.; Park, N. Hepatoprotective Effects of Radish (*Raphanus sativus* L.) on Acetaminophen-Induced Liver Damage via Inhibiting Oxidative Stress and Apoptosis. *Nutrients* **2022**, *14*, 5082. [CrossRef]
200. Du, K.; Ramachandran, A.; McGill, M.R.; Mansouri, A.; Asselah, T.; Farhood, A.; Woolbright, B.L.; Ding, W.X.; Jaeschke, H. Induction of mitochondrial biogenesis protects against acetaminophen hepatotoxicity. *Food Chem. Toxicol.* **2017**, *108*, 339–350.

livers

MDPI

Review

Mitochondria in Acetaminophen-Induced Liver Injury and Recovery: A Concise Review

Anup Ramachandran * and Hartmut Jaeschke

Department of Pharmacology, Toxicology, and Therapeutic, University of Kansas Medical Center, Kansas City, KS 66160, USA; hjaeschke@kumc.edu

* Correspondence: aramachandran@kumc.edu; Tel.: +1-913-588-9842

Abstract: Mitochondria are critical organelles responsible for the maintenance of cellular energy homeostasis. Thus, their dysfunction can have severe consequences in cells responsible for energy-intensive metabolic function, such as hepatocytes. Extensive research over the last decades have identified compromised mitochondrial function as a central feature in the pathophysiology of liver injury induced by an acetaminophen (APAP) overdose, the most common cause of acute liver failure in the United States. While hepatocyte mitochondrial oxidative and nitrosative stress coupled with induction of the mitochondrial permeability transition are well recognized after an APAP overdose, recent studies have revealed additional details about the organelle's role in APAP pathophysiology. This concise review highlights these new advances, which establish the central role of the mitochondria in APAP pathophysiology, and places them in the context of earlier information in the literature. Adaptive alterations in mitochondrial morphology as well as the role of cellular iron in mitochondrial dysfunction and the organelle's importance in liver recovery after APAP-induced injury will be discussed.

Keywords: acetaminophen; mitochondria; paracetamol; iron; morphology; spheroid; biogenesis

1. Introduction

Mitochondria are unique organelles that evolved from the integration of an endosymbiotic alphaproteobacterium into a host eukaryotic cell of the Archaea group [1]. This symbiotic relationship was refined over millions of years of evolution, and these organelles are now critical to eukaryotic cell function. Mitochondria are essential to several cellular functions and have been extensively studied over the years, with emphasis on their role in cellular energy maintenance through ATP generation. In addition, mitochondria are critical hubs of cellular metabolism, being involved in glucose metabolism to produce acetyl CoA, as well as fatty acid oxidation and redox homeostasis [2], among others. These critical functions are possible due to the unique structural features of mitochondria, which are double membrane structures with inner membrane folds called cristae that increase their surface area and accommodate the protein complexes of the electron transport chain (ETC) [3]. This dual membrane structure and localization of the ETC components on the inner mitochondrial membrane are important for the establishment of a proton motive force during electron transport for ATP synthesis [3]. The outer mitochondrial membrane, on the other hand, functions as a diffusion barrier for small molecules and helps create rate-dependent concentration gradients for metabolic function [4]. Additionally, outer membrane proteins also play critical roles in mitochondrial fusion and fission as well as mitophagy [5]. Another unique feature of mitochondria is the presence of mitochondrial DNA in the matrix within the organelle. Several copies of this double-stranded circular genome are present within the matrix, encoding 13 proteins of the ETC along with mitochondria-specific ribosomal RNA and tRNA [6].

In recent decades, the role of mitochondria in cellular signaling and its control of the cellular response to various pathophysiological conditions have been intensely investigated.

While this was initially focused on cell death pathways such as apoptosis, it is now evident that mitochondria are essential organelles in almost all facets of cellular homeostasis and signaling, especially in specialized cells with energy-intensive functions and abundant mitochondria such as hepatocytes. This is especially important from the standpoint of drug metabolism and its consequences since it is recognized that critical enzymes in the process such as cytochrome P450 2E1 can localize to mitochondria [7,8]. While CYP450 enzymes are essential mediators of drug metabolism and xenobiotic scavenging under homeostasis, the inadvertent formation of reactive metabolites during metabolism plays a critical role in drug-induced pathophysiology. One of the most clinically relevant examples is hepatotoxicity induced by an acetaminophen (APAP) overdose, which is the most common cause of acute liver failure (ALF) in the United States and many western countries [9,10], where hepatocyte mitochondria play a central role in pathophysiology [11]. This concise review examines recent evidence that has uncovered the nuanced role played by this critical organelle in regulating cellular decision-making in response to an APAP overdose.

2. Acetaminophen Metabolism and Early Mitochondrial Insults

Generally, therapeutic doses of APAP are not toxic due to rapid metabolism in hepatocytes to glucuronide or sulphate metabolites by UDP-glucuronosyl transferases or sulfotransferases, respectively [12]. While a minor percentage of a therapeutic APAP dose is also metabolized by cytochrome P450 enzymes such as Cyp2E1, Cyp1A2, and Cyp3A4 to form a reactive metabolite, N-acetyl-p-benzoquinone imine (NAPQI) [12], this is efficiently scavenged by hepatic glutathione and hence does not induce cellular damage. A minor formation of protein adducts by therapeutic doses is effectively removed by autophagy [13,14]. However, some conditions, such as fatty liver disease, could predispose patients to APAP hepatotoxicity [15]. In fact, patients with pre-existing conditions such as severe acute viral hepatitis or those on antitubercular drugs have been shown to exhibit features of liver injury even after therapeutic doses of APAP [16]. A recent study from France indicated that patients with excess drinking and/or fasting exhibited liver injury on therapeutic doses of APAP (defined as <6 g/d in the study) [17]. The increased susceptibility to injury in alcoholics is probably due to the compromised mitochondrial structure and function evident in this population [18–20] while fasting interferes with glutathione resynthesis and thus facilitates injury. In addition to these vulnerable populations, a randomized controlled trial also indicated transient elevations in aminotransferase levels in healthy adults receiving a therapeutic dose of 4 g APAP daily [21]. However, there was never any severe liver injury or ALF in these patients [21]. The possible mechanisms involved in this benign ALT elevation are not very clear, and this is an area that deserves to be investigated in detail. Biomarkers are being identified that can distinguish between hazardous and benign ALT elevations, and some of them are derived from mitochondria, e.g., argininosuccinate synthase 1 [22].

While the rate of glucuronidation can be significantly upregulated in response to an APAP overdose [23], this seems to be insufficient to prevent shunting of APAP towards cytochrome P450-mediated reactive metabolite formation after an overdose, probably due to limitations in the availability of UDP-glucuronic acid. The enhanced cytochrome P450-mediated formation of NAPQI is central to APAP pathophysiology in the liver [24], and the subsequent depletion of hepatic glutathione stores initiates a complex signaling cascade where the mitochondria take center stage. Even though reactive metabolites such as NAPQI could presumably react with a multitude of cellular cysteine- or lysine-containing proteins after glutathione depletion [12], the formation of mitochondrial protein adducts is critical for APAP-induced hepatotoxicity [25,26]. While it was generally believed that the formation of mitochondrial protein adducts immediately initiated hepatocytes on a slippery slope of cell death signaling culminating in hepatocyte necrosis, recent evidence indicates that the mitochondrial response is much more nuanced, with the initial response being attempts at adaptation prior to commitment towards cell death.

3. Adaptive Mitochondrial Response and Changes in Mitochondrial Morphology

Excessive formation of NAPQI targets hepatocyte mitochondrial proteins for adduct formation, which severely compromises protein function and subsequently induces mitochondrial oxidative stress [27]. However, initial superoxide formation due to adducts on complex III is directed away from the mitochondrial matrix and inner membrane towards the intermembrane space and cytosol, preserving mitochondrial respiratory chain function [28]. Subsequent JNK activation and mitochondrial translocation in hepatocytes amplifies mitochondrial oxidative stress, as will be detailed in the next section, but the initial decrease in mitochondrial membrane potential only seems to activate a mitochondrial adaptation by change in morphology. Changes in mitochondrial morphology and dynamics have been well recognized as being important during various phases of cellular metabolism, and their role in APAP-induced hepatocyte necrosis is also recognized [29]. While most changes in mitochondrial morphology contributing to mitochondrial dynamics (mitochondrial fission and fusion) are controlled by proteins such as mitofusins and Drp1 [29], it is recognized that changes in mitochondrial morphology can also occur independently of these canonical pathways [30–32]. These studies have identified donut-like or spheroid mitochondria, which seem to be produced in response to changes in mitochondrial membrane potential or mitochondrial oxidative stress [30,33]. Our work on early mitochondrial changes in hepatocytes after APAP exposure also revealed the formation of donut-like mitochondria accompanied by loss of mitochondrial membrane potential without a significant effect on mitochondrial respiratory rates [34]. Interestingly, these changes were reversible on removal of APAP [34], such as those seen after hypoxia-induced reoxygenation in cardiomyocytes [33]. Similar transitions from tubular to donut-shaped mitochondria were also reversible when lung epithelial cells were treated with inhibitors of mitochondrial respiration with the generation of reactive oxygen species [35]. While mitochondrial generation of reactive oxygen species has been implicated for decades in APAP-induced hepatocyte necrosis [36], it is now revealed that early superoxide generation, which probably accompanies the loss of mitochondrial membrane and formation of donut-like mitochondria, occurs without proton leak from the mitochondrial respiratory chain or alteration in mitochondrial electron transport.

A detailed study using confocal microscopy and 3D electron microscopic tomography of this mitochondrial morphology change induced by loss of mitochondrial membrane potential revealed that these donut-like mitochondria have central indentations forming discoid forms while lacking holes in the center [30]. The mechanisms involved in the formation of such discoid mitochondria have not been characterized, but it has been suggested to occur through physical membrane mechanisms to attain a final structure with the lowest free energy [27], though membrane phospholipids could also play a role [37]. Computational analysis also indicates that formation of the discoid shape is facilitated by the release of osmotic potential energy through a decrease in total Gibbs free energy, with the bending energy being the barrier for donut formation [38]. Another factor that has been implicated in mitochondrial discoid formation is cellular calcium dynamics, with the transition to the donut shape being mediated by the mitochondrial Miro1 protein in a calcium-dependent manner [32]. Interestingly, increases in cytosolic calcium have been noted in cultured hepatocytes after treatment with APAP [39] within time frames where donut-shaped mitochondria were also detected [34]. This change in intracellular calcium has also been implicated in APAP-induced hepatotoxicity [40], suggesting that the effect of intracellular calcium on this adaptive mitochondrial morphology response could have consequences for downstream cellular signaling, though that is an area for further investigation. Additionally, adaptive changes in mitochondrial bioenergetics such as those induced by enhanced respiratory chain flux in mice deficient in pyruvate dehydrogenase kinase 4 (PDK4) can render them highly efficient in handling APAP-induced oxidant stress, probably through modulation of UCP2 levels [41].

Given the central role of hepatocyte mitochondria in the injury process, additional adaptive mechanisms that mitigate this effect have been recognized. Most important is the process of autophagy or, more specifically, mitophagy, which can remove damaged mitochondria and thereby limit the progression of the cell death mechanisms during APAP hepatotoxicity [42]. Damaged mitochondria are identified through the PINK1/Parkin pathway [43–45] but may also involve Parkin-independent mechanisms [46,47]. It was shown that autophagy is activated after a single APAP overdose and that removal of damaged mitochondria [48] and protein adducts [13] attenuated APAP-induced liver injury. However, autophagy appears to be most effective in cells located at the outer area of necrosis, where the severity of the insult is more limited and adaptive mechanisms have a chance to successfully intervene [49]. Consistent with this hypothesis is the observation that the removal of cytosolic and mitochondrial protein adducts by autophagy is most effective in preventing liver injury at therapeutic or moderately supratherapeutic doses of APAP [14]. Because even these low doses of APAP can cause protein adduct formation in humans [50], the consistent removal of these adducts by autophagy makes it possible that therapeutic doses of APAP can be used chronically for years without adverse effects. In animal studies, it was shown that therapeutic doses of APAP mainly cause soluble protein adduct formation, while repeated supratherapeutic doses or a severe overdose also cause mitochondrial adduct formation [14]. However, any inhibition of autophagy can rapidly trigger liver injury after multiple therapeutic or supratherapeutic doses, demonstrating the vital importance of the autophagy/mitophagy processes for cell survival [14].

4. Activation of the MAP Kinase Cascade and Amplification of Mitochondrial Injury Cause Hepatocyte Necrosis

Persistent activation of JNK in the cytosol and the translocation of phosphorylated JNK to the mitochondria overcomes the adaptive mitochondrial mechanisms to ultimately amplify mitochondrial oxidative stress and compromise mitochondrial respiration. Phosphorylated JNK binds to the mitochondrial outer membrane protein Sab [51] and inhibits the electron transport chain (ETC) through a Src-dependent process [52]. Among the JNK isoforms, experiments with anti-sense oligonucleotides targeting them individually indicate that JNK2 is probably more important in APAP hepatotoxicity, though JNK1 can take over in its absence, indicating both isoforms are involved. JNK activation is also important to APAP pathophysiology in primary human hepatocytes [53], though it seems to be inconsequential to cell death pathways after APAP exposure in the human hepatoma HepaRG cell line [53,54], which exhibit all other signaling characteristics after APAP [53]. The demonstration of JNK phosphorylation in human liver tissue, however, is complicated by the timing of sample availability since liver biopsies are typically contraindicated in APAP overdose patients in the clinic due to the risk of bleeding. The few studies examining liver biopsies from APAP overdose patients only collect them after coagulation parameters have stabilized [55,56], but these may not be very useful since JNK activation after APAP is transient [57] and unlikely to be detected at these later time points.

JNK interaction with mitochondrial Sab and the inhibition of the ETC then results in elevated mitochondrial free radical generation, which is now also derived from complex I [58], unlike the initial superoxide generation from complex III [28]. Mitochondrial respiratory complex II (succinate dehydrogenase) has been identified as a sensitive target for NAPQI-mediated inhibition of activity [59], which would have significant effects on energy homeostasis through modulation of the TCA cycle since succinate dehydrogenase participates in both the TCA cycle and ETC [60]. However, this is likely a later event after JNK translocation, based on studies in cultured cells and in vivo experiments [27]. This would be especially important considering the recent report suggesting that mitochondrial complex I is dispensable for the homeostasis of the adult mouse liver, which compensates through alternate electron donors to fuel the mitochondrial ETC [61]. Thus, inhibition of a predominant alternative electron donor such as complex II by APAP could have dramatic effects on hepatic mitochondrial function. This is highlighted by the demonstration that use of methylene blue to accept electrons from NAPQI-modified complex II and transfer them to cytochrome c, bypassing this inhibition, prevented hepatocyte necrosis [62]. However, complex II inhibition was not detected by in vitro respiratory measurements in human liver biopsies exposed to APAP [63], and the clinical use of methylene blue would require tight control of dosage due to the severe risk of methemoglobinemia as a side effect of this drug [64].

To prevent cellular injury in the event of enhanced free radical generation from the organelle, mitochondria have active antioxidant systems such as the manganese superoxide dismutase (MnSOD), which typically scavenge excess free radicals. These systems are critical to APAP pathophysiology since partial deficiency of MnSOD exacerbates APAP-induced liver injury [65,66]. Mitochondrial dysfunction is amplified when these anti-oxidant systems are compromised by the formation of the potent oxidant peroxynitrite [67] after the reaction of superoxide with nitric oxide (NO) within the cellular compartment [68]. Interestingly, the initial superoxide generation from mitochondria into the cytosol is not accompanied by peroxynitrite formation [28], which is only evident after JNK translocation to the mitochondria with active inhibition of the mitochondrial respiratory chain [69,70]. This further suggests that the source of NO for the formation of peroxynitrite in the context of APAP pathophysiology is likely within the mitochondria, since nitrotyrosine adducts are only detected inside mitochondria [68] and peroxynitrite formation is not evident when superoxide is shunted towards the cytosol [28]. The most likely contributor of NO within mitochondria seems to be neuronal nitric oxide synthase (nNOS), since its deficiency prevented APAP-induced liver injury without affecting metabolism [67] and it has been suggested to be localized to mitochondria [71,72], though this is controversial [73]. Irrespective of the source of NO, mitochondrial peroxynitrite formation is central to APAP pathophysiology, as demonstrated by the robust protection provided by interventions targeting its formation, such as the use of the SOD mimetic Mito-TEMPO [74,75] or its scavenging with GSH [76]. An additional role for cellular iron in peroxynitrite toxicity in mitochondria in the context of APAP pathophysiology has now been revealed by recent research [77]. While the role of cellular iron in APAP pathophysiology has been controversial [77], its nuanced contribution has been indicated in more recent studies examining lysosomal instability after APAP overdose [78]. Release of lysosomal iron into the cytosol [79] and its uptake into mitochondria [80] were noted, and the importance of these phenomena to the pathophysiology was evidenced by the protection against cell necrosis conferred by chelation of lysosomal iron or blocking its mitochondrial uptake [79–81]. We recently showed that treatment with deferoxamine and minocycline did not influence activation and translocation of JNK but prevented the formation of nitrotyrosine protein adducts from peroxynitrite and subsequent steps such as induction of the mitochondrial permeability transition [77]. Since iron can facilitate the formation of nitrotyrosine from peroxynitrite in a milieu of GSH depletion [82], this indicates that mitochondrial iron accumulation from the lysosome facilitates mitochondrial amplification of injury.

An important consequence of mitochondrial peroxynitrite formation is the damage to mitochondrial DNA, seen within 3 h after a dose of 300 mg/kg APAP [68]. This causes substantial depletion of mtDNA within the liver [68] and release of mtDNA fragments into the circulation in mice and humans [83]. These DNA fragments could function as damage-associated molecular patterns (DAMPs) to initiate the innate immune response necessary for liver recovery and regeneration [83]. The loss of mtDNA would have catastrophic effects on the maintenance of mitochondrial homeostasis in damaged hepatocytes, not only impacting ATP synthesis but also decreasing fatty acid oxidation [6]. This has been evident after an APAP overdose [84] and was initially identified in serum metabolomic studies that revealed marked elevations in serum acylcarnitine early after an APAP overdose in mice, which were prevented in Cyp2E1-deficient mice [85]. Interestingly, these changes were not evident at a lower (200 mg/kg) overdose of APAP, which induces all other signaling pathways and liver necrosis [86], but only evident at the higher 400 mg/kg overdose of APAP in 129/Sv mice [85]. This indicates that severe mitochondrial dysfunction is probably required for these changes in lipid metabolism to occur after APAP. However, there seems to be strain-dependent differences in this effect since B6C3F1 mice showed early elevations in circulating acylcarnitines even at the 200 mg/kg dose [87], similar to C57BL6/J mice [88]. The role of this inhibition of fatty acid oxidation in APAP pathophysiology was also highlighted by a recent study, which showed that hepatocyte-specific activation of the G protein-coupled receptor Mas, involved in the renin-angiotensin system, enhanced lipophagy and fatty acid oxidation to protect against APAP-induced hepatotoxicity in mice [89]. The APAP-induced inhibition of fatty acid oxidation also seems to occur in humans, where elevations in circulating acylcarnitines could be biomarkers of mitochondrial dysfunction [88], but only if measured prior to administration of NAC [88,90].

Enhanced mitochondrial peroxynitrite formation coupled with the inhibition of mitochondrial antioxidant systems due to protein nitration ultimately induces the mitochondrial permeability transition (MPT), whose early inhibition provided transient protection that was however not sustainable [91]. Ultimately, the persistent loss of mitochondrial membrane potential sustains the MPT [86,91,92], accompanied by mitochondrial fission mediated by canonical proteins involved in mitochondrial dynamics such as Drp1 [93]. The induction of the MPT allows the release of mitochondrial proteins such as endonuclease G (Endo G) and apoptosis-inducing factor (AIF) into the cytosol and their subsequent translocation to the nucleus [94,95]. Once within the nucleus, AIF induces chromatin condensation [96] and, in co-operation with Endo G, cleaves nuclear DNA, causing its fragmentation [96,97]. The partial protection against APAP-induced hepatocyte necrosis in AIF-deficient mice [98] highlights the role played by this mitochondrial protein in APAP pathophysiology. In addition to the MPT triggering the release of AIF and Endo G through matrix swelling and rupture of the outer membrane, mitochondrial Bax translocation and the formation of a Bax pore in the outer mitochondrial membrane can also induce the early release of these intermembrane proteins and cause DNA fragmentation [99]. In general, this type of mitochondria-dependent DNA fragmentation is the point-of-no-return in the intracellular signaling pathways to cell necrosis [100]. Thus, the mitochondria play a central role in APAP-induced hepatocyte necrosis, with the complex interplay of various signaling pathways converging on this organelle being continuously revealed by ongoing research in the field. However, the role of the mitochondria is not restricted to APAP-induced injury, as will be discussed in the following section.

5. Mitochondria in Liver Recovery and Regeneration

In addition to their central role in liver injury after APAP overdose, mitochondria also play critical roles in liver recovery after APAP-induced hepatocyte necrosis, with mitochondrial biogenesis being central to the process [101]. Acetaminophen-induced hepatocyte necrosis is characteristically centrilobular in nature, predominantly affecting hepatocytes surrounding the central vein, with mitochondrial spheroid formation and autophagy in cells beyond that, and mitochondrial biogenesis in cells farthest from the central vein [49]. Our earlier study demonstrated that mitochondrial biogenesis is induced in cells surrounding the area of necrosis beginning at 24 h after a 300 mg/kg overdose of APAP, accompanied by a substantial recovery in hepatic mtDNA levels [102]. The importance of the process for liver recovery after this moderate APAP overdose was illustrated by the enhanced recovery when mice were treated with the mitochondrial biogenesis inducer SRT1720 [102]. Mice deficient in fibroblast growth factor 21 (FGF21), which induces hepatocyte expression of PGC1α, the central regulator of mitochondrial biogenesis, also showed exacerbated liver injury after APAP overdose [103]. Induction of PGC-1α with inducers such as diphenyl diselenide was also able to enhance mitochondrial bioenergetics after APAP overdose [104]. Though mitochondrial biogenesis was not explicitly measured in these studies, the effects on PGC-1α will presumably influence mitochondrial biogenesis. Thus, induction of mitochondrial biogenesis in the discrete population of surviving hepatocytes surrounding areas of necrosis plays an essential role in liver recovery and regeneration after APAP overdose.

Another well-recognized factor in recovery and regeneration after APAP-induced liver injury is the innate immune response induced by the release of damage-associated molecular patterns (DAMPs) from necrotic hepatocytes, such as the high molecular weight group box 1 (HMGB1) protein [24,105]. These signals activate cytokine and chemokine formation in resident macrophages such as Kupffer cells, which then activate and recruit neutrophils, monocytes, and other leukocytes into the liver [105], which facilitate tissue repair and regeneration at moderate overdoses but can also aggravate the injury at severe overdoses [106]. Macrophages have high immune plasticity and their polarization is influenced by the microenvironment [107]. In the context of APAP, these monocyte-derived macrophages, though initially having a pro-inflammatory phenotype, mature after hepatic recruitment into a pro-regenerative phenotype with increased phagocytosis capacity and expression of anti-inflammatory genes [105]. It is recognized that parameters of cellular metabolism differ depending on macrophage phenotype, with pro-inflammatory macrophages mostly using glycolysis to meet their energetic needs, while anti-inflammatory macrophages rely on mitochondrial respiration, with changes in cellular metabolism influencing the cytokine secretion profile and expression of key inflammatory genes [107]. A recent study also found that myeloid-specific deletion of mitochondrial Complex I protein Ndufs4 (mKO) induced a proinflammatory metabolic profile in macrophages with a blunted transition to the reparative phase [108], reiterating the importance of macrophage mitochondrial function in the phenotype change. Our recent in vitro and in vivo experiments also demonstrated that Kupffer cells regulate CXCR2 expression and pro-regenerative gene expression in surviving hepatocytes around the areas of necrosis through the production of IL-10 to support the transition of these hepatocytes around the areas of necrosis to a proliferative state [109]. We further demonstrated that these recovered hepatocytes then promote macrophage apoptosis through CXCR4 signaling to resolve the inflammatory response and return to homeostasis [110]. Interestingly, it has also been demonstrated that neutrophils promote the development of reparative macrophages through ROS production to facilitate liver repair after an APAP overdose [111], and the role of mitochondria in controlling several facets of neutrophil physiology, including maturation and behavior, is now being recognized [112]. Thus, in addition to its role within hepatocytes through the induction of biogenesis, mitochondria could potentially have important roles within the infiltrating immune cells in controlling recovery and regeneration after an APAP overdose. Though information on these aspects is currently scarce, it is an important area for future investigation.

6. Conclusions

Taken together, it is now evident that mitochondria play central roles in both liver injury and recovery after an APAP overdose (Figure 1). While these aspects were recognized earlier, recent evidence revealed the nuanced response of the organelle to increased generation of the reactive metabolite NAPQI and indicates that significant attempts at adaptation to the insult are initiated. It is only when the persistent formation of mitochondrial protein adducts and JNK-mediated inhibition of electron transport overwhelm these adaptive mechanisms that the organelle undergoes MPT, triggers nuclear DNA fragmentation, and finally causes hepatocyte necrosis. From a therapeutic standpoint, enhancing these adaptive mechanisms could be an approach to delay the cascade of necrotic cell death and prevent progression to acute liver failure after APAP overdose. Additionally, further studies on the role of macrophage and neutrophil mitochondria in modulating the innate immune response would uncover additional avenues that could be targeted to facilitate recovery and regeneration after APAP overdose.

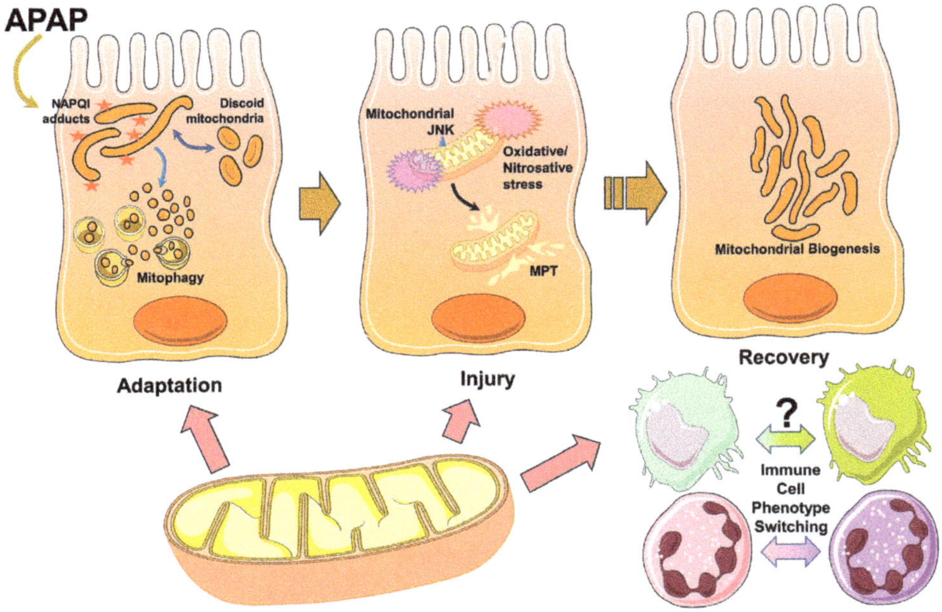

Figure 1. Mitochondria are involved in multiple phases of APAP pathophysiology. Formation of protein adducts on mitochondria due to generation of the reactive metabolite NAPQI from an acetaminophen (APAP) overdose initiates cellular stress. This induces early adaptive changes in mitochondrial morphology due to a decrease in membrane potential, which are reversible. Additional adaptive mechanisms include mitophagy, which allows the removal of dysfunctional mitochondria after their fragmentation. Persistence of adduct formation and activation of the MAP kinase JNK after APAP would then cause mitochondrial JNK translocation accompanied by oxidative and nitrosative stress in the organelle with induction of the mitochondrial permeability transition (MPT), which ultimately causes hepatocyte necrosis. In addition to these roles in adaptation and injury, mitochondria are also involved in liver recovery with the induction of mitochondrial biogenesis in surviving hepatocytes, facilitating liver regeneration. The organelle may also be involved in phenotype switching of infiltrating immune cells to the reparative phenotype to aid in liver recovery.

Author Contributions: A.R. wrote the first draft of the manuscript and generated the graphic. H.J. contributed sections and edited the manuscript. All authors have read and agreed to the published version of the manuscript.

Funding: Work in the authors' laboratory was supported by grants from the National Institute of Diabetes and Digestive and Kidney Diseases (NIDDK), grants R01 DK102142 (H.J.) and DK125465 (A.R.), and National Institute of General Medicine (NIGMS)-funded Liver Disease COBRE grants P20 GM103549 and P30 GM118247.

Conflicts of Interest: The authors declare no conflict of interest.

References

1. Roger, A.J.; Munoz-Gomez, S.A.; Kamikawa, R. The Origin and Diversification of Mitochondria. *Curr. Biol.* **2017**, *27*, R1177–R1192. [CrossRef] [PubMed]
2. Pessayre, D.; Fromenty, B.; Berson, A.; Robin, M.A.; Letteron, P.; Moreau, R.; Mansouri, A. Central role of mitochondria in drug-induced liver injury. *Drug Metab. Rev.* **2012**, *44*, 34–87. [CrossRef] [PubMed]
3. Glancy, B.; Kim, Y.; Katti, P.; Willingham, T.B. The Functional Impact of Mitochondrial Structure Across Subcellular Scales. *Front. Physiol.* **2020**, *11*, 541040. [CrossRef] [PubMed]
4. Gellerich, F.N.; Trumbeckaite, S.; Opalka, J.R.; Seppet, E.; Rasmussen, H.N.; Neuhoff, C.; Zierz, S. Function of the mitochondrial outer membrane as a diffusion barrier in health and diseases. *Biochem. Soc. Trans.* **2000**, *28*, 164–169. [CrossRef]

5. Xian, H.; Liou, Y.C. Functions of outer mitochondrial membrane proteins: Mediating the crosstalk between mitochondrial dynamics and mitophagy. *Cell Death Differ.* **2021**, *28*, 827–842. [CrossRef]
6. Fromenty, B. Alteration of mitochondrial DNA homeostasis in drug-induced liver injury. *Food Chem. Toxicol.* **2020**, *135*, 110916. [CrossRef]
7. Massart, J.; Begriche, K.; Hartman, J.H.; Fromenty, B. Role of Mitochondrial Cytochrome P450 2E1 in Healthy and Diseased Liver. *Cells* **2022**, *11*, 288. [CrossRef]
8. Anandatheerthavarada, H.K.; Addya, S.; Dwivedi, R.S.; Biswas, G.; Mullick, J.; Avadhani, N.G. Localization of multiple forms of inducible cytochromes P450 in rat liver mitochondria: Immunological characteristics and patterns of xenobiotic substrate metabolism. *Arch. Biochem. Biophys.* **1997**, *339*, 136–150. [CrossRef]
9. Bernal, W.; Williams, R. Acute Liver Failure. *Clin. Liver Dis.* **2020**, *16*, 45–55. [CrossRef]
10. Stravitz, R.T.; Lee, W.M. Acute liver failure. *Lancet* **2019**, *394*, 869–881. [CrossRef]
11. Ramachandran, A.; Jaeschke, H. Acetaminophen hepatotoxicity: A mitochondrial perspective. *Adv. Pharmacol.* **2019**, *85*, 195–219. [CrossRef]
12. McGill, M.R.; Jaeschke, H. Metabolism and disposition of acetaminophen: Recent advances in relation to hepatotoxicity and diagnosis. *Pharm. Res.* **2013**, *30*, 2174–2187. [CrossRef]
13. Ni, H.M.; McGill, M.R.; Chao, X.; Du, K.; Williams, J.A.; Xie, Y.; Jaeschke, H.; Ding, W.X. Removal of acetaminophen protein adducts by autophagy protects against acetaminophen-induced liver injury in mice. *J. Hepatol.* **2016**, *65*, 354–362. [CrossRef]
14. Nguyen, N.T.; Akakpo, J.Y.; Weemhoff, J.L.; Ramachandran, A.; Ding, W.X.; Jaeschke, H. Impaired protein adduct removal following repeat administration of subtoxic doses of acetaminophen enhances liver injury in fed mice. *Arch. Toxicol.* **2021**, *95*, 1463–1473. [CrossRef]
15. Begriche, K.; Penhoat, C.; Bernabeu-Gentey, P.; Massart, J.; Fromenty, B. Acetaminophen-Induced Hepatotoxicity in Obesity and Nonalcoholic Fatty Liver Disease: A Critical Review. *Livers* **2023**, *3*, 33–53. [CrossRef]
16. Jalan, R.; Williams, R.; Bernuau, J. Paracetamol: Are therapeutic doses entirely safe? *Lancet* **2006**, *368*, 2195–2196. [CrossRef]
17. Louvet, A.; Wandji, L.C.N.; Lemaitre, E.; Khaldi, M.; Lafforgue, C.; Artru, F.; Quesnel, B.; Lassailly, G.; Dharancy, S.; Mathurin, P. Acute Liver Injury with Therapeutic Doses of Acetaminophen: A Prospective Study. *Hepatology* **2021**, *73*, 1945–1955. [CrossRef]
18. Lauterburg, B.H.; Liang, D.; Schwarzenbach, F.A.; Breen, K.J. Mitochondrial dysfunction in alcoholic patients as assessed by breath analysis. *Hepatology* **1993**, *17*, 418–422. [CrossRef]
19. Mansouri, A.; Demeilliers, C.; Amsellem, S.; Pessayre, D.; Fromenty, B. Acute ethanol administration oxidatively damages and depletes mitochondrial dna in mouse liver, brain, heart, and skeletal muscles: Protective effects of antioxidants. *J. Pharmacol. Exp. Ther.* **2001**, *298*, 737–743.
20. Mansouri, A.; Gaou, I.; De Kerguenec, C.; Amsellem, S.; Haouzi, D.; Berson, A.; Moreau, A.; Feldmann, G.; Letteron, P.; Pessayre, D.; et al. An alcoholic binge causes massive degradation of hepatic mitochondrial DNA in mice. *Gastroenterology* **1999**, *117*, 181–190. [CrossRef]
21. Watkins, P.B.; Kaplowitz, N.; Slattery, J.T.; Colonese, C.R.; Colucci, S.V.; Stewart, P.W.; Harris, S.C. Aminotransferase elevations in healthy adults receiving 4 grams of acetaminophen daily: A randomized controlled trial. *JAMA* **2006**, *296*, 87–93. [CrossRef] [PubMed]
22. Vazquez, J.H.; Clemens, M.M.; Allard, F.D.; Yee, E.U.; Kennon-McGill, S.; Mackintosh, S.G.; Jaeschke, H.; Hambuchen, M.D.; McGill, M.R. Identification of Serum Biomarkers to Distinguish Hazardous and Benign Aminotransferase Elevations. *Toxicol. Sci.* **2020**, *173*, 244–254. [CrossRef] [PubMed]
23. Gelotte, C.K.; Auiler, J.F.; Lynch, J.M.; Temple, A.R.; Slattery, J.T. Disposition of acetaminophen at 4, 6, and 8 g/day for 3 days in healthy young adults. *Clin. Pharmacol. Ther.* **2007**, *81*, 840–848. [CrossRef] [PubMed]
24. Jaeschke, H.; Adelusi, O.B.; Akakpo, J.Y.; Nguyen, N.T.; Sanchez-Guerrero, G.; Umbaugh, D.S.; Ding, W.X.; Ramachandran, A. Recommendations for the use of the acetaminophen hepatotoxicity model for mechanistic studies and how to avoid common pitfalls. *Acta Pharm. Sin. B* **2021**, *11*, 3740–3755. [CrossRef]
25. Jollow, D.J.; Mitchell, J.R.; Potter, W.Z.; Davis, D.C.; Gillette, J.R.; Brodie, B.B. Acetaminophen-induced hepatic necrosis. II. Role of covalent binding in vivo. *J. Pharmacol. Exp. Ther.* **1973**, *187*, 195–202.
26. Tirmenstein, M.A.; Nelson, S.D. Subcellular binding and effects on calcium homeostasis produced by acetaminophen and a nonhepatotoxic regioisomer, 3′-hydroxyacetanilide, in mouse liver. *J. Biol. Chem.* **1989**, *264*, 9814–9819. [CrossRef]
27. Ramachandran, A.; Jaeschke, H. A mitochondrial journey through acetaminophen hepatotoxicity. *Food Chem. Toxicol.* **2020**, *140*, 111282. [CrossRef]
28. Nguyen, N.T.; Du, K.; Akakpo, J.Y.; Umbaugh, D.S.; Jaeschke, H.; Ramachandran, A. Mitochondrial protein adduct and superoxide generation are prerequisites for early activation of c-jun N-terminal kinase within the cytosol after an acetaminophen overdose in mice. *Toxicol. Lett.* **2021**, *338*, 21–31. [CrossRef]
29. Ramachandran, A.; Umbaugh, D.S.; Jaeschke, H. Mitochondrial Dynamics in Drug-Induced Liver Injury. *Livers* **2021**, *1*, 102–115. [CrossRef]
30. Miyazono, Y.; Hirashima, S.; Ishihara, N.; Kusukawa, J.; Nakamura, K.I.; Ohta, K. Uncoupled mitochondria quickly shorten along their long axis to form indented spheroids, instead of rings, in a fission-independent manner. *Sci. Rep.* **2018**, *8*, 350. [CrossRef]
31. Ding, W.X.; Guo, F.; Ni, H.M.; Bockus, A.; Manley, S.; Stolz, D.B.; Eskelinen, E.L.; Jaeschke, H.; Yin, X.M. Parkin and mitofusins reciprocally regulate mitophagy and mitochondrial spheroid formation. *J. Biol. Chem.* **2012**, *287*, 42379–42388. [CrossRef]

32. Nemani, N.; Carvalho, E.; Tomar, D.; Dong, Z.; Ketschek, A.; Breves, S.L.; Jana, F.; Worth, A.M.; Heffler, J.; Palaniappan, P.; et al. MIRO-1 Determines Mitochondrial Shape Transition upon GPCR Activation and Ca^{2+} Stress. *Cell Rep.* **2018**, *23*, 1005–1019. [CrossRef]
33. Liu, X.; Hajnoczky, G. Altered fusion dynamics underlie unique morphological changes in mitochondria during hypoxia-reoxygenation stress. *Cell Death Differ.* **2011**, *18*, 1561–1572. [CrossRef]
34. Umbaugh, D.S.; Nguyen, N.T.; Jaeschke, H.; Ramachandran, A. Mitochondrial Membrane Potential Drives Early Change in Mitochondrial Morphology After Acetaminophen Exposure. *Toxicol. Sci.* **2021**, *180*, 186–195. [CrossRef]
35. Ahmad, T.; Aggarwal, K.; Pattnaik, B.; Mukherjee, S.; Sethi, T.; Tiwari, B.K.; Kumar, M.; Micheal, A.; Mabalirajan, U.; Ghosh, B.; et al. Computational classification of mitochondrial shapes reflects stress and redox state. *Cell Death Dis.* **2013**, *4*, e461. [CrossRef]
36. Jaeschke, H. Glutathione disulfide formation and oxidant stress during acetaminophen-induced hepatotoxicity in mice in vivo: The protective effect of allopurinol. *J. Pharmacol. Exp. Ther.* **1990**, *255*, 935–941.
37. Basu Ball, W.; Neff, J.K.; Gohil, V.M. The role of nonbilayer phospholipids in mitochondrial structure and function. *FEBS Lett.* **2018**, *592*, 1273–1290. [CrossRef]
38. Long, Q.; Zhao, D.; Fan, W.; Yang, L.; Zhou, Y.; Qi, J.; Wang, X.; Liu, X. Modeling of Mitochondrial Donut Formation. *Biophys. J.* **2015**, *109*, 892–899. [CrossRef]
39. Bruschi, S.A.; Priestly, B.G. Implication of alterations in intracellular calcium ion homoeostasis in the advent of paracetamol-induced cytotoxicity in primary mouse hepatocyte monolayer cultures. *Toxicol. Vitr.* **1990**, *4*, 743–749. [CrossRef]
40. Shen, W.; Kamendulis, L.M.; Ray, S.D.; Corcoran, G.B. Acetaminophen-induced cytotoxicity in cultured mouse hepatocytes: Correlation of nuclear Ca^{2+} accumulation and early DNA fragmentation with cell death. *Toxicol. Appl. Pharmacol.* **1991**, *111*, 242–254. [CrossRef]
41. Duan, L.; Ramachandran, A.; Akakpo, J.Y.; Woolbright, B.L.; Zhang, Y.; Jaeschke, H. Mice deficient in pyruvate dehydrogenase kinase 4 are protected against acetaminophen-induced hepatotoxicity. *Toxicol. Appl. Pharmacol.* **2020**, *387*, 114849. [CrossRef] [PubMed]
42. Chao, X.; Wang, H.; Jaeschke, H.; Ding, W.X. Role and mechanisms of autophagy in acetaminophen-induced liver injury. *Liver Int.* **2018**, *38*, 1363–1374. [CrossRef] [PubMed]
43. Williams, J.A.; Ni, H.M.; Haynes, A.; Manley, S.; Li, Y.; Jaeschke, H.; Ding, W.X. Chronic Deletion and Acute Knockdown of Parkin Have Differential Responses to Acetaminophen-induced Mitophagy and Liver Injury in Mice. *J. Biol. Chem.* **2015**, *290*, 10934–10946. [CrossRef] [PubMed]
44. Williams, J.A.; Ding, W.X. Targeting Pink1-Parkin-mediated mitophagy for treating liver injury. *Pharmacol. Res.* **2015**, *102*, 264–269. [CrossRef]
45. Wang, H.; Ni, H.M.; Chao, X.; Ma, X.; Rodriguez, Y.A.; Chavan, H.; Wang, S.; Krishnamurthy, P.; Dobrowsky, R.; Xu, D.X.; et al. Double deletion of PINK1 and Parkin impairs hepatic mitophagy and exacerbates acetaminophen-induced liver injury in mice. *Redox Biol.* **2019**, *22*, 101148. [CrossRef]
46. Williams, J.A.; Ding, W.X. Mechanisms, pathophysiological roles and methods for analyzing mitophagy—Recent insights. *Biol. Chem.* **2018**, *399*, 147–178. [CrossRef]
47. Qian, H.; Bai, Q.; Yang, X.; Akakpo, J.Y.; Ji, L.; Yang, L.; Rulicke, T.; Zatloukal, K.; Jaeschke, H.; Ni, H.M.; et al. Dual roles of p62/SQSTM1 in the injury and recovery phases of acetaminophen-induced liver injury in mice. *Acta Pharm. Sin. B* **2021**, *11*, 3791–3805. [CrossRef]
48. Ni, H.M.; Bockus, A.; Boggess, N.; Jaeschke, H.; Ding, W.X. Activation of autophagy protects against acetaminophen-induced hepatotoxicity. *Hepatology* **2012**, *55*, 222–232. [CrossRef]
49. Ni, H.M.; Williams, J.A.; Jaeschke, H.; Ding, W.X. Zonated induction of autophagy and mitochondrial spheroids limits acetaminophen-induced necrosis in the liver. *Redox Biol.* **2013**, *1*, 427–432. [CrossRef]
50. Heard, K.J.; Green, J.L.; James, L.P.; Judge, B.S.; Zolot, L.; Rhyee, S.; Dart, R.C. Acetaminophen-cysteine adducts during therapeutic dosing and following overdose. *BMC Gastroenterol.* **2011**, *11*, 20. [CrossRef]
51. Win, S.; Than, T.A.; Han, D.; Petrovic, L.M.; Kaplowitz, N. c-Jun N-terminal kinase (JNK)-dependent acute liver injury from acetaminophen or tumor necrosis factor (TNF) requires mitochondrial Sab protein expression in mice. *J. Biol. Chem.* **2011**, *286*, 35071–35078. [CrossRef]
52. Win, S.; Than, T.A.; Min, R.W.; Aghajan, M.; Kaplowitz, N. c-Jun N-terminal kinase mediates mouse liver injury through a novel Sab (SH3BP5)-dependent pathway leading to inactivation of intramitochondrial Src. *Hepatology* **2016**, *63*, 1987–2003. [CrossRef]
53. Xie, Y.; McGill, M.R.; Dorko, K.; Kumer, S.C.; Schmitt, T.M.; Forster, J.; Jaeschke, H. Mechanisms of acetaminophen-induced cell death in primary human hepatocytes. *Toxicol. Appl. Pharmacol.* **2014**, *279*, 266–274. [CrossRef]
54. Michaut, A.; Le Guillou, D.; Moreau, C.; Bucher, S.; McGill, M.R.; Martinais, S.; Gicquel, T.; Morel, I.; Robin, M.A.; Jaeschke, H.; et al. A cellular model to study drug-induced liver injury in nonalcoholic fatty liver disease: Application to acetaminophen. *Toxicol. Appl. Pharmacol.* **2016**, *292*, 40–55. [CrossRef]
55. Lesna, M.; Watson, A.J.; Douglas, A.P.; Hamlyn, A.N.; James, O.F. Evaluation of paracetamol-induced damage in liver biopsies. Acute changes and follow-up findings. *Virchows Arch. A Pathol. Anat. Histol.* **1976**, *370*, 333–344. [CrossRef]
56. Portmann, B.; Talbot, I.C.; Day, D.W.; Davidson, A.R.; Murray-Lyon, I.M.; Williams, R. Histopathological changes in the liver following a paracetamol overdose: Correlation with clinical and biochemical parameters. *J. Pathol.* **1975**, *117*, 169–181. [CrossRef]

57. Gunawan, B.K.; Liu, Z.X.; Han, D.; Hanawa, N.; Gaarde, W.A.; Kaplowitz, N. c-Jun N-terminal kinase plays a major role in murine acetaminophen hepatotoxicity. *Gastroenterology* **2006**, *131*, 165–178. [CrossRef]
58. Du, K.; Ramachandran, A.; Weemhoff, J.L.; Chavan, H.; Xie, Y.; Krishnamurthy, P.; Jaeschke, H. Editor's Highlight: Metformin Protects Against Acetaminophen Hepatotoxicity by Attenuation of Mitochondrial Oxidant Stress and Dysfunction. *Toxicol. Sci.* **2016**, *154*, 214–226. [CrossRef]
59. Burcham, P.C.; Harman, A.W. Acetaminophen toxicity results in site-specific mitochondrial damage in isolated mouse hepatocytes. *J. Biol. Chem.* **1991**, *266*, 5049–5054. [CrossRef]
60. Martinez-Reyes, I.; Chandel, N.S. Mitochondrial TCA cycle metabolites control physiology and disease. *Nat. Commun.* **2020**, *11*, 102. [CrossRef]
61. Lesner, N.P.; Wang, X.; Chen, Z.; Frank, A.; Menezes, C.J.; House, S.; Shelton, S.D.; Lemoff, A.; McFadden, D.G.; Wansapura, J.; et al. Differential requirements for mitochondrial electron transport chain components in the adult murine liver. *Elife* **2022**, *11*, e80919. [CrossRef] [PubMed]
62. Lee, K.K.; Imaizumi, N.; Chamberland, S.R.; Alder, N.N.; Boelsterli, U.A. Targeting mitochondria with methylene blue protects mice against acetaminophen-induced liver injury. *Hepatology* **2015**, *61*, 326–336. [CrossRef] [PubMed]
63. Chrois, K.M.; Larsen, S.; Pedersen, J.S.; Rygg, M.O.; Boilsen, A.E.B.; Bendtsen, F.; Dela, F. Acetaminophen toxicity induces mitochondrial complex I inhibition in human liver tissue. *Basic Clin. Pharmacol. Toxicol.* **2020**, *126*, 86–91. [CrossRef] [PubMed]
64. Jaeschke, H.; Akakpo, J.Y.; Umbaugh, D.S.; Ramachandran, A. Novel Therapeutic Approaches Against Acetaminophen-induced Liver Injury and Acute Liver Failure. *Toxicol. Sci.* **2020**, *174*, 159–167. [CrossRef]
65. Ramachandran, A.; Lebofsky, M.; Weinman, S.A.; Jaeschke, H. The impact of partial manganese superoxide dismutase (SOD2)-deficiency on mitochondrial oxidant stress, DNA fragmentation and liver injury during acetaminophen hepatotoxicity. *Toxicol. Appl. Pharmacol.* **2011**, *251*, 226–233. [CrossRef]
66. Fujimoto, K.; Kumagai, K.; Ito, K.; Arakawa, S.; Ando, Y.; Oda, S.; Yamoto, T.; Manabe, S. Sensitivity of liver injury in heterozygous Sod2 knockout mice treated with troglitazone or acetaminophen. *Toxicol. Pathol.* **2009**, *37*, 193–200. [CrossRef]
67. Agarwal, R.; Hennings, L.; Rafferty, T.M.; Letzig, L.G.; McCullough, S.; James, L.P.; MacMillan-Crow, L.A.; Hinson, J.A. Acetaminophen-induced hepatotoxicity and protein nitration in neuronal nitric-oxide synthase knockout mice. *J. Pharmacol. Exp. Ther.* **2012**, *340*, 134–142. [CrossRef]
68. Cover, C.; Mansouri, A.; Knight, T.R.; Bajt, M.L.; Lemasters, J.J.; Pessayre, D.; Jaeschke, H. Peroxynitrite-induced mitochondrial and endonuclease-mediated nuclear DNA damage in acetaminophen hepatotoxicity. *J. Pharmacol. Exp. Ther.* **2005**, *315*, 879–887. [CrossRef]
69. Knight, T.R.; Kurtz, A.; Bajt, M.L.; Hinson, J.A.; Jaeschke, H. Vascular and hepatocellular peroxynitrite formation during acetaminophen toxicity: Role of mitochondrial oxidant stress. *Toxicol. Sci.* **2001**, *62*, 212–220. [CrossRef]
70. Xie, Y.; Ramachandran, A.; Breckenridge, D.G.; Liles, J.T.; Lebofsky, M.; Farhood, A.; Jaeschke, H. Inhibitor of apoptosis signal-regulating kinase 1 protects against acetaminophen-induced liver injury. *Toxicol. Appl. Pharmacol.* **2015**, *286*, 1–9. [CrossRef]
71. Brookes, P.S. Mitochondrial nitric oxide synthase. *Mitochondrion* **2004**, *3*, 187–204. [CrossRef]
72. Ghafourifar, P.; Cadenas, E. Mitochondrial nitric oxide synthase. *Trends Pharmacol. Sci.* **2005**, *26*, 190–195. [CrossRef]
73. Lacza, Z.; Snipes, J.A.; Zhang, J.; Horvath, E.M.; Figueroa, J.P.; Szabo, C.; Busija, D.W. Mitochondrial nitric oxide synthase is not eNOS, nNOS or iNOS. *Free Radic. Biol. Med.* **2003**, *35*, 1217–1228. [CrossRef]
74. Du, K.; Farhood, A.; Jaeschke, H. Mitochondria-targeted antioxidant Mito-Tempo protects against acetaminophen hepatotoxicity. *Arch. Toxicol.* **2017**, *91*, 761–773. [CrossRef]
75. Du, K.; Ramachandran, A.; Weemhoff, J.L.; Woolbright, B.L.; Jaeschke, A.H.; Chao, X.; Ding, W.X.; Jaeschke, H. Mito-tempo protects against acute liver injury but induces limited secondary apoptosis during the late phase of acetaminophen hepatotoxicity. *Arch. Toxicol.* **2019**, *93*, 163–178. [CrossRef]
76. Knight, T.R.; Ho, Y.S.; Farhood, A.; Jaeschke, H. Peroxynitrite is a critical mediator of acetaminophen hepatotoxicity in murine livers: Protection by glutathione. *J. Pharmacol. Exp. Ther.* **2002**, *303*, 468–475. [CrossRef]
77. Adelusi, O.B.; Ramachandran, A.; Lemasters, J.J.; Jaeschke, H. The role of Iron in lipid peroxidation and protein nitration during acetaminophen-induced liver injury in mice. *Toxicol. Appl. Pharmacol.* **2022**, *445*, 116043. [CrossRef]
78. Woolbright, B.L.; Ramachandran, A.; McGill, M.R.; Yan, H.M.; Bajt, M.L.; Sharpe, M.R.; Lemasters, J.J.; Jaeschke, H. Lysosomal instability and cathepsin B release during acetaminophen hepatotoxicity. *Basic Clin. Pharmacol. Toxicol.* **2012**, *111*, 417–425. [CrossRef]
79. Kon, K.; Kim, J.S.; Uchiyama, A.; Jaeschke, H.; Lemasters, J.J. Lysosomal iron mobilization and induction of the mitochondrial permeability transition in acetaminophen-induced toxicity to mouse hepatocytes. *Toxicol. Sci.* **2010**, *117*, 101–108. [CrossRef]
80. Hu, J.; Kholmukhamedov, A.; Lindsey, C.C.; Beeson, C.C.; Jaeschke, H.; Lemasters, J.J. Translocation of iron from lysosomes to mitochondria during acetaminophen-induced hepatocellular injury: Protection by starch-desferal and minocycline. *Free Radic. Biol. Med.* **2016**, *97*, 418–426. [CrossRef]
81. Hu, J.; Lemasters, J.J. Suppression of iron mobilization from lysosomes to mitochondria attenuates liver injury after acetaminophen overdose in vivo in mice: Protection by minocycline. *Toxicol. Appl. Pharmacol.* **2020**, *392*, 114930. [CrossRef]
82. Campolo, N.; Bartesaghi, S.; Radi, R. Metal-catalyzed protein tyrosine nitration in biological systems. *Redox Rep.* **2014**, *19*, 221–231. [CrossRef] [PubMed]

83. McGill, M.R.; Sharpe, M.R.; Williams, C.D.; Taha, M.; Curry, S.C.; Jaeschke, H. The mechanism underlying acetaminophen-induced hepatotoxicity in humans and mice involves mitochondrial damage and nuclear DNA fragmentation. *J. Clin. Investig.* **2012**, *122*, 1574–1583. [CrossRef] [PubMed]
84. Fromenty, B. Inhibition of mitochondrial fatty acid oxidation in drug-induced hepatic steatosis. *Liver Res.* **2019**, *3*, 157–169. [CrossRef]
85. Chen, C.; Krausz, K.W.; Shah, Y.M.; Idle, J.R.; Gonzalez, F.J. Serum metabolomics reveals irreversible inhibition of fatty acid beta-oxidation through the suppression of PPARalpha activation as a contributing mechanism of acetaminophen-induced hepatotoxicity. *Chem. Res. Toxicol.* **2009**, *22*, 699–707. [CrossRef]
86. Ramachandran, A.; Lebofsky, M.; Baines, C.P.; Lemasters, J.J.; Jaeschke, H. Cyclophilin D deficiency protects against acetaminophen-induced oxidant stress and liver injury. *Free Radic. Res.* **2011**, *45*, 156–164. [CrossRef]
87. Bhattacharyya, S.; Pence, L.; Beger, R.; Chaudhuri, S.; McCullough, S.; Yan, K.; Simpson, P.; Hennings, L.; Hinson, J.; James, L. Acylcarnitine profiles in acetaminophen toxicity in the mouse: Comparison to toxicity, metabolism and hepatocyte regeneration. *Metabolites* **2013**, *3*, 606–622. [CrossRef]
88. McGill, M.R.; Li, F.; Sharpe, M.R.; Williams, C.D.; Curry, S.C.; Ma, X.; Jaeschke, H. Circulating acylcarnitines as biomarkers of mitochondrial dysfunction after acetaminophen overdose in mice and humans. *Arch. Toxicol.* **2014**, *88*, 391–401. [CrossRef]
89. Chen, S.; Lu, Z.; Jia, H.; Yang, B.; Liu, C.; Yang, Y.; Zhang, S.; Wang, Z.; Yang, L.; Li, S.; et al. Hepatocyte-specific Mas activation enhances lipophagy and fatty acid oxidation to protect against acetaminophen-induced hepatotoxicity in mice. *J. Hepatol.* **2023**, *78*, 543–557. [CrossRef]
90. Bhattacharyya, S.; Yan, K.; Pence, L.; Simpson, P.M.; Gill, P.; Letzig, L.G.; Beger, R.D.; Sullivan, J.E.; Kearns, G.L.; Reed, M.D.; et al. Targeted liquid chromatography-mass spectrometry analysis of serum acylcarnitines in acetaminophen toxicity in children. *Biomark. Med.* **2014**, *8*, 147–159. [CrossRef]
91. Kon, K.; Kim, J.S.; Jaeschke, H.; Lemasters, J.J. Mitochondrial permeability transition in acetaminophen-induced necrosis and apoptosis of cultured mouse hepatocytes. *Hepatology* **2004**, *40*, 1170–1179. [CrossRef]
92. Masubuchi, Y.; Suda, C.; Horie, T. Involvement of mitochondrial permeability transition in acetaminophen-induced liver injury in mice. *J. Hepatol.* **2005**, *42*, 110–116. [CrossRef]
93. Ramachandran, A.; McGill, M.R.; Xie, Y.; Ni, H.M.; Ding, W.X.; Jaeschke, H. Receptor interacting protein kinase 3 is a critical early mediator of acetaminophen-induced hepatocyte necrosis in mice. *Hepatology* **2013**, *58*, 2099–2108. [CrossRef]
94. Bajt, M.L.; Cover, C.; Lemasters, J.J.; Jaeschke, H. Nuclear translocation of endonuclease G and apoptosis-inducing factor during acetaminophen-induced liver cell injury. *Toxicol. Sci.* **2006**, *94*, 217–225. [CrossRef]
95. Norberg, E.; Orrenius, S.; Zhivotovsky, B. Mitochondrial regulation of cell death: Processing of apoptosis-inducing factor (AIF). *Biochem. Biophys. Res. Commun.* **2010**, *396*, 95–100. [CrossRef]
96. Boujrad, H.; Gubkina, O.; Robert, N.; Krantic, S.; Susin, S.A. AIF-mediated programmed necrosis: A highly regulated way to die. *Cell Cycle* **2007**, *6*, 2612–2619. [CrossRef]
97. Widlak, P.; Garrard, W.T. Discovery, regulation, and action of the major apoptotic nucleases DFF40/CAD and endonuclease G. *J. Cell. Biochem.* **2005**, *94*, 1078–1087. [CrossRef]
98. Bajt, M.L.; Ramachandran, A.; Yan, H.M.; Lebofsky, M.; Farhood, A.; Lemasters, J.J.; Jaeschke, H. Apoptosis-inducing factor modulates mitochondrial oxidant stress in acetaminophen hepatotoxicity. *Toxicol. Sci.* **2011**, *122*, 598–605. [CrossRef]
99. Bajt, M.L.; Farhood, A.; Lemasters, J.J.; Jaeschke, H. Mitochondrial bax translocation accelerates DNA fragmentation and cell necrosis in a murine model of acetaminophen hepatotoxicity. *J. Pharmacol. Exp. Ther.* **2008**, *324*, 8–14. [CrossRef]
100. Jaeschke, H.; Murray, F.J.; Monnot, A.D.; Jacobson-Kram, D.; Cohen, S.M.; Hardisty, J.F.; Atillasoy, E.; Hermanowski-Vosatka, A.; Kuffner, E.; Wikoff, D.; et al. Assessment of the biochemical pathways for acetaminophen toxicity: Implications for its carcinogenic hazard potential. *Regul. Toxicol. Pharmacol.* **2021**, *120*, 104859. [CrossRef]
101. Jaeschke, H.; Duan, L.; Nguyen, N.; Ramachandran, A. Mitochondrial Damage and Biogenesis in Acetaminophen-induced Liver Injury. *Liver Res.* **2019**, *3*, 150–156. [CrossRef] [PubMed]
102. Du, K.; Ramachandran, A.; McGill, M.R.; Mansouri, A.; Asselah, T.; Farhood, A.; Woolbright, B.L.; Ding, W.X.; Jaeschke, H. Induction of mitochondrial biogenesis protects against acetaminophen hepatotoxicity. *Food Chem. Toxicol.* **2017**, *108*, 339–350. [CrossRef] [PubMed]
103. Ye, D.; Wang, Y.; Li, H.; Jia, W.; Man, K.; Lo, C.M.; Wang, Y.; Lam, K.S.; Xu, A. Fibroblast growth factor 21 protects against acetaminophen-induced hepatotoxicity by potentiating peroxisome proliferator-activated receptor coactivator protein-1alpha-mediated antioxidant capacity in mice. *Hepatology* **2014**, *60*, 977–989. [CrossRef] [PubMed]
104. Carvalho, N.R.; Tassi, C.C.; Dobraschinski, F.; Amaral, G.P.; Zemolin, A.P.; Golombieski, R.M.; Dalla Corte, C.L.; Franco, J.L.; Mauriz, J.L.; Gonzalez-Gallego, J.; et al. Reversal of bioenergetics dysfunction by diphenyl diselenide is critical to protection against the acetaminophen-induced acute liver failure. *Life Sci.* **2017**, *180*, 42–50. [CrossRef]
105. Jaeschke, H.; Ramachandran, A. Mechanisms and pathophysiological significance of sterile inflammation during acetaminophen hepatotoxicity. *Food Chem. Toxicol.* **2020**, *138*, 111240. [CrossRef]
106. Nguyen, N.T.; Umbaugh, D.S.; Smith, S.; Adelusi, O.B.; Sanchez-Guerrero, G.; Ramachandran, A.; Jaeschke, H. Dose-dependent Pleiotropic Role of Neutrophils during Acetaminophen-induced Liver Injury in Male and Female Mice. *Arch. Toxicol.* **2023**, *in press*. [CrossRef]

107. Thibaut, R.; Orliaguet, L.; Ejlalmanesh, T.; Venteclef, N.; Alzaid, F. Perspective on direction of control: Cellular metabolism and macrophage polarization. *Front. Immunol.* **2022**, *13*, 918747. [CrossRef]
108. Cai, S.; Zhao, M.; Zhou, B.; Yoshii, A.; Bugg, D.; Villet, O.; Sahu, A.; Olson, G.S.; Davis, J.; Tian, R. Mitochondrial dysfunction in macrophages promotes inflammation and suppresses repair after myocardial infarction. *J. Clin. Investig.* **2023**, *133*, e159498. [CrossRef]
109. Nguyen, N.T.; Umbaugh, D.S.; Sanchez-Guerrero, G.; Ramachandran, A.; Jaeschke, H. Kupffer cells regulate liver recovery through induction of chemokine receptor CXCR2 on hepatocytes after acetaminophen overdose in mice. *Arch. Toxicol.* **2022**, *96*, 305–320. [CrossRef]
110. Nguyen, N.T.; Umbaugh, D.S.; Huang, E.L.; Adelusi, O.B.; Sanchez Guerrero, G.; Ramachandran, A.; Jaeschke, H. Recovered Hepatocytes Promote Macrophage Apoptosis Through CXCR4 After Acetaminophen-Induced Liver Injury in Mice. *Toxicol. Sci.* **2022**, *188*, 248–260. [CrossRef]
111. Yang, W.; Tao, Y.; Wu, Y.; Zhao, X.; Ye, W.; Zhao, D.; Fu, L.; Tian, C.; Yang, J.; He, F.; et al. Neutrophils promote the development of reparative macrophages mediated by ROS to orchestrate liver repair. *Nat. Commun.* **2019**, *10*, 1076. [CrossRef]
112. Peng, S.; Gao, J.; Stojkov, D.; Yousefi, S.; Simon, H.U. Established and emerging roles for mitochondria in neutrophils. *Immunol. Rev.* **2023**. *Online ahead of print*. [CrossRef]

livers

MDPI

Review

Regeneration and Recovery after Acetaminophen Hepatotoxicity

Bharat Bhushan [1,2,*] and Udayan Apte [3]

1 Department of Pathology, University of Pittsburgh School of Medicine, Pittsburgh, PA 15261, USA
2 Pittsburgh Liver Research Center, University of Pittsburgh Medical Center, University of Pittsburgh School of Medicine, Pittsburgh, PA 15261, USA
3 Department of Pharmacology, Toxicology and Therapeutics, University of Kansas Medical Center, Kansas City, KS 66160, USA; uapte@kumc.edu
* Correspondence: bhb14@pitt.edu; Tel.: +1-412-648-2021

Abstract: Liver regeneration is a compensatory response to tissue injury and loss. It is known that liver regeneration plays a crucial role in recovery following acetaminophen (APAP)-induced hepatotoxicity, which is the major cause of acute liver failure (ALF) in the US. Regeneration increases proportional to the extent of liver injury upon APAP overdose, ultimately leading to regression of injury and spontaneous recovery in most cases. However, severe APAP overdose results in impaired liver regeneration and unchecked progression of liver injury, leading to failed recovery and mortality. Inter-communication between various cell types in the liver is important for effective regenerative response following APAP hepatotoxicity. Various non-parenchymal cells such macrophages, stellate cells, and endothelial cells produce mediators crucial for proliferation of hepatocytes. Liver regeneration is orchestrated by synchronized actions of several proliferative signaling pathways involving numerous kinases, nuclear receptors, transcription factors, transcriptional co-activators, which are activated by cytokines, growth factors, and endobiotics. Overt activation of anti-proliferative signaling pathways causes cell-cycle arrest and impaired liver regeneration after severe APAP overdose. Stimulating liver regeneration by activating proliferating signaling and suppressing anti-proliferative signaling in liver can prove to be important in developing novel therapeutics for APAP-induced ALF.

Keywords: hepatotoxicity; liver regeneration; proliferation; drug-induced liver injury; Cyclin D1; p21; TGFβ1; β-catenin

1. Introduction

The liver has an extraordinary capacity to regenerate upon surgical resection, infection, and toxicant- or chemical-induced liver injury. The liver is the only organ that restores exactly to its original mass even after two-thirds of tissue loss [1]. Each cell type in the liver including hepatocytes, cholangiocytes, hepatic stellate cells, and endothelial cells usually proliferate to replace their own cell type ultimately attaining original liver mass and function. The phenomenon that regulates liver size in normal physiology and especially during compensatory regeneration has been termed as the hepatostat [1,2]. Liver regeneration is orchestrated by synchronized actions of several proliferative signaling pathways involving numerous kinases, nuclear receptors, transcription factors, transcriptional co-activators, which are governed by cytokines, growth factors, endobiotics such as bile acids, and hormones [3]. Typical regenerative response of healthy liver is very robust, and the elimination of any one signaling pathway does not usually have a major impact on overall outcome due to redundancy of the signaling mechanisms [1].

Extensive studies have shown that liver regeneration plays a crucial role in recovery after acetaminophen (APAP) overdose, a major clinical problem [4–9]. APAP is one of the most used over-the-counter analgesics and is considered very safe at therapeutic doses. However, APAP overdose results in acute liver injury involving hepatocyte cell death and centrilobular necrosis, which in severe cases leads to acute liver failure (ALF). APAP overdose is the topmost cause of ALF in the United States and the Western world [10]. APAP-induced hepatocyte death and centrilobular necrosis is initiated by its toxic metabolite NAPQI (N-acetyl-p-benzoquinone imine), which is normally excreted after conjugation with cellular glutathione (GSH). Excess NAPQI accumulated after APAP overdose depletes cellular GSH stores and forms adducts with cellular proteins (majorly with mitochondrial proteins), ultimately leading to mitochondrial damage, release of cell death mediators from mitochondria, and necrosis [11,12]. Interestingly, most of the APAP overdose patients recover spontaneously due to robust compensatory regenerative response. During this compensatory regenerative response, dead hepatocytes are replaced by newly formed cells, originating from viable hepatocytes surrounding the necrotic zones leading to restoration of normal liver mass and function. However, in severe cases, spontaneous recovery does not occur because of delayed and inhibited liver regeneration leading to mortality. Numerous studies have correlated robust liver regenerative response with better outcome in APAP-induced ALF patients [13,14]. Thus, timely stimulation of liver regeneration is a potential therapeutic option for APAP-induced ALF, and understanding the mechanisms of liver regeneration is important for developing potential therapeutic targets. Regenerative therapies can be especially beneficial considering liver injury is already established in most of the patients by the time they seek medical attention and is difficult to manipulate. This is evident from the fact that N-acetyl cysteine (NAC), the only pharmacological therapy of APAP-induced ALF, which is based on intervening early stages of liver injury, is not effective in late presenting patients [15]. In contrast, regenerative interventions can be potentially applied even at a later stage.

In the past, most of the studies to understand the mechanisms of liver regeneration have been focused on a partial hepatectomy model, which involves resection of healthy liver [16]. However, APAP hepatotoxicity is complicated by presence of massive cell death and subsequent persistent inflammation. These processes and associated signaling mediators intricately regulate the liver regeneration response after APAP hepatotoxicity. Recent studies have shown that liver regeneration response and the underlying mechanisms are very different in this toxic environment compared to the healthy liver [17]. Further, other underlying pathological conditions such as alcoholic or non-alcoholic fatty liver disease can also impact liver regeneration response. Liver regeneration is much more synchronized after partial hepatectomy of healthy liver compared to regeneration in response to APAP hepatotoxicity, where several injury related factors can actively impede proliferation [17]. Thus, in recent years, studies have focused on delineating liver regeneration mechanisms specifically in an APAP-induced liver injury model. The mechanisms that promote or inhibit liver regeneration specifically after APAP hepatotoxicity, their dose–response characteristics, and the role of various hepatic cell types in the liver regeneration response are discussed in this review. Additionally, factors to consider while designing studies to investigate liver regeneration following APAP hepatotoxicity are also discussed.

2. Dose–Response Characteristics of Liver Regeneration after APAP Hepatotoxicity

Hepatocyte proliferation and liver regeneration occur as a compensatory response to exposure of any injurious chemical toxicants [18]. These include toxicants that cause injury to different zones of liver, including centrilobular hepatotoxicants (such as carbon tetrachloride, thioacetamide, and APAP) and periportal hepatotoxicants (such as allyl alcohol) [9,18–21]. Detailed dose–response characteristics of liver regeneration following these toxicant-induced liver damage have been extensively studied and have been reviewed earlier [18]. These studies have established that liver regeneration increases proportional to the liver injury upon increasing the dose of toxicant [18,20]. There is also a progressive delay in liver regeneration response with increasing the dose. However, the incremental liver regeneration response more than offsets the delay in regenerative response up to a certain dose, ultimately inducing regression of liver injury and recovery. Thus, up to a threshold dose, stimulation of liver regeneration occurs proportionate to the extent of injury. Beyond this threshold dose, there is a sharp decline and delay in liver regeneration response upon increasing the dose further. This results in unchecked progression of liver injury leading to failed recovery and mortality [9,18]. For instance, this dose–response relationship of liver regeneration has been well characterized for thioacetamide, utilizing several different doses (50, 150, 300, and 600 mg/kg) over a time-course of 0–96 h in rats. Liver regeneration increases proportionate to liver injury up to 300 mg/kg dose of thioacetamide leading to complete recovery. However, liver regeneration is severely compromised and delayed at a 600 mg/kg dose leading to significant mortality [20]. Further, if proliferation is blocked by administering anti-mitotic agents (such as colchicine) after doses of toxicants that normally result in robust liver regeneration and spontaneous recovery, it also results in progression of injury and failed recovery [18,22]. These studies further emphasize the importance of liver regeneration for recovery and regression of injury.

Studies utilizing incremental doses of APAP in mice have shown similar dose–response characteristics of liver regeneration after APAP hepatotoxicity [9]. A moderately toxic dose of APAP (300 mg/kg) in mice causes extensive liver injury but also timely and robust compensatory liver regeneration, ultimately leading to regression of injury, spontaneous recovery, and survival. In contrast, severe APAP overdose (600 mg/kg) in mice results in comparable initial liver injury but disproportionately impaired and delayed liver regeneration, resulting in unchecked progression of injury, failed recovery, and significant mortality [9]. Other doses of APAP such as 350, 450, and 525 mg/kg of APAP have also been utilized for investigating liver regeneration [23]. However, a more comprehensive dose–response relationship of liver regeneration in the APAP model, including several different doses of APAP, and all temporal phases of APAP hepatotoxicity and compensatory regeneration still needs to be documented. Lastly, the mechanisms involved in liver injury and compensatory regeneration vary greatly with the dose of APAP. Thus, it is important to study the mechanisms of liver injury and regeneration utilizing multiple doses, especially severely toxic doses of APAP, which are not well studied as the majority of previously published studies utilize only moderately toxic doses of APAP, where animals regenerate spontaneously. Understanding these mechanisms at severely toxic doses of APAP is also clinically relevant to mimic pathophysiology of APAP-induced ALF patients who fail to recover spontaneously and require liver transplantation. Thus, it is important to consider if doses utilized in a study investigating liver regeneration are relevant for exposure observed in APAP overdose patients, especially in those who do not recover spontaneously. Overall, the dose–response relationship of liver regeneration following APAP hepatotoxicity is very important to consider for any study design focusing on understanding the mechanisms of liver regeneration or developing regenerative therapeutics for APAP-induced ALF.

3. Multiple Proliferative Signaling Mediators Contribute to Orchestrate Liver Regeneration Following APAP Hepatotoxicity

Liver regeneration is orchestrated by complex interplay of several cytokines, mitogens, and other proliferative signaling pathways following APAP hepatotoxicity [1]. While cytokines (such as tumor necrosis factor alpha: TNF-α and Interleukin 6: IL-6) are considered auxiliary mitogens for liver as they alone do not induce hepatocyte proliferation in vivo or in vitro, growth factors such as hepatocyte growth factor (HGF) and epidermal growth factor (EGF) receptor ligands (e.g., EGF and transforming growth factor alpha: TGF-α) are considered primary mitogens for liver as they can alone induce hepatocyte proliferation in vivo or in vitro even in serum free chemically defined medium [1,3]. Further, the EGF receptor (EGFR) and HGF receptor (i.e., c-MET) are the only known cell membrane receptors whose signaling disruption in combination results in complete elimination of liver regeneration response after partial hepatectomy, highlighting importance of these receptor tyrosine kinases [24]. Elimination of any other upstream signaling pathway causes only delay in liver regeneration response after partial hepatectomy, but the liver eventually regenerates to attain hepatostat. Temporal and dose-dependent dynamics of activation of growth factors, cytokines, and other important pro-regenerative signaling have also been comprehensively investigated in the context of APAP-induced liver injury as discussed in the following part of this section [9].

Both c-MET and EGFR are robustly activated dose-dependently after APAP overdose in mice and might play an important role in liver regeneration following APAP hepatotoxicity [9]. Interestingly, these receptors are activated very early following APAP overdose in mice, even prior to any observable liver injury. EGFR is activated within the first 30 min of APAP administration in mice and remains activated in sustained manner even during the recovery phase (up to 96 h after APAP) [8,9]. EGFR activation during the recovery phase might be crucial for driving regenerative response as late administration of EGFR inhibitor (after liver injury is already established) not only impairs liver regeneration but also leads to failed recovery and significant mortality after a moderately toxic dose of APAP (300 mg/kg) that normally culminates in spontaneous recovery in mice [8]. Paradoxically, EGFR activation during the injury initiation phase might be linked to cell death signaling as early EGFR inhibition (prior to injury development) results in almost complete attenuation of liver injury following APAP overdose in mice, eliminating any need for compensatory liver regeneration [8]. c-MET is also activated very early (within 3 h) after APAP overdose in mice, but its causal role in liver regeneration in the APAP-induced ALF model has not yet explored [9]. Further, the role of both EGFR and c-MET in liver injury or regeneration after APAP overdose needs to be established using specific genetic deletion approaches considering the potential off-target effects of chemical inhibition.

The role of cytokine signaling (TNF-α/NFκB and IL-6/STAT3) is relatively more extensively studied in the APAP model utilizing transgenic mice. Both TNF-α and IL-6 expression levels in liver increase after APAP overdose in mice [9,25]. Further, the deletion of TNF receptor 1 (TNF-R1) and IL6 in mice results in impaired liver regeneration after APAP hepatotoxicity [6,26,27]. Moreover, the administration of IL-6 in IL-6 knock-out mice results in restoration of the liver regeneration response [6]. Interestingly in our previous study, TNFα/NFκB signaling activation, downstream nuclear translocation of NFκB, and its binding to the promoter of core cell cycle genes (such as Cyclin D1, which governs entry into cell cycle) were greater after moderate APAP overdose, which was accompanied by robust liver regeneration response. However, TNFα/NFκB signaling activation was remarkably inhibited after severe APAP overdose which correlated with impaired liver regeneration [9]. In contrast, IL-6/STAT-3 signaling activation was dose-dependently higher after severe APAP overdose in mice [9]. This suggests dose-dependent differential role of these cytokines in liver regeneration after APAP hepatotoxicity, which needs further exploration.

Other than growth factors and cytokine signaling, Wnt/β-catenin signaling is also considered to be very important for hepatocyte proliferation and liver regeneration [1]. The role of the Wnt/β-catenin signaling pathway has also been studied in the APAP model of liver regeneration using transgenic and pharmacological approaches. Similar to the TNFα/NFκB signaling pathway, β-catenin signaling activation, nuclear translocation of β-catenin, and its binding to the Cyclin D1 promoter occurs robustly at a regenerating dose of APAP in mice but is inhibited at doses where liver regeneration is impaired [9]. B-catenin signaling activation is also correlated with higher liver regeneration and survival in ALF patients [14]. Utilization of the β-catenin deletion strategy to demonstrate its causal link with liver regeneration in the APAP model has been hampered as these mice exhibit very low expression of Cyp2e1, the main enzyme involved in metabolic activation of APAP, and thus exhibit low hepatotoxicity compared to wild-type (WT) mice [14]. However, β-catenin deletion in the liver results in impaired liver regeneration when different doses of APAP are utilized in WT and β-catenin KO mice to achieve equal liver injury (i.e., equitoxic dose strategy), and consistent overexpression of β-catenin results in significant stimulation of liver regeneration [9,14]. β-catenin signaling has also been targeted pharmacologically to develop regenerative therapy for APAP-induced ALF by using the inhibitor of glycogen synthase kinase 3 (GSK3), which is an upstream inhibitor of β-catenin. However, pharmacological activation of β-catenin signaling by inhibiting GSK3 results only in early onset of a proliferative response after severe APAP overdose, without significantly affecting the peak regenerative response or overall outcome/survival [28]. Although several studies have established β-catenin to be a critical regulator of liver regeneration following APAP hepatotoxicity, the specific Wnt ligands that activate β-catenin and the source of these Wnt ligands remain elusive in this model.

Apart from the Wnt/β-catenin signaling pathway, the Hippo/YAP signaling pathway has been also emerged as a critical regulator of hepatocyte proliferation and liver size in recent years [1]. YAP signaling activation, which is normally associated with higher proliferation and hepatomegaly in liver, is also rapidly activated during APAP overdose in mice [29,30]. However, in the context of APAP hepatotoxicity, YAP appears to inflict the opposite effect as hepatocyte-specific YAP deletion results in faster hepatocyte proliferation and rapid recovery after APAP hepatotoxicity in mice [29]. Further, rapid recovery from APAP overdose in the hepatocyte specific YAP knockout mice is related to faster activation of the Wnt/β-catenin pathway [29]. Lastly, several endobiotics such as bile acids and hormones can also potentially regulate liver regeneration following APAP hepatotoxicity based on knowledge from the partial hepatectomy model. Indeed, signaling via bile acids can contribute to liver regeneration response following APAP hepatotoxicity as both cholic acid and FGF19 (a downstream mediator of bile acid signaling) treatment result in improved liver regeneration after APAP overdose in mice [31,32].

4. Signaling Mechanisms Involved in Inhibiting Liver Regeneration Following APAP Hepatotoxicity

One of the most interesting findings with regard to liver regeneration in the APAP model is that many of the proliferative signaling pathways considered very critical for liver regeneration remain highly activated even after severe APAP overdose in mice, but liver regeneration is still severely impaired at these high doses [9]. For example, primary mitogen signaling via HGF/c-MET and EGF/EGFR pathways and their downstream ERK signaling are more activated after severe APAP overdose, where liver regeneration is impaired [8,9]. Similar is the case of cytokine signaling via the IL-6/STAT-3 pathway [9]. Interestingly, the majority of the hepatocytes are still viable even after severe APAP overdose in mice, but they fail to respond to these proliferative signals [9]. This indicates the possible contribution of mediators that actively inhibit cell cycle, leading to cell cycle arrest at severe APAP overdose, where liver regeneration is impaired. Although activation of cell cycle inhibitory mechanisms is important for balanced proliferative response and effective DNA repair, overt activation of these pathways after severe APAP overdose may result in impaired liver regeneration and failed recovery. Indeed, studies have shown striking activation of key cell cycle inhibitors such as p21 and p53 after severe APAP overdose in mice [9,33]. Further, the deletion of p21 and p53 results in higher or faster liver regeneration after APAP overdose in mice [23,34]. Excessive double strand DNA damage and limited DNA repair pathways activation in peri-necrotic regions might be responsible for the activation of cell cycle arrest signaling after severe APAP overdose [33]. Clinical relevance of all these findings can be appreciated by studies showing association of hepatic DNA damage, increased expression of cell cycle inhibitors such as p21, and cell cycle arrest with impaired liver regeneration response in APAP-induced ALF patients [23,35].

Transforming growth factor beta (TGFβ) appears to be one of the important upstream signaling pathways to be involved in induction of p21 and senescence in perinecrotic areas after severe APAP overdose [23]. TGFβ signaling is activated in perinecrotic areas after APAP overdose in mice/humans correlating to p21 induction and the deletion of the *Tgfb1* gene, or treatment with the TGFβ receptor 1 inhibitor in mice decreases p21 expression and improves liver regeneration/survival [23]. Macrophages were found to be an important source of TGFβ driving anti-proliferative effects in the above study [23]. Treatment with the TGFβ1 inhibitor can be a potential therapeutic option for stimulating regeneration after APAP overdose. Apart from TGFβ, extracellular matrix signaling transduction via integrin-linked kinase (ILK) is also important for producing anti-proliferative effects on hepatocytes, maintaining a quiescent state, and in the termination of liver regeneration following partial hepatectomy [36]. A similar role of ILK in inflicting inhibitory effects on hepatocyte proliferation and liver regeneration has also reported in the APAP overdose model as a liver-specific ILK deletion resulted in striking increase in hepatocyte proliferation disproportionate to the extent of liver injury after APAP overdose in mice [37].

5. Liver Regeneration after APAP Hepatotoxicity Involves Complex Interplay of Hepatic Parenchymal and Non-Parenchymal Cells

As mentioned previously in this review, each hepatic cell type usually proliferates to replace its own cell type during the process of liver regeneration [3]. However, each hepatic cell type can produce mediators which are important for proliferation of other cell types in liver [1]. Moreover, extrahepatic tissues can also produce some of the important growth factors involved in liver regeneration. For instance, Brunner glands of the duodenum are the major source of EGF exposed to liver via portal circulation, which is an important primary mitogen for hepatocytes. Stellate cells are the major source of HGF in liver, which is another major primary mitogen for hepatocytes. Stellate cell depletion or treatment with stellate cell-derived conditioned medium produces the opposite effect of inhibited or improved hepatocyte proliferation/liver regeneration, respectively, after APAP hepatotoxicity in mice [38,39]. Similarly, endothelial cell proliferation is not only important for restoring hepatic vasculature but also for hepatocyte proliferation as vascular endothelial growth factor (VEGF)-stimulated endothelial cells also produce HGF. Indeed, treatment with the VEGF inhibitor or deletion of VEGF receptor 1 (Vegfr-1) in mice results in impaired hepatocyte proliferation after APAP hepatotoxicity, and treatment with recombinant VEGF results in increased hepatocyte proliferation following APAP hepatotoxicity [5,40,41]. Lastly, macrophages recruited to centrilobular necrotic areas after APAP hepatotoxicity are not only important for removal of cell debris to house newly formed hepatocytes, but they are known to produce both cytokines (TNF-α, and IL-6) and mitogens (HGF and TGF-α) important for hepatocyte proliferation. Liver resident macrophages (Kupffer cells) can promote proliferative signaling in hepatocytes via induction of chemokine receptor CXCR2 [42]. The therapeutic potential of targeting macrophages has been also demonstrated by a recent study where cell-based therapy involving administration of alternatively activated macrophages promoted hepatocyte proliferation and resolution of APAP-induced liver injury [43]. Thus, inter-communication between different cell types in liver is important for an effective regenerative response following APAP hepatotoxicity. Recent temporal and spatially resolved single-cell RNA sequencing (sc-RNA seq) studies have further revealed importance of coordinated and zonal response via various liver cell types in orchestrating liver regeneration and maintenance of essential liver function following APAP hepatotoxicity, which need further exploration [44,45].

6. Factors to Consider while Designing Studies to Investigate Liver Regeneration Following APAP Hepatotoxicity

One of the most important factors to consider while studying liver regeneration following APAP hepatotoxicity is that the extent of liver regeneration response is dependent on the amount of initial liver injury [9]. Thus, any interventions altering initial liver injury can indirectly affect liver regeneration secondary to altered injury making it difficult to delineate a direct role of any intervention/mediator in liver regeneration. If the focus of a study is to investigate a direct role of a mediator on liver regeneration, intervention should be done at a late time point such that liver injury is already established. For instance, in our previous study, early treatment with the EGFR inhibitor drastically decreased initial liver injury making it unfeasible to investigate a direct role of EGFR in liver regeneration using this experimental strategy. Therefore, we utilized a strategy of late treatment with EGFR inhibitor (after liver injury was fully established), so that we can study a direct role of EGFR in liver regeneration [8]. Late interventions are especially relevant clinically as NAC is already available as a gold-standard therapy that is highly effective upon early intervention. If late intervention is not possible due to experimental constraints (such as utilization of transgenic mice model), the effect on liver injury should also be fully characterized, and any alteration of liver regeneration indirectly due to effect on liver injury should be considered. For example, in our previous study, investigation of a direct role of ILK or β-catenin in liver regeneration was hampered using the KO mice strategy as deletion of these genes decreased expression of Cyp2e1 and thus decreased metabolic activation and initial liver injury after APAP overdose [14,37]. Further, it is also important to study the complete time course of liver regeneration phase as some of the interventions/mediators might only produce temporal effects such as delay or early onset of liver regeneration without altering the peak of liver regeneration or the final outcome. For instance, in our previous study, GSK3 inhibition resulted in early initiation of regeneration response following APAP hepatotoxicity, but analysis of complete time-course of regeneration phase revealed that peak regenerative response, overall recovery, and survival were not affected [28]. For studies that are solely focused on investigating the effect of any intervention on the APAP hepatotoxicity phase, the inclusion of regeneration phase time points should also be considered to rule out any deleterious effects of that intervention on liver regeneration and overall recovery. For example, in our previous study, EGFR inhibition showed striking protection against liver injury after APAP overdose in mice; however, it impaired regeneration upon late intervention during the regeneration phase, diminishing the scope of its potential therapeutic utility [8]. Further, as discussed previously, it is critical to consider the use of multiple doses of APAP in a study, considering characteristics and mechanisms of liver injury/regeneration greatly vary in a dose-dependent manner. Especially if the aim of a study is to find interventions to stimulate liver regeneration, higher doses of APAP should be considered. This is because, at moderately toxic doses of APAP, the liver undergoes robust spontaneous regeneration, and only at severe APAP overdose is liver regeneration impaired, reflecting clinical APAP-induced ALF, which requires transplantation. While designing studies using high doses of APAP (such as 600 mg/kg) in mice, it is important to properly control the extent of fasting prior to APAP administration as excessive fasting (more than 12 h) may result in high mortality such that analysis of late time points might be difficult. Lastly, for complete analysis of liver regeneration in APAP-induced ALF model, multiple proliferative markers should be investigated encompassing all the phases of the cell cycle from initiation of cell cycle to mitosis. Further, hepatocyte proliferation parameters should be corroborated other parameters such as regression of injury, final recovery, and survival to demonstrate clinical significance of the interventions on final outcome.

7. Concluding Remarks

Timely liver regeneration is an important determinant of final recovery after acetaminophen hepatotoxicity. Liver regeneration after APAP overdose is orchestrated by various signaling pathways activated by myriad of cytokines, growth factors, and endobiotics. Effective communication between hepatic parenchymal and non-parenchymal cells is crucial for regenerative response following APAP-induced liver injury. A summary of the process of liver regeneration and recovery following acetaminophen (APAP)-hepatotoxicity is presented in Figure 1. Liver regeneration after APAP overdose is a dose-dependent compensatory response. The mechanisms involved in regulating regeneration vary greatly with the dose of APAP with overt activation of anti-proliferative signaling pathways after severe APAP overdose. It is important to consider dose–response characteristics of liver regeneration while designing regenerative studies using the APAP model. There is still a need to fully understand the mechanisms that regulate liver regeneration, especially after severe APAP overdose, which is associated with failed spontaneous recovery and adverse outcome. Since liver regeneration can be targeted even after liver injury has been fully developed, regenerative therapies can be especially promising for late presenting APAP-induced ALF patients.

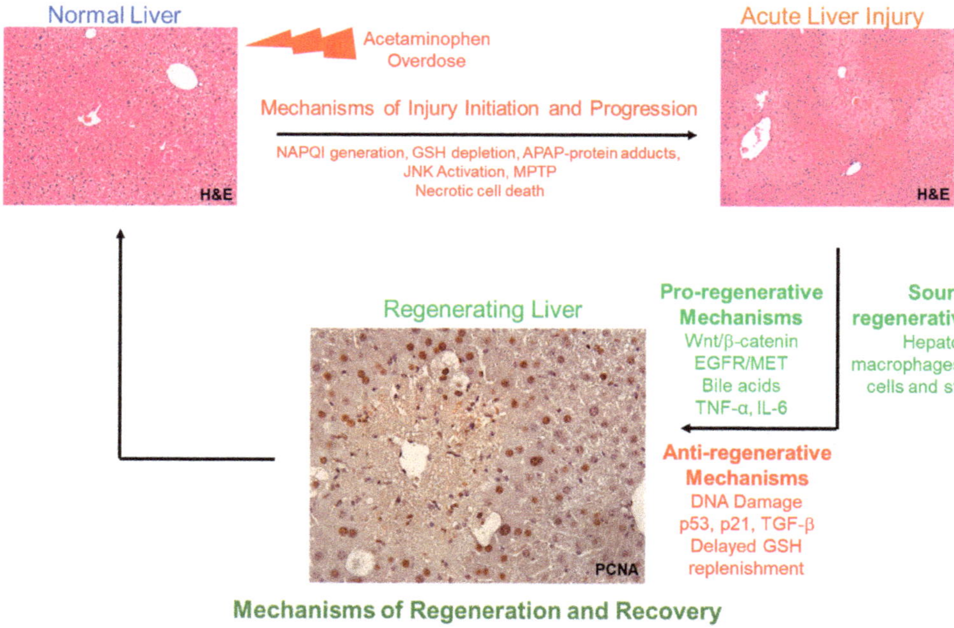

Figure 1. Schematics showing an overview of the process of liver regeneration and recovery following acetaminophen (APAP)-hepatotoxicity: APAP overdose initiates a cascade of events resulting in centrilobular liver necrosis. Pro-regenerative signals from various hepatic cell types stimulate hepatocyte proliferation and liver regeneration resulting in regression of liver injury and spontaneous recovery after moderate APAP overdose. Various anti-regenerative signals are also activated for balanced proliferative response and effective repair. However, overt activation of anti-proliferative pathways after severe APAP overdose results in impaired liver regeneration and failed recovery. GSH, glutathione; MPTP, mitochondrial permeability transition pore; NAPQI, N-acetyl-p-benzoquinone imine. Normal liver (**top, left**) and necrotic liver after acetaminophen-induced acute liver injury (**top, right**) are represented by respective hematoxylin and eosin (H&E)-stained liver sections; Regenerating liver (bottom) is represented by liver section with proliferating cell nuclear antigen (PCNA) positive hepatocytes (brown staining).

Author Contributions: All authors contributed equally. All authors have read and agreed to the published version of the manuscript.

Funding: Supported by NIH R01 DK135566; NIH R01 DK98414; NIH R01 DK122990; Additional support provided by NIH grant P30 DK120531 to Pittsburgh Liver Research Center (PLRC).

Institutional Review Board Statement: Not applicable.

Informed Consent Statement: Not applicable.

Data Availability Statement: Not applicable.

Conflicts of Interest: The authors declare no conflict of interest.

References

1. Michalopoulos, G.K.; Bhushan, B. Liver regeneration: Biological and pathological mechanisms and implications. *Nat. Rev. Gastroenterol. Hepatol.* **2021**, *18*, 40–55. [CrossRef] [PubMed]
2. Michalopoulos, G.K. Hepatostat: Liver regeneration and normal liver tissue maintenance. *Hepatology* **2017**, *65*, 1384–1392. [CrossRef]
3. Michalopoulos, G.K. Principles of liver regeneration and growth homeostasis. *Compr. Physiol.* **2013**, *3*, 485–513. [CrossRef]

4. Bhushan, B.; Apte, U. Liver Regeneration after Acetaminophen Hepatotoxicity: Mechanisms and Therapeutic Opportunities. *Am. J. Pathol.* **2019**, *189*, 719–729. [CrossRef]
5. Donahower, B.C.; McCullough, S.S.; Hennings, L.; Simpson, P.M.; Stowe, C.D.; Saad, A.G.; Kurten, R.C.; Hinson, J.A.; James, L.P. Human recombinant vascular endothelial growth factor reduces necrosis and enhances hepatocyte regeneration in a mouse model of acetaminophen toxicity. *J. Pharmacol. Exp. Ther.* **2010**, *334*, 33–43. [CrossRef]
6. James, L.P.; Lamps, L.W.; McCullough, S.; Hinson, J.A. Interleukin 6 and hepatocyte regeneration in acetaminophen toxicity in the mouse. *Biochem. Biophys. Res. Commun.* **2003**, *309*, 857–863. [CrossRef]
7. Hu, B.; Colletti, L.M. Stem cell factor and c-kit are involved in hepatic recovery after acetaminophen-induced liver injury in mice. *Am. J. Physiol. Gastrointest. Liver Physiol.* **2008**, *295*, G45–G53. [CrossRef] [PubMed]
8. Bhushan, B.; Chavan, H.; Borude, P.; Xie, Y.; Du, K.; McGill, M.R.; Lebofsky, M.; Jaeschke, H.; Krishnamurthy, P.; Apte, U. Dual Role of Epidermal Growth Factor Receptor in Liver Injury and Regeneration after Acetaminophen Overdose in Mice. *Toxicol. Sci.* **2017**, *155*, 363–378. [CrossRef]
9. Bhushan, B.; Walesky, C.; Manley, M.; Gallagher, T.; Borude, P.; Edwards, G.; Monga, S.P.; Apte, U. Pro-regenerative signaling after acetaminophen-induced acute liver injury in mice identified using a novel incremental dose model. *Am. J. Pathol.* **2014**, *184*, 3013–3025. [CrossRef] [PubMed]
10. Stravitz, R.T.; Lee, W.M. Acute liver failure. *Lancet* **2019**, *394*, 869–881. [CrossRef]
11. Bhushan, B.; Apte, U. Acetaminophen Test Battery (ATB): A Comprehensive Method to Study Acetaminophen-Induced Acute Liver Injury. *Gene Expr.* **2020**, *20*, 125–138. [CrossRef]
12. Ramachandran, A.; Jaeschke, H. Acetaminophen Toxicity: Novel Insights Into Mechanisms and Future Perspectives. *Gene Expr.* **2018**, *18*, 19–30. [CrossRef] [PubMed]
13. Schmidt, L.E.; Dalhoff, K. Alpha-fetoprotein is a predictor of outcome in acetaminophen-induced liver injury. *Hepatology* **2005**, *41*, 26–31. [CrossRef] [PubMed]
14. Apte, U.; Singh, S.; Zeng, G.; Cieply, B.; Virji, M.A.; Wu, T.; Monga, S.P. Beta-catenin activation promotes liver regeneration after acetaminophen-induced injury. *Am. J. Pathol.* **2009**, *175*, 1056–1065. [CrossRef]
15. Larson, A.M. Acetaminophen hepatotoxicity. *Clin. Liver Dis.* **2007**, *11*, 525–548. [CrossRef]
16. Forbes, S.J.; Newsome, P.N. Liver regeneration—Mechanisms and models to clinical application. *Nat. Rev. Gastroenterol. Hepatol.* **2016**, *13*, 473–485. [CrossRef]
17. Bhushan, B.; Gunewardena, S.; Edwards, G.; Apte, U. Comparison of liver regeneration after partial hepatectomy and acetaminophen-induced acute liver failure: A global picture based on transcriptome analysis. *Food Chem. Toxicol.* **2020**, *139*, 111186. [CrossRef] [PubMed]
18. Mehendale, H.M. Tissue repair: An important determinant of final outcome of toxicant-induced injury. *Toxicol. Pathol.* **2005**, *33*, 41–51. [CrossRef]
19. Anand, S.S.; Murthy, S.N.; Vaidya, V.S.; Mumtaz, M.M.; Mehendale, H.M. Tissue repair plays pivotal role in final outcome of liver injury following chloroform and allyl alcohol binary mixture. *Food Chem. Toxicol.* **2003**, *41*, 1123–1132. [CrossRef] [PubMed]
20. Mangipudy, R.S.; Chanda, S.; Mehendale, H.M. Tissue repair response as a function of dose in thioacetamide hepatotoxicity. *Environ. Health Perspect.* **1995**, *103*, 260–267. [CrossRef]
21. Rao, P.S.; Mangipudy, R.S.; Mehendale, H.M. Tissue injury and repair as parallel and opposing responses to CCl4 hepatotoxicity: A novel dose-response. *Toxicology* **1997**, *118*, 181–193. [CrossRef]
22. Mangipudy, R.S.; Rao, P.S.; Mehendale, H.M. Effect of an antimitotic agent colchicine on thioacetamide hepatotoxicity. *Environ. Health Perspect.* **1996**, *104*, 744–749. [CrossRef]
23. Bird, T.G.; Muller, M.; Boulter, L.; Vincent, D.F.; Ridgway, R.A.; Lopez-Guadamillas, E.; Lu, W.Y.; Jamieson, T.; Govaere, O.; Campbell, A.D.; et al. TGFbeta inhibition restores a regenerative response in acute liver injury by suppressing paracrine senescence. *Sci. Transl. Med.* **2018**, *10*, eaan1230. [CrossRef] [PubMed]
24. Paranjpe, S.; Bowen, W.C.; Mars, W.M.; Orr, A.; Haynes, M.M.; DeFrances, M.C.; Liu, S.; Tseng, G.C.; Tsagianni, A.; Michalopoulos, G.K. Combined systemic elimination of MET and epidermal growth factor receptor signaling completely abolishes liver regeneration and leads to liver decompensation. *Hepatology* **2016**, *64*, 1711–1724. [CrossRef] [PubMed]
25. Masubuchi, Y.; Bourdi, M.; Reilly, T.P.; Graf, M.L.; George, J.W.; Pohl, L.R. Role of interleukin-6 in hepatic heat shock protein expression and protection against acetaminophen-induced liver disease. *Biochem. Biophys. Res. Commun.* **2003**, *304*, 207–212. [CrossRef]
26. Chiu, H.; Gardner, C.R.; Dambach, D.M.; Durham, S.K.; Brittingham, J.A.; Laskin, J.D.; Laskin, D.L. Role of tumor necrosis factor receptor 1 (p55) in hepatocyte proliferation during acetaminophen-induced toxicity in mice. *Toxicol. Appl. Pharmacol.* **2003**, *193*, 218–227. [CrossRef] [PubMed]
27. James, L.P.; Kurten, R.C.; Lamps, L.W.; McCullough, S.; Hinson, J.A. Tumour necrosis factor receptor 1 and hepatocyte regeneration in acetaminophen toxicity: A kinetic study of proliferating cell nuclear antigen and cytokine expression. *Basic Clin. Pharmacol. Toxicol.* **2005**, *97*, 8–14. [CrossRef]
28. Bhushan, B.; Poudel, S.; Manley, M.W., Jr.; Roy, N.; Apte, U. Inhibition of Glycogen Synthase Kinase 3 Accelerated Liver Regeneration after Acetaminophen-Induced Hepatotoxicity in Mice. *Am. J. Pathol.* **2017**, *187*, 543–552. [CrossRef]

29. Poudel, S.; Cabrera, D.P.; Bhushan, B.; Manley, M.W.; Gunewardena, S.; Jaeschke, H.; Apte, U. Hepatocyte-Specific Deletion of Yes-Associated Protein Improves Recovery From Acetaminophen-Induced Acute Liver Injury. *Toxicol. Sci.* **2021**, *184*, 276–285. [CrossRef]
30. Bhushan, B.; Stoops, J.W.; Mars, W.M.; Orr, A.; Bowen, W.C.; Paranjpe, S.; Michalopoulos, G.K. TCPOBOP-induced hepatomegaly & hepatocyte proliferation is attenuated by combined disruption of MET & EGFR signaling. *Hepatology* **2018**, *69*, 1702–1718. [CrossRef]
31. Bhushan, B.; Borude, P.C.; Edwards, G.; Walesky, C.M.; Apte, U. Role of bile acids in liver injury and regeneration following acetaminophen overdose. *Am. J. Pathol.* **2013**, *183*, 1518–1526. [CrossRef]
32. Alvarez-Sola, G.; Uriarte, I.; Latasa, M.U.; Jimenez, M.; Barcena-Varela, M.; Santamaria, E.; Urtasun, R.; Rodriguez-Ortigosa, C.; Prieto, J.; Corrales, F.J.; et al. Engineered fibroblast growth factor 19 protects from acetaminophen-induced liver injury and stimulates aged liver regeneration in mice. *Cell Death Dis.* **2017**, *8*, e3083. [CrossRef] [PubMed]
33. Borude, P.; Bhushan, B.; Apte, U. DNA Damage Response Regulates Initiation of Liver Regeneration Following Acetaminophen Overdose. *Gene Expr.* **2018**, *18*, 115–123. [CrossRef]
34. Borude, P.; Bhushan, B.; Gunewardena, S.; Akakpo, J.; Jaeschke, H.; Apte, U. Pleiotropic Role of p53 in Injury and Liver Regeneration after Acetaminophen Overdose. *Am. J. Pathol.* **2018**, *188*, 1406–1418. [CrossRef]
35. Viswanathan, P.; Sharma, Y.; Gupta, P.; Gupta, S. Replicative stress and alterations in cell cycle checkpoint controls following acetaminophen hepatotoxicity restrict liver regeneration. *Cell Prolif.* **2018**, *51*, e12445. [CrossRef]
36. Apte, U.; Gkretsi, V.; Bowen, W.C.; Mars, W.M.; Luo, J.H.; Donthamsetty, S.; Orr, A.; Monga, S.P.; Wu, C.; Michalopoulos, G.K. Enhanced liver regeneration following changes induced by hepatocyte-specific genetic ablation of integrin-linked kinase. *Hepatology* **2009**, *50*, 844–851. [CrossRef] [PubMed]
37. Bhushan, B.; Edwards, G.; Desai, A.; Michalopoulos, G.K.; Apte, U. Liver-Specific Deletion of Integrin-Linked Kinase in Mice Attenuates Hepatotoxicity and Improves Liver Regeneration After Acetaminophen Overdose. *Gene Expr.* **2016**, *17*, 35–45. [CrossRef] [PubMed]
38. Chang, W.; Song, L.; Chang, X.; Ji, M.; Wang, H.; Qin, X.; Niu, W. Early activated hepatic stellate cell-derived paracrine molecules modulate acute liver injury and regeneration. *Lab. Investig.* **2017**, *97*, 318–328. [CrossRef]
39. Shen, K.; Chang, W.; Gao, X.; Wang, H.; Niu, W.; Song, L.; Qin, X. Depletion of activated hepatic stellate cell correlates with severe liver damage and abnormal liver regeneration in acetaminophen-induced liver injury. *Acta Biochim. Biophys. Sin.* **2011**, *43*, 307–315. [CrossRef]
40. Kato, T.; Ito, Y.; Hosono, K.; Suzuki, T.; Tamaki, H.; Minamino, T.; Kato, S.; Sakagami, H.; Shibuya, M.; Majima, M. Vascular endothelial growth factor receptor-1 signaling promotes liver repair through restoration of liver microvasculature after acetaminophen hepatotoxicity. *Toxicol. Sci.* **2011**, *120*, 218–229. [CrossRef]
41. Donahower, B.; McCullough, S.S.; Kurten, R.; Lamps, L.W.; Simpson, P.; Hinson, J.A.; James, L.P. Vascular endothelial growth factor and hepatocyte regeneration in acetaminophen toxicity. *Am. J. Physiol. Gastrointest. Liver Physiol.* **2006**, *291*, G102–G109. [CrossRef] [PubMed]
42. Nguyen, N.T.; Umbaugh, D.S.; Sanchez-Guerrero, G.; Ramachandran, A.; Jaeschke, H. Kupffer cells regulate liver recovery through induction of chemokine receptor CXCR2 on hepatocytes after acetaminophen overdose in mice. *Arch. Toxicol.* **2022**, *96*, 305–320. [CrossRef]
43. Starkey Lewis, P.; Campana, L.; Aleksieva, N.; Cartwright, J.A.; Mackinnon, A.; O'Duibhir, E.; Kendall, T.; Vermeren, M.; Thomson, A.; Gadd, V.; et al. Alternatively activated macrophages promote resolution of necrosis following acute liver injury. *J. Hepatol.* **2020**, *73*, 349–360. [CrossRef] [PubMed]
44. Ben-Moshe, S.; Veg, T.; Manco, R.; Dan, S.; Papinutti, D.; Lifshitz, A.; Kolodziejczyk, A.A.; Bahar Halpern, K.; Elinav, E.; Itzkovitz, S. The spatiotemporal program of zonal liver regeneration following acute injury. *Cell Stem. Cell* **2022**, *29*, 973–989.e910. [CrossRef]
45. Walesky, C.M.; Kolb, K.E.; Winston, C.L.; Henderson, J.; Kruft, B.; Fleming, I.; Ko, S.; Monga, S.P.; Mueller, F.; Apte, U.; et al. Functional compensation precedes recovery of tissue mass following acute liver injury. *Nat. Commun.* **2020**, *11*, 5785. [CrossRef] [PubMed]

livers

MDPI

Review

The Evolution of Circulating Biomarkers for Use in Acetaminophen/Paracetamol-Induced Liver Injury in Humans: A Scoping Review

Mitchell R. McGill [1,2,3,*] and Steven C. Curry [4,5]

1 Department of Environmental Health Sciences, Fay W. Boozman College of Public Health, University of Arkansas for Medical Sciences, Little Rock, AR 72205, USA
2 Department of Pharmacology and Toxicology, College of Medicine, University of Arkansas for Medical Sciences, Little Rock, AR 72205, USA
3 Department of Pathology, College of Medicine, University of Arkansas for Medical Sciences, Little Rock, AR 72205, USA
4 Division of Clinical Data Analytics and Decision Support, University of Arizona College of Medicine—Phoenix, Phoenix, AZ 85006, USA; steven.curry@bannerhealth.com
5 Department of Medical Toxicology, Banner—University Medical Center Phoenix, Phoenix, AZ 85006, USA
* Correspondence: mmcgill@uams.edu

Abstract: Acetaminophen (APAP) is a widely used drug, but overdose can cause severe acute liver injury. The first reports of APAP hepatotoxicity in humans were published in 1966, shortly after the development of alanine aminotransferase (ALT) and aspartate aminotransferase (AST) as the first biomarkers of liver injury as opposed to liver function. Thus, the field of liver injury biomarkers has evolved alongside the growth in APAP hepatotoxicity incidence. Numerous biomarkers have been proposed for use in the management of APAP overdose patients in the intervening years. Here, we comprehensively review the development of these markers from the 1960s to the present day and briefly discuss possible future directions.

Keywords: adducts; cell death; diagnosis; GLDH; hepatotoxicity; keratin-18; LDH; miR-122; overdose; prognosis

1. Introduction

Acetaminophen (APAP; also known as paracetamol) toxicity was recognized as a clinical problem around 1966, when the first two cases of APAP overdose in patients were described by D.G. Davidson—then associated with the storied Ward 3, Regional Poisoning Treatment Center at the Royal Infirmary in Edinburgh [1]—and W. Noel Eastham [2]. APAP-induced liver and renal damage had been observed in cats [3] several years before and in rodents earlier in the same year [4], but APAP had not been thought of as a significant risk to humans. Indeed, many considered it safer than other analgesics available at that time (for example, see [5]). However, more reports of APAP toxicity soon followed [6–14] as its incidence rapidly increased throughout the UK and Europe [15]. Within a decade, APAP overdose arrived in North America as well, with the first reports appearing in 1971 [8]. Today, APAP overdose is a major cause of acute liver failure (ALF) in the US and UK, and a lesser cause in other countries [15]. In the US, for example, approximately 50,000 to 80,000 emergency department visits per year are attributable to APAP overdose [16–18], and APAP hepatotoxicity accounts for roughly half of all ALF cases [19].

The first reports by Davidson and Eastham are as notable for what they did not include as for what they did. In addition to presentation and symptomology, the authors provided detailed descriptions of the gross and microscopic histopathology of the liver and kidney that laid the foundation for later mechanistic investigations into modes of cell death and inflammation in APAP hepatotoxicity. They also provided results from

11 (Case 1) and 18 (Case 2) clinical chemistry, hematology, and coagulation tests, and suggested ways in which these data might be used to differentiate APAP toxicity from other causes of liver damage. Conspicuously lacking for the modern reader, however, was any mention of the serum transaminases, alanine aminotransferase (ALT; also known as SGPT, for serum glutamate-pyruvate transaminase) and aspartate aminotransferase (AST; also known as SGOT, for serum glutamate-oxaloacetate transaminase). These two enzymes were described as liver injury biomarkers only a decade earlier [20–22]. Although AST was routinely measured in serum in many clinical laboratories by 1960, ALT evidently took longer to catch on. Though ALT reagent kits [23] were becoming available around that time and were even available for the newly developed automated analyzers of the time [24,25], they were not as ubiquitous as they are today. Thus, the history of APAP toxicity has run parallel with the evolution of liver injury biomarkers. Furthermore, because APAP overdose is common, it is relatively easy to obtain serum and plasma specimens from APAP toxicity patients. As a result, many recent advances in liver injury biomarker development have come from studies on APAP overdose.

Here, we review APAP toxicity biomarkers in more-or-less chronological order. We begin by briefly discussing the broad categories of use of biomarkers in APAP overdose patients; then, we describe the earliest tests for liver injury, like ALT and AST, in the context of APAP overdose; continue with development of APAP toxicity diagnostics based on APAP and APAP metabolite levels; describe advances in both protein and microRNA (miRNA)-based markers; and conclude with a discussion of the lessons we can learn from these data and possible future directions in APAP biomarker research. Note that some prior knowledge of APAP metabolism, mechanisms of toxicity, and treatments is assumed. The reader is directed to other reviews for more information on these topics [26–28].

2. Uses of Biomarkers in APAP Overdose

Biomarkers in APAP overdose can be broadly grouped into (1) biomarkers for diagnosis, (2) biomarkers for prognosis, and (3) mechanistic biomarkers. Biomarkers for diagnosis should be elevated early enough after overdose to permit detection in early-presenting patients and should be specific enough for APAP that they can distinguish between liver injury caused by the drug and liver injury due to other etiologies in a broad set of liver injury patients. The latter is especially difficult as we will see in our discussion of APAP-protein adducts, which one might reasonably expect to have high specificity for APAP overdose. More biomarkers of prognosis are available, but the evaluation of those markers is complicated, due, in part, to variations in endpoints. For example, one study may be designed to identify biomarkers that predict elevated peak prothrombin time (PT), while another study is designed to look for biomarkers that predict death. While there is an association between peak PT and death, the correlation is imperfect, and so these different designs can yield different results. In another example, studies may be designed to discover biomarkers that identify patients who are at risk of developing high ALT elevations (and therefore in need of treatment) despite presenting with ALT values in the normal range. This may seem straightforward until one considers that ALT elevation is defined in some studies as anything >50 U/L (in other words, any release of ALT from the liver above roughly the upper limit of normal), while in others it is defined as only values >1000 U/L (which are more likely to lead to poor outcomes). In other words, the clinical utility of a biomarker depends on the particular outcome one wants to predict, and many different outcomes have been used in the literature. We can simplify things by sub-dividing prognostic biomarkers into (A) biomarkers intended to predict hepatotoxicity in patients who initially present without evidence of liver injury and (B) biomarkers intended to predict poor clinical outcomes, like encephalopathy or death. We will use this convention roughly throughout the manuscript. However, the reader should consider exactly what outcome the authors of a study are trying to predict and whether or not that outcome is clinically meaningful or optimal.

3. ALT, AST, and Other Enzymes

3.1. The Kinetics of Serum Aminotransferases after APAP Overdose

ALT and AST are transaminases present in both the cytosol (ALT1 and AST1) and mitochondria (ALT2 and AST2) of hepatocytes. Both ALT1 and AST1 activity are present in circulation at baseline (with lesser contributions from ALT2 and AST2) [29,30]—generally believed to be due to normal hepatocyte turnover, though other mechanisms may be involved. Although the hepatic AST/ALT ratio is approximately 2.5:1, AST1 has a shorter half-life in blood, resulting in a roughly 1:1 ratio in circulation under normal conditions [31]. Karmen et al. and De Ritis et al. independently reported elevations of ALT and AST activity in serum from patients with liver injury in 1955 [20,22,32,33]. By the mid-to-late 1960s, ALT (measured using the coupled enzyme reaction approach developed by Karmen for AST [20] and later applied to ALT [21]) had become the standard blood biomarker of hepatocellular damage for both clinical and experimental use, and has remained so ever since [33]. Thomson and Prescott briefly mentioned ALT and AST values in the range of 100–200 "units" in one APAP overdose patient in 1966 [6], just after the reports from Davidson and Eastham, but the first complete time courses of these enzymes in an APAP patient were published by a group in Australia two years later [34]. These investigators observed peak values on day 4 of hospitalization followed by a sharp decline in AST the next day and a more gradual recess of ALT over the next several days. Similar kinetics have been reported by other groups since then [35–40], and it is now generally agreed that both transaminases begin to rise with a 1:1 AST/ALT ratio within 24 h of overdose, peak between 48 and 72 h with a 1:1 to 3:1 ratio, and fall thereafter, with a faster drop in AST in the absence of preexisting liver disease. The serum half-lives for AST and ALT during the latter phase are around 15–20 h and 40–50 h, respectively [37]. A typical ALT time course in humans is shown in Figure 1.

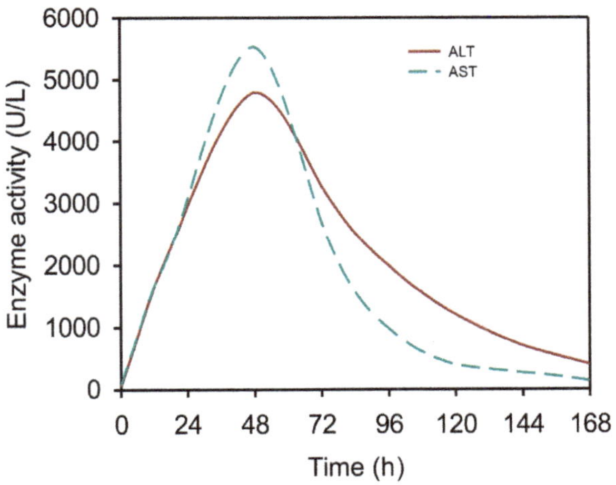

Figure 1. Typical time course of ALT and AST in APAP overdose patients. The solid line represents ALT while the dashed line represents AST.

3.2. Uses and Limitations of Serum Aminotransferases in APAP Toxicity

Elevated aminotransferases can occur for a number of reasons, so they cannot be used to diagnose APAP overdose specifically. However, they are useful for the detection of potential liver injury that should elicit further investigations. It has been reported that ALT values also have some prognostic value to predict hepatotoxicity and therefore guide N-acetyl-l-cysteine (NAC) treatment. James Dear and colleagues reviewed the charts of 410 APAP overdose patients from their institution to determine if an initial ALT above 50 U/L could predict later injury, as indicated primarily by peak ALT $\geq$ 1000 U/L or prothrombin time >2 [41]. While the positive predictive value (PPV) of ALT > 50 was low, the negative predictive value (NPV) was around 100%. Of course, this was likely because the patients with ALT < 50 presented before the development of liver injury and received prompt NAC treatment (even if the patients' clinical histories may have indicated later presentation). Curry and others reported that among 160 APAP overdose patients in whom NAC was commenced within 4 h of having an ALT $\leq$ 50 U/L, just 10 (6%) developed a peak ALT > 1000 U/L. Of 127 patients with an initial ALT > 100 U/L near the time of beginning NAC therapy, 29 developed hepatic encephalopathy, and 12 died. No patient died if NAC therapy was commenced when ALT was <200 U/L [42].

As for patients who present after the onset of injury, a decline in either ALT or AST in serial measurements along with improvements in hepatic synthetic function and a lack of, or improving, encephalopathy likely indicate that the patient has passed the peak of injury and may no longer benefit from NAC, which targets only the early induction of APAP toxicity. AST may be especially useful for this purpose because it falls faster than ALT and could theoretically allow treatment discontinuation and patient discharge earlier [37]. Taking this idea a step further, it has been suggested that a AST/ALT ratio < 0.4 can identify patients who are beyond the window for NAC treatment without the need for serial measurements [32]. Ideas such as these have been criticized, however, based on evidence that NAC improves survival even when administered very late post-overdose. Two papers [43,44] by the late Roger Williams are often cited to support this view [45]. In one of these studies [43], the investigators included patients treated with NAC within 10–36 h post-overdose, with a median time of 17 h—well within the early phase of APAP toxicity in humans, when the transaminases are still rising, as discussed above. The second study [44], however, is more compelling. In that experiment, the investigators randomized patients with liver failure into two groups, NAC and no NAC, and looked at patient survival over the next 21 days. Importantly, the patients who received NAC were treated $\geq$30 h after overdose, though the authors did not describe how the exact time of ingestion was determined. Approximately 60% of the NAC patients survived compared to 20% of the controls [44]. While the investigators relied on small sample sizes, with only 25 patients per group, the results are supported by data from mice and primary human hepatocytes. It has been demonstrated that NAC protects against APAP-induced liver injury in mice even up to 2 h after overdose [46] and as late as 6 h after initial APAP exposure in primary human hepatocytes [47]. Both time points are after APAP metabolism is complete [46,48] and when there is already evidence of oxidative stress and mitochondrial damage [46,47]. However, all of these time points—30 h in humans, 2 h in mice, and 6 h in human hepatocytes—are still before the typical peak of transaminases, around 48–72 h in humans and human hepatocytes and 12 h in mice. By the time transaminases have peaked and begun to fall at even later time points, it seems likely correct that NAC is not useful.

In addition to guiding NAC treatment, ALT and AST may have some prognostic utility to predict poor outcomes. Although large ALT and AST elevations, by themselves, do not predict death in APAP hepatotoxicity or any other forms of liver injury [38,39,49], combining ALT and AST together or with other markers may improve their value for this purpose. For example, patients who died after APAP overdose tended to have a greater AST/ALT ratio at the time of NAC treatment in one cohort [37]. However, that study included only six patients who died. Larger studies are needed to further explore and validate this use of the AST/ALT ratio. In another example, it has been noted that patients with shorter doubling times for ALT and AST from the approximate time of APAP ingestion to peak injury usually have higher peak INR values [40], with the latter having an association with liver failure and death in the most severe cases. Based on the latter study and on the observation that slower declines in serum APAP concentration are associated with faster onset of toxicity, Sivilotti et al. [50] proposed the parameter "APAP $\times$ AT" to predict liver injury that is both rapid and severe after APAP overdose (defined as reaching ALT values $\geq$1000 U/L within 24 h of ingestion and high peak INR, respectively) despite NAC treatment. APAP $\times$ AT is the multiplication product of the earliest paired serum

APAP and aminotransferase values available—in other words, the product of APAP and either ALT or AST nearest to the time of patient presentation or treatment. Because serum APAP declines due to metabolism while aminotransferases proportionally increase due to liver damage, this product is more-or-less stable over time until about the peak of injury [50], making it somewhat independent of the time elapsed since APAP ingestion. However, INR is only a surrogate for death, and the ability of APAP × AT to actually predict death after APAP overdose has not yet been tested. Overall, then, the utility of ALT and AST to predict poor clinical outcomes remains limited.

3.3. Other Early Enzymes

About the same time that serum ALT and AST were found to increase in patients with liver injury, some of the same investigators noted that high lactate dehydrogenase (LDH) activities "were observed in patients with myocardial infarction, diabetic acidosis, acute stem cell leukemia, chronic myelogenous leukemia and hepatitis" [51]. These results were quickly confirmed by others [52]. However, LDH is expressed in other organs at or near the level in the liver [51,53,54], so serum values are not specific for liver damage. Indeed, serum LDH is elevated in numerous diseases [55]. As a result, it is not widely viewed as an important liver injury marker and has no diagnostic value for APAP overdose beyond what ALT and AST provide. But, recent data have demonstrated that it does have prognostic value. We used an untargeted proteomics approach to analyze serum samples from 58 transplant-free survivors and non-survivors of APAP-induced ALF [49]. Much to our surprise, LDH displayed the greatest ability to predict death out of >1600 proteins that we were able to measure [49]. We then confirmed the prognostic value of LDH in this context through a retrospective review of laboratory data from 238 patients hospitalized with ALF at our institution over a 12-year period [39]. Importantly, LDH performed about as well as, or better than, the current prognostic tools, the Model for End-Stage Liver Disease (MELD) score and the King's College Criteria, in both studies [39,49], with a preliminary cutoff of 2000 U/L. Furthermore, only a single laboratory value is needed to use LDH, whereas the Model for End-stage Liver Disease (MELD) score, the King's College Criteria (KCC), the Acute Liver Failure Study Group Prognostic Index (ALFSGPI), and other prognostic scores include multiple laboratory results and/or demographic factors. Interestingly, the isoform of LDH that is dominant in the liver, LDH-M, was elevated in these patients, while the non-liver form, LDH-H, decreased [49]. The latter may have offset some of the total LDH elevation caused by liver injury, so specific measurements of LDH-M may have had an even greater prognostic value than total LDH activity. Although LDH can be increased by hemolysis, which may be common in ischemic hepatitis, the effect is negligible at serum LDH values > 1000 U/L [56], so interference due to hemolysis is generally not a concern in ALF patients—especially when the 2000 U/L LDH cutoff is used. Finally, while serum LDH elevations occur in many conditions, the increases seen in acute liver injury are much greater, so these high values provide some specificity. Thus, LDH appears to be a promising prognostic biomarker to predict the need for a liver transplant in ALF, including APAP-induced ALF. In addition, the combination of LDH with the MELD score (our so-called MELD-LDH score)—or with other parameters still to be tested—may improve utility further [39,49].

It was also noted early on that malate dehydrogenase increases in serum after liver injury [57], and recent work revealed that it correlates with serum ALT and other markers of liver injury [58]. In addition, we found that MDH1 was elevated in non-survivors of APAP-induced ALF compared to survivors [49], indicating that it may have prognostic value for poor outcomes. However, additional studies are needed to fully characterize the clinical or regulatory utility of MDH.

4. Serum APAP and the Rumack–Matthew Nomogram

Arguably, the first biomarker to be measured in APAP hepatotoxicity after or around the same time as the aminotransferases was serum APAP. The earliest methods to estimate

APAP in biological specimens predate the initial cases of APAP toxicity in humans [59,60], and even the first reports of APAP overdose by Davidson and Eastham included values for serum total p-aminophenol, a product of the hydrolysis of APAP and APAP metabolites [2]. Today, clinical assays use a variety of methods to measure APAP, including conversion to p-aminophenol followed by a reaction with the chromogen o-cresol and the enzyme multiplied immunoassay technique (EMIT). However, it was quickly realized that serum p-aminophenol and even parent APAP values alone have limited value for the diagnosis or prediction of APAP hepatotoxicity, overall, and other parameters like serum APAP half-life were suggested instead [61]. This issue was addressed to some degree by the Rumack–Matthew nomogram, which introduced a time dimension to help interpret serum APAP. In 1973, Henry Matthew, the medical director of the Regional Poisoning Treatment Center in Edinburgh, and Barry Rumack, a clinician visiting from the US, began working on a nomogram for APAP overdose inspired by the Done nomogram for salicylate poisoning [62] (Rumack, personal communication). Rumack and Matthew plotted the logarithm of serum APAP levels from 64 Ward 3 patients with acute APAP ingestions (30 of whom were included in a publication by Laurie Prescott [61]) on the *y*-axis against time-after-ingestion on the *x*-axis, and then drew a straight line dividing those who developed ALT >1000 U/L from those with lower peak ALT values. The final graph was published in 1975 [63]. Patients above the line are likely to develop clinically significant hepatotoxicity and should therefore be treated with NAC, while those below the line generally do not require treatment (Figure 2). The Rumack–Matthew line began at 200 µg/mL APAP at four hours post-ingestion, but when clinical trials of NAC began, the US FDA required a line 25% lower, beginning at 150 µg/mL. The latter is now referred to sometimes as the "treatment line" in the US. Other modifications of the Rumack–Matthew nomogram have been introduced in the intervening years, but the basic premise is the same and the graph is still useful in emergency departments today. In addition, new ways to use the nomogram have been introduced, such as the APAP ratio, which is the first APAP value measured between 4 and 24 h post-ingestion divided by the APAP concentration on the standard nomogram line at the same time point [64–66]. Unfortunately, it is difficult to use the nomogram when the time of APAP ingestion cannot be determined or in cases of cumulative overdose from multiple supratherapeutic ingestions over time. Curry found that in 335 subjects with definite APAP poisoning (both acute and chronic), the history of the time of ingestion was thought to be reliable only 12% of the time [67]. Furthermore, the *x*-axis of the nomogram ends at 24 h, so it cannot be used for later-presenting patients who may still benefit somewhat from NAC. Some APAP assays used in clinical laboratories are also susceptible to false results due to bilirubin [68–72] and even NAC [72,73] interference, which would both be expected to be an issue in hospitalized patients with very high serum bilirubin or NAC levels after APAP-induced liver injury or treatment (though this is not an issue with all such assays). Thus, some serum APAP results may be misleading.

Another challenge with the nomogram is that it does not explicitly take into account the lag time from APAP ingestion to NAC treatment, which is a major factor in the development of hepatotoxicity and adverse outcomes [74–76], presumably because greater delays in treatment allow more time for the formation of the reactive metabolite of APAP, *N*-acetyl-*p*-benzoquinone imine (NAPQI). To address this, Sivilotti et al. introduced the psi parameter [77]. Psi is essentially the area under the serum APAP concentration curve from an approximate time of hepatic glutathione depletion post-ingestion (usually set as 4 or 6 h) to the time of NAC initiation, and so theoretically reflects the window of time in which NAPQI formation exceeds detoxification by glutathione before glutathione can be restored by NAC [77]. This parameter was found to be a strong predictor of hepatotoxicity development in early-presenting patients with ALT <100 U/L at admission [78–80]. However, like the Rumack–Matthew nomogram, it is difficult to use when the time of ingestion is unknown. Extrapolation of the curve is necessary and may not be accurate.

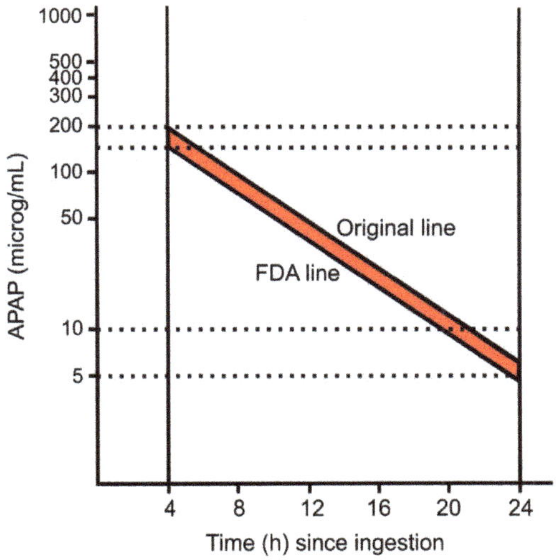

Figure 2. The Rumack–Matthew nomogram. Both the original line and the FDA-modified line are shown. Other modifications are not shown for simplicity.

5. APAP-Protein Adducts

5.1. Diagnostic Utility of APAP-Protein Adducts as a Biomarker

APAP-protein adducts, measured as protein-derived APAP-cysteine (APAP-CYS) after the removal of free cysteine and proteolysis of the specimen, overcome some major shortcomings of serum APAP, APAP × AT, psi, and similar endpoints that are based on, or incorporate, serum APAP levels. Like APAP, adducts can become detectable in circulation as early as 1 h after a therapeutic dose, with a peak between 3 and 12 h after therapeutic or sub-hepatotoxic doses [81,82] and between 24 and 72 h after overdose [65] (similar to ALT), but they are more stable than APAP and decline slowly, with a half-life of 1–2 days [82–85] (Figure 3). Thus, serum adducts provide a longer diagnostic window than APAP alone. Furthermore, bilirubin and NAC have no effect on the HPLC-electrochemical detection (HPLC-EC) method of adduct measurement that is currently used clinically. Generally, values >1 nmol/mL are associated with overdose and serum ALT > 1000 U/L [83,85,86]. Note, however, that some critical considerations are outlined in Section 5.3 of this paper.

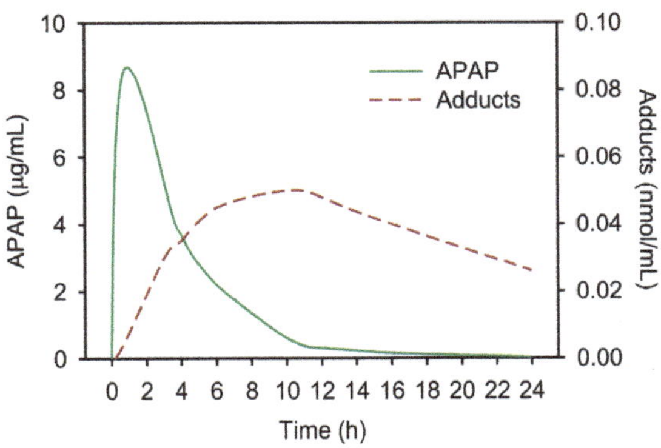

Figure 3. Relative kinetics of APAP and APAP-protein adducts. Simulated data for non-hepatotoxic APAP doses. Derived from publications [65,81–85] and from known half-lives. With liver injury, longer half-lives for both analytes are expected, with the APAP-protein adducts' half-life still exceeding that of APAP.

5.2. Evolution of APAP-Protein Adduct Methods

The first studies to explore the fundamental mechanisms of APAP hepatotoxicity were undertaken by Bernard Brodie, David Jollow, Jerry Mitchell, and others at the US National Institutes of Health and published in 1973–1974 [27,87–91]. In those papers, the authors discovered that APAP is converted to a reactive metabolite that can deplete hepatic glutathione and bind to proteins. The original methods to measure APAP-protein adducts in these early studies required the administration of radiolabeled APAP followed by multiple sample extraction steps to remove non-protein-bound drug and metabolites, and, finally, the measurement of radioactivity [88]. These methods were laborious and could not be easily applied to serum. The first convenient methods to measure adducts were antibody-based [92]. The development of the original antibodies against APAP-protein adducts came about through a collaboration between Jack Hinson and Dean Roberts while they were working at the National Center for Toxicological Research (NCTR) of the US Food and Drug Administration in the mid-1980s [92]. The two met carpooling to work due to the remote location of the NCTR in a rural area of central Arkansas in the US. During a drive, Hinson described his work on APAP metabolism and protein alkylation to Roberts, who then offered to make an antibody to recognize APAP-cysteine adducts in proteins. According to Hinson:

"It resulted from a conversation we had while we were commuting to NCTR. I described the APAP toxicity mechanism. I clearly remember [Dean] saying, 'I can make an antibody to that'. Following the development of the anti-APAP antibody, we studied the presence of APAP-protein adducts in mice. As expected, we found adducts in liver. An unexpected finding was adducts in serum. The appearance of serum adducts correlated with the appearance of liver enzymes in the serum (ALT) and were determined to be of hepatic origin. We immediately recognized that serum of APAP overdose victims would have APAP-protein adducts too. We collaborated with Dr. Henrik Poulsen from the University of Copenhagen, Denmark, to assay clinical samples from APAP overdose patients that he had stockpiled in his freezer. This resulted in a publication in the Lancet."

Hinson later discovered the more sensitive and specific HPLC-EC method [93]:

"The HPLC-EC assay came about by our attempts to assay for 3-nitrotyrosine in APAP samples. We were working with Phil Mayeux and a medical student who had taken a year off to perform research, Ken Muldrew. We had observed nitrotyrosine in livers of APAP-treated mice by immunohistochemical methods. We had also observed it in homogenates from APAP-treated livers using Western blot. Following a published procedure for 3-nitrotyrosine, Ken did not observe any nitrotyrosine but did observe a peak coming out of the HPLC column very late. It was observed only in the liver homogenates from the APAP-treated livers. I postulated that it may be the APAP-cysteine adduct. I then synthesized the 3-cysteinyl-acetaminophen conjugate and confirmed the synthesis by NMR spectral analysis of the product. The peak [in the HPLC-EC assay] was subsequently confirmed to be APAP-cysteine".

The physician-scientist Laura James joined Hinson and Roberts shortly before the development of the HPLC-EC method and helped to collect the first human samples for HPLC-EC analyses. In her words:

"In subsequent studies, serum samples obtained from patients with APAP overdose were assayed using the HPLC assay. APAP adducts were detected in patients with a documented history of APAP overdose and resulting liver injury. Collectively, these findings were published in the 2002 Muldrew manuscript. Publication of this manuscript caught the attention of hepatologists funded by the National Institute of Diabetes and Digestive and Kidney Diseases (NIDDK) of the US National Institutes of Health through the Acute Liver Failure Study Group. Subsequent research collaborations with this NIDDK-funded network defined the range and magnitude of APAP adducts in multiple clinical scenarios, including 'low-dose' exposure, acute overdose with early NAC treatment and acute overdose with delayed or no NAC treatment. Ultimately, the collaborations demonstrated that measurement of adducts in human serum samples could accurately identify patients with

APAP-induced ALF and found that approximately 20% of patients with ALF of unknown etiology were secondary to APAP-induced injury. This understanding prompted the development of AcetaSTAT, a rapid, lateral flow diagnostic assay for the semi-qualitative detection of APAP-protein adducts in human sera".

The development of the HPLC-EC method for adducts was followed by mass spectrometry-based methods [94,95], but HPLC-EC is currently the only method used clinically in the US. As alluded to in the quote above, a lateral flow immunoassay called AcetaSTAT has also been developed and is pending the completion of various studies before FDA review. A prototype of this device reportedly had 100% sensitivity and 96% specificity for APAP-induced liver injury in one small clinical study [86].

5.3. Limitations of APAP-Protein Adducts for Diagnosis and Proposed Solutions

APAP-protein adducts can be detected in circulation during sub-toxic and therapeutic use. Mice treated with 75 mg/kg, which is 5× greater than the equivalent therapeutic dose in humans of approximately 14–15 mg/kg (1 g divided by 70 kg for an average healthy adult, for example) but still sub-toxic, have detectable serum adducts around 0.2 nmol/mL [48]. More importantly, some human volunteers taking therapeutic doses have had adduct values as high as 0.9 to 1.0 nmol/mL [96]—around the proposed diagnostic threshold. Although the diagnosis of APAP overdose may require both an adduct level >1.0 and elevated ALT, there is evidence that co-incidental liver injury leading to ALT elevations can increase APAP-protein adduct concentrations in blood during therapeutic APAP use. For example, we treated mice with the sub-toxic 75 mg/kg dose of APAP, induced co-incidental liver injury by ischemia-reperfusion (IR), or performed sham surgery, and then compared plasma adducts between the IR and sham groups [48]. IR increased plasma adducts by approximately 9-fold, from far below the 1.0 nmol/mL threshold in sham animals to just under it [48]. More significantly, for clinical use, Curry et al. found that some patients classified as having liver injury "definitely not" due to APAP had adduct levels > 1.0 nmol/mL and even as high as 2.86 nmol/mL, which is consistent with elevated adducts due to co-incidental liver damage in patients using sub-toxic APAP doses [67]. To address this issue, Curry proposed the use of 95% probability intervals. That is, the areas on a graph in which 95% of paired serum APAP and serum APAP-protein adduct values from patients with liver injury due to APAP overdose or due to another cause are predicted to fall when adducts are plotted on the *y*-axis against ALT on the *x*-axis [67] (Figure 4). Using this approach, the authors noted, for example, that "finding a serum APAP-CYS [APAP-protein] concentration of 1.4 μM [nmol/mL] when corresponding ALT activity was 12,000 IU/L would be unexpected in APAP-induced hepatic necrosis". (See example case in Figure 4.) In other words, even though adducts would be >1.0 nmol/mL and ALT > 1000 U/L, the clinician could still discern that APAP is not a likely cause of the liver injury in such a case because the elevated adduct levels are still low compared to the very high ALT. Importantly, Curry's data also indicate that there is a zone of overlap between APAP overdose and non-APAP overdose patients. In cases that fall within this zone, as always, the clinician must look at the complete clinical picture to determine a likely diagnosis or etiology. The 95% prediction interval requires further testing and validation, but moving forward 1.0 nmol/mL may serve as the generally recommended diagnostic cutoff in straightforward APAP overdose cases while the 95% prediction intervals may be helpful when considering overdose in patients with more complicated or uncertain presentations or histories. Finally, it is notable that kidney failure, which is often present in APAP-induced ALF [97], is associated with a more prolonged elimination half-life of serum APAP-CYS, probably from a larger apparent volume of distribution [98]. The latter may also affect the clinical interpretation of adduct values.

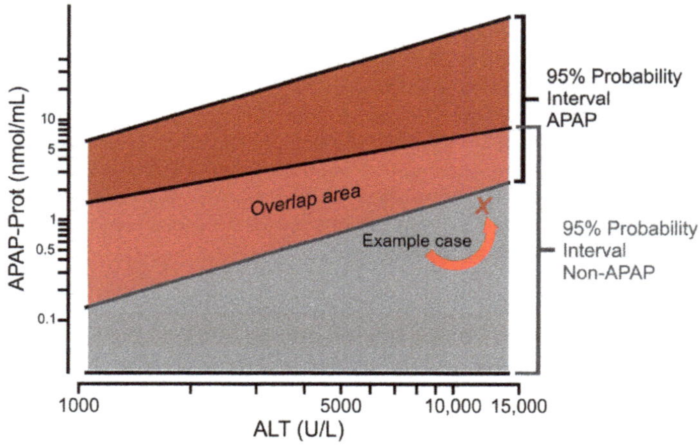

Figure 4. The 95% prediction interval. The prediction intervals are the areas in which 95% of values from patients with liver injury due to APAP overdose (APAP interval, top) or to something other than APAP (non-APAP interval, lower) are predicted to fall. Calculated probability intervals were based on 908 paired adduct-ALT points in 335 subjects with definite APAP overdose, and 95 data points from 32 subjects who definitely did not have APAP overdose (mainly ischemic hepatitis) [67]. The X shows where the example case described in the main text falls.

5.4. *Factors Affecting Serum Adduct Levels at Therapeutic Doses of Acetaminophen*

Data from clinical trials indicate that APAP-protein adducts are detectable in serum in most people during therapeutic APAP use [82,96,99]. While the adduct concentrations are generally low, a few subjects in these studies have had values that reached or exceeded the proposed diagnostic threshold for APAP overdose of 1 nmol/mL, as mentioned above. Andrew Monte and colleagues have explored possible mechanisms for this inter-individual variation in adduct levels using 'omics approaches. For example, in a manuscript describing a small, exploratory study in which they performed genomics analysis on samples from eight subjects administered therapeutic doses of APAP, they reported that there were 194 variants in 65 genes that were associated with adduct concentration [100]. They further reported that patients with higher adduct levels were more likely to have damaging variants in genes involved in signal transduction, and singled out *ARHGAP11A* and *MUC20* as examples. Although these observations are interesting, their causal significance is currently unclear. Nevertheless, they point to potential genetic or otherwise personal factors affecting APAP-protein adduct levels.

Finally, postmortem blood APAP-protein adduct concentrations do not reflect antemortem levels. They can be dramatically elevated in patients who have taken APAP, but have no evidence of APAP-induced hepatotoxicity [101]. This should be kept in mind when investigating causes of liver injury or death in deceased subjects.

6. The Rise of Mechanism-Based Biomarkers

6.1. *Mitotoxicity Biomarkers*

Mitochondrial protein alkylation was noted by Jollow et al. in the early mouse studies published in 1973 [88], and mitochondrial swelling was observed in liver sections from APAP overdose patients as early as 1979 [102]. However, the importance of mitochondria in APAP toxicity was not recognized at that time. In the late 1980s and early 1990s, research groups led by Steve Cohen at the University of Connecticut, Hartmut Jaeschke at Baylor University, and others, demonstrated that mitochondria are damaged during APAP hepatotoxicity, leading to reduced respiration and increased mitochondrial oxidative stress [103,104]. Additional studies in the 2000s, mostly from Dr. Jaeschke's group, further demonstrated that these are critical events in the toxicity, driving much of the liver damage [36,105–111]. Also, in the 2000s, Neil Kaplowitz and colleagues revealed that the c-Jun N-terminal kinases 1/2 are important in the pathogenesis of APAP-induced liver injury [112–115].

We became interested in translating these mechanisms from rodent models to humans while working together with Dr. Jaeschke around 2009. It is difficult to obtain liver tissue from APAP overdose patients, but blood samples are drawn from those patients daily, so we took up the challenge of studying these mechanisms in patients using blood as a window to peer into the liver. We initially focused on the mitochondrial damage and reasoned that because one can see mitochondrial content spilling into the cytosol after APAP overdose [116], the same mitochondrial macromolecules must also spill into blood when plasma membrane integrity is lost and other large molecules like ALT are released. Consistent with that, when we measured mitochondrial matrix components like glutamate dehydrogenase (GLDH) (by activity) and mitochondrial DNA (mtDNA; by PCR) in plasma from APAP overdose patients, we found that they were elevated [36]. However, it was not enough to simply show that these mitochondrial markers increased during APAP toxicity. We needed a model of liver injury without mitochondrial damage to demonstrate that the molecules are only present, or at least present at higher levels, in blood when mitochondrial damage has occurred. Our solution came when we found a paper in which the authors compared the mechanisms of furosemide and bromobenzene hepatotoxicity and found that furosemide, specifically, caused liver damage without altering mitochondrial respiration [117]. When we then compared plasma or serum GLDH and mtDNA in mice with furosemide and APAP toxicity, they were much higher in the APAP mice [36], indicating that these markers do indeed have some specificity for mitochondrial injury. The GLDH data were recently reproduced by another group [118]. Although they framed their results as a challenge to our work, their data confirmed our fundamental observation that mitochondrial markers like GLDH are higher in blood from mice with APAP toxicity compared to furosemide toxicity [118,119]. We later published similar results for long-chain acylcarnitines in mice [120]. While we were unable to detect an increase in acylcarnitines in adult humans after APAP overdose, another group reported elevations in a pediatric overdose population [121], further supporting the hypothesis that mitochondrial damage occurs in humans as it does in mice. Importantly, data from both studies indicated that early NAC treatment can explain why we did not observe elevated acylcarnitines in our patient population. NAC mitigated the acylcarnitine increase in mice, and acylcarnitine elevations were more apparent in pediatric patients with delayed NAC treatment. We also found that GLDH and mtDNA are higher in serum from non-survivors of APAP-induced ALF than in survivors [38], indicating that mitochondrial damage not only occurs but is a driver of APAP hepatotoxicity in humans. We supported these conclusions with additional data from human HepaRG cells and primary human hepatocytes, which further demonstrated the central role of mitochondrial damage in APAP-induced liver injury in humans [47,94,122].

Another marker that may reflect mitotoxicity in the context of APAP overdose is nuclear DNA fragments. In mice, nuclear DNA fragmentation in the liver occurs partly as a result of the translocation of endonucleases from damaged mitochondria to the nucleus [108], so the presence of high levels of fragmented DNA (or nucleosomes) in the circulation may reflect mitochondrial destruction. We and others were able to measure nuclear DNA fragments in the circulation of APAP overdose patients with liver injury using an anti-histone ELISA [36,38,123], again lending credence to the idea that mitochondrial damage occurs in humans as in mice.

Unfortunately, the clinical value of GLDH, mtDNA, nuclear DNA fragments, and acylcarnitines to predict poor outcomes in APAP overdose patients appears limited at best [38,123]. However, another mitochondrial marker, carbamoyl phosphate synthetase 1 (CPS1), is also elevated in APAP hepatotoxicity [124,125] and may have both mechanistic and prognostic value. A study from 2006 demonstrated that circulating CPS1 values increased at 8 and 24 h after surgery in the cecal ligation and puncture model of sepsis-induced liver damage [126]. Importantly, this increase was co-incident with the loss of mitochondria in the liver and changes in mitochondrial morphology, while ALT release occurred much later. The authors interpreted this to mean that CPS1 appeared in serum as a result of mitochondrial destruction specifically, rather than simply necrosis [126]. Bishr Omary and coworkers later reported that CPS1 is elevated in the culture medium and circulation from primary mouse hepatocytes and mice, respectively, during APAP-induced injury, and in serum from APAP overdose patients [124]. They also found that serum CPS1 levels were greater in non-survivors of APAP-induced ALF and in transplant recipients than in spontaneous survivors [125], indicating that these levels can predict poor outcomes. Notably, CPS1 levels modestly improved the MELD score for prognosis [125].

6.2. Cell Death Mode Markers

While we were working on mitochondrial biomarkers, other groups were exploring the mode of cell death in human APAP hepatotoxicity by measuring keratin 18 (K18) and high mobility group box 1 (HMGB1) protein in blood. An antibody ("M30") against a caspase-cleaved form of K18 (ccK18) had been developed in the 1990s and was used to label apoptotic cells in sections from colonic carcinoma tissue and cancer cell lines [127]. It was later applied to serum from cancer patients using an ELISA [128,129]. Rutherford et al. [130] then measured ccK18 in serum from patients with ALF of various etiologies and noted that median levels were higher in APAP overdose patients than in healthy controls. However, they did not measure total K18 for comparison, so it was not possible to determine the relative contributions of apoptosis and necrosis. At about the same time, Bechmann et al. [131] measured ccK18 in the circulation of one patient with APAP-induced ALF and reported only minor elevations in comparison to total K18 ("M65"), indicating "a low rate of apoptosis". Since then, most studies have demonstrated that only about 10–20% of total K18 is in the caspase-cleaved form. For example, Volkmann et al. [132] reported ccK18 values around 8–9000 and total K18 values around 50–55,000 U/L (~15–16%) in APAP patients while Craig et al. reported median values of 9646 and 45,615, respectively (21%) [123]. Importantly, even these percentages likely overestimate the amount of apoptotic vs. necrotic cell death in the human liver after APAP overdose. Very few apoptotic cells appear in the liver after APAP overdose in mice, and caspase inhibitors do not protect against the injury at all [47,94,133–135]. Furthermore, we could not detect any caspase 3 activity in plasma from APAP overdose patients with liver injury, even though we observed very high levels in plasma from mice with hepatocyte apoptosis due to galactosamine/LPS treatment [36]. Finally, histological studies have revealed that only ~0.6% of hepatocytes display characteristic morphological features of apoptosis during APAP hepatotoxicity in humans compared to >60% with necrotic appearance [135], though the authors of that study insisted on an interpretation of the data that likely exaggerates the importance of apoptosis. In any case, even when considering only the ccK18 and K18 data, necrosis is the dominant mode of cell death during APAP hepatotoxicity.

There are conflicting data regarding the prognostic value of K18 and ccK18 to predict death. On the one hand, Rutherford et al. measured serum ccK18 in the earliest available samples from a subset of 52 patients with ALF of various etiologies and reported that the median levels were significantly greater in non-survivors and transplant recipients compared to spontaneous survivors [130]. Consistent with these data, Church et al. [136] measured K18 and ccK18 in samples from patients with non-APAP DILI from the DILI Network (DILIN) and reported that K18 levels were significantly greater in patients who died or required a transplant. On the other hand, Craig et al. measured K18 and ccK18 in serum from APAP overdose patients specifically and reported that there were no significant differences in either biomarker between those who spontaneously survived ($n = 14$) and those who died or received a liver transplant ($n = 12$), at the time of admission [117]. Results from ROC analyses, sensitivity and specificity, and the diagnostic odds ratio were unimpressive (AUCs ≤ 0.67 and 95% CIs for odds ratios overlapping one, for example) [123]. Regarding the prediction of hepatotoxicity in early-presenting APAP overdose patients,

Dear and colleagues measured K18, ccK18, microRNA-122 (miR-122), and GLDH in admission samples from APAP overdose patients who presented with normal ALT values < 50 U/L and reported that K18 was one of the best markers to predict later injury in these early presenters [137]. GLDH was also associated with later injury, but not as strongly [137].

Like K18, HMGB1 has also been interpreted as a marker of necrotic cell death. Scaffidi et al. [138] stained for HMGB1 in HeLa cells undergoing TNF-α/cyclohexamide-stimulated apoptosis and observed that it localized to and remained within the nucleus throughout the apoptotic process. Additionally, there was little release of HMGB1 into the cell culture medium during apoptosis compared to necrosis induced by CCCP and other compounds [138]. Finally, they reported that an anti-HMGB1 antibody decreased inflammatory cell recruitment in the liver (as assessed by myeloperoxidase) after APAP-induced hepatocyte necrosis in mice, implying that HMGB1 was released into serum by necrosis and had a pro-inflammatory effect [138]. Importantly, HMGB1 release has been reported in APAP overdose patients as well, further supporting necrosis as the primary mode of cell death in APAP hepatotoxicity in humans [123,137]. Additionally, like K18 and GLDH, HMGB1 levels can forecast APAP hepatotoxicity in early-presenting APAP overdose patients with normal ALT values [137], though they likely cannot predict death [123,139].

6.3. Other Mechanistic Biomarkers

The results from an intriguing recent study indicate that bile acids leak out of bile canaliculi early in APAP hepatotoxicity and are taken up by hepatocytes, where they accumulate and contribute to hepatocyte death [140]. While this hypothesis requires confirmation, especially in light of prior data demonstrating that bile acid depletion worsens APAP-induced injury [141], we and others previously reported that bile acids increase in the serum in APAP hepatotoxicity in both mice and humans [142,143]. Furthermore, we found that glycodeoxycholic acid, in particular, can predict death in APAP overdose patients [142]. Thus, bile acids may also be considered mechanistic biomarkers in APAP patients, pending independent replication of the mechanistic studies mentioned. In addition, some bile acids appear to increase earlier than ALT, indicating that they may have value as prognostic markers to predict later injury in early-presenting patients with normal ALT.

Additional studies have addressed the utility of these and other biomarkers for the diagnosis of APAP-induced liver injury [144]. While such studies may be useful when extrapolating the results to DILI more generally, for which diagnosis is a greater challenge [145], in most cases, their kinetics mirror the kinetics of ALT (see [36] for example). It is not clear what value they might add to diagnosis or prognosis if they cannot detect injury earlier.

7. Inflammation Biomarkers

The role of inflammation in APAP hepatotoxicity and liver repair is complex, multiphasic, and controversial [27,146–148]. Early studies in the 1980s found that Kupffer cells are activated in rats during APAP toxicity [149,150], and that inactivation with gadolinium chloride protects against APAP in mice [151]. However, later work revealed that total Kupffer cell ablation, instead of simply inactivation, with a single dose of liposomal clodronate either worsens injury in mice [152] or has no effect [153]. More recently, we demonstrated that two doses of liposomal clodronate actually protect against APAP, in contrast to the single dose regimen, but also that the protective effect was likely due to Nrf2 activation rather than anything directly having to do with Kupffer cells [153]. Furthermore, NADPH oxidase and C-C chemokine receptor 2 (CCR2) KO mice are not protected against APAP [154,155]. Thus, overall, it appears that Kupffer cells do not contribute significantly to APAP hepatotoxicity. Similar conflicting data exist for neutrophils [27,156–158], though recent data indicate that the role of neutrophils may depend upon the APAP dose or extent of injury [159], which may explain some discrepancies in the literature. Studies are currently ongoing to investigate other inflammatory cell types in the context of APAP overdose.

Regardless, a number of cytokines and other pro- and anti-inflammatory markers have been measured in APAP overdose patients. In 2001, James et al. reported increased interleukin-8 (IL-8; aka CXCL8) in the circulation of pediatric overdose patients, but no elevations in IL-6 or IL-10, compared to healthy controls [160]. They also reported that patients with high peak IL-8 had higher peak prothrombin times, suggesting some prognostic utility, despite the possible confounding effects of time-to-NAC treatment in their analysis (delayed NAC treatment may result in both higher IL-8 and worse outcomes independent of each other, and a novel marker like IL-8 is probably not needed to determine if presentation was delayed) [160]. A 2003 study by another group reproduced the observation that IL-8 is elevated in APAP-induced liver injury in humans and revealed that IL-8 and hyaluronic acid serum levels were higher in non-survivors of APAP overdose compared to survivors [161]. Similarly, we observed a trend toward increased IL-8 in non-survivors, though it did not achieve statistical significance [162].

In contrast to their 2001 study, James et al. later observed that IL-6 is significantly elevated after APAP overdose, but only in patients with more severe liver injury than those included in their initial work [163]. They also found in that study that monocyte chemoattractant protein 1 (MPC1; aka CCL2) was elevated in APAP toxicity patients, and, like IL-8, was associated with peak prothrombin time [163]. Consistent with those observations, we recently reported that both IL-6 and MCP1 are significantly higher in serum from non-survivors of APAP-induced ALF compared to spontaneous survivors at some early time points [162]. However, in contrast to James et al., we also observed elevated IL-10, and it too was associated with poor outcomes [162]. Elevations in IL-6, IL-8, and IL-10 have also been reported in other DILI patients [163,164]. Overall, it appears that IL-6, IL-8, and MCP1 are consistently elevated in serum from APAP overdose patients with liver injury and may have prognostic value to predict poor outcomes. IL-10 may also be prognostic but requires further investigation. Other inflammation markers including pentraxin 3 [165], Lect2 [166], and neopterin [167] also seem to be elevated in APAP-induced liver injury and associated with patient outcome, but have not been explored as thoroughly as the cytokines and chemokines already mentioned.

8. miRNA-Based Biomarkers

Wang et al. 2009 [168] first reported that serum levels of multiple miRNAs are altered in mice with APAP-induced liver injury, and these data were extended to APAP overdose patients by the research group of Kevin Park at the University of Liverpool two years later [169]. Since then, many miRNAs have been shown to increase or decrease in circulation in APAP hepatotoxicity [169–174], but miR-122 seems to display the largest and most consistent changes [175].

The most promising application of miR-122 at this point still appears to be in the prediction of hepatotoxicity in APAP overdose patients presenting with normal ALT and liver function test results. It is rare for patients presenting with ALT < 50 U/L to later develop injury (as described in Section 3.2, above), and those who do rarely develop severe hepatotoxicity. This is even clear from the studies supporting miR-122 use themselves, as pointed out in a letter to the editor [176]. However, others argue that if the potential for hepatotoxicity, despite NAC, can be ruled out in these early presenters using a marker specifically for that purpose, then NAC treatment can be tailored, unnecessary hospitalizations can be avoided, and patients who require care can still be identified and promptly treated. K18, HMGB1, and—to a lesser extent—GLDH may have some value for this purpose, as mentioned in Section 6 [137], but miR-122 and perhaps K18 appear to be uniquely positioned for this because they seem to be more sensitive to hepatocellular stress. For example, we observed that K18 was elevated in patients with compensated cirrhosis, despite normal ALT [82]. Furthermore, serum miR-122 was significantly elevated in 18 human subjects after a moderate alcohol binge that had no effect on ALT or GGT [177]. Dear et al. demonstrated that miR-122 at admission has high sensitivity and specificity to predict peak ALT >100 U/L in patients who present with an initial ALT value < 50 [137].

While there are concerns about the biological variation in miR-122 [136] as well as technical challenges with current measurement methods (e.g., PCR), new analytical approaches are in development that may help to overcome some of the relevant problems [178–180]. In addition, an alternative approach may be to measure the levels of proteins encoded by genes that are miR-122 targets. miR-122 decreases in the liver during APAP-induced injury in mice [168], so it is theoretically possible that miR-122 targets are upregulated in the liver and could be released into the circulation. Finally, despite the likely utility of miR-122 as a prognostic marker for later injury in early-presenters, it appears that it is only modestly associated with death in APAP-induced ALF [181,182], if at all. Overall, the necessity of new markers to predict hepatotoxicity in early presenters has been questioned, but if one were to be used clinically then miR-122 appears to be a reasonable candidate.

Specific miRNA profiles have also been linked to liver regeneration and survival [182,183]. For example, Salehi et al. [183] described miRNA profiles in patients who underwent auxiliary liver transplantation. In this procedure, the patient's damaged liver is left in place and allowed to regenerate, while the transplanted liver takes over the normal liver functions. After successful regeneration, immunosuppression is withdrawn and the transplanted liver is allowed to atrophy, leaving the patient's recovered liver. This unique scenario allowed the researchers to monitor miRNA changes in biopsy samples from the native liver at multiple time points during the regeneration period. Of the 11 total patients enrolled in the study, 7 experienced successful regeneration leading to the complete withdrawal of immunosuppression, while 4 failed to regenerate. The investigators isolated RNA from their biopsies and performed microarray analysis to measure numerous miRNAs, followed by pathway analysis to determine what signaling pathways would be expected to be altered due to the detected changes in miRNA. The authors reported decreased levels of miRNAs that can suppress the expression of pro-proliferative genes (e.g., *CCND2*)—miR-23a, miR-150, miR-503, and miR-663—and increased levels of miRNAs that can activate expression of pro-proliferative genes (e.g., *VEGF*)—miR-20a, miR-126, miR-130a, and miR-520e—over time from the day of transplantation to later phases of regeneration in patients whose native livers successfully regenerated. They later measured some of these miRNAs in the serum from patients with APAP-induced ALF and found that miR-23a, miR-150, and miR-503a (the miRNAs associated with suppressed proliferation) were lower in patients who survived compared to those who died or received a liver transplant, consistent with the idea that these miRNAs are biomarkers of liver regeneration [184]. Finally, they measured these same miRNAs plus additional regeneration-linked species in the serum from 192 patients with APAP-induced ALF and explored their abilities to differentiate between survivors and non-survivors individually, in combination, and when combined with conventional clinical endpoints [181]. While they again observed an association between patient outcome and miR-150, as well as several other miRNAs, the discriminatory powers of the individual miRNA species were modest. However, the prognostic value improved when some of the miRNAs were combined, and further improved when these miRNA species were considered with the MELD score and vasopressor use [181]. Unfortunately, the authors of the latter study also discovered that there was considerable within- and between-person variation in miRNA levels over time. Some species that were elevated in non-survivors compared to survivors at an early time point, for example, were lower compared to survivors at the later time point, and vice versa. Furthermore, the inclusion of multiple miRNAs increases test complexity and cost. These are significant barriers to clinical use that will need to be overcome.

9. Liver Regeneration and Repair Biomarkers

Circulating miRNA profiles are not the only regeneration-associated biomarkers. Arguably, the oldest markers of liver function that are still in use today, namely bilirubin and prothrombin time, are really markers of liver regeneration. Bilirubin undergoes conjugation in the liver to facilitate its excretion, so the accumulation of bilirubin in serum after injury indicates impaired metabolic or excretory liver function. Prothrombin time, on the other hand, is a measure of blood clotting. As most clotting factors are synthesized in the liver, long prothrombin times after injury indicate impaired synthetic function. As the liver regenerates and liver function recovers, values for these tests return to normal. It is not surprising then that these markers correlate well with patient outcome in liver failure. Indeed, the MELD score, the KCC, and the ALF Study Group Prognostic Index (ALFSG PI) include both [185–187]. However, these markers often cannot be used to forecast regeneration because their kinetics are more-or-less parallel to the kinetics of regeneration. That is, liver function improves as regeneration occurs, not before, though there is evidence that remnant hepatocytes induce basal function to partially offset the liver damage [188]. Because function markers mostly parallel regeneration, changes in these markers may not be useful to predict recovery vs. death. Schmidt and Dalhoff [189] also reported that circulating α-fetoprotein (AFP), a marker of hepatocyte proliferation, is increased in the serum from survivors of APAP-induced ALF compared to non-survivors. AFP is already measured clinically as a tumor marker and as part of the screening tests for chromosomal abnormalities during gestation, so it could have immediate clinical application. Like bilirubin and prothrombin time, however, AFP values do not increase until after the peak of liver injury. Several other biomarkers of regeneration have been proposed but require further validation. Serum phosphate is elevated in non-survivors of APAP-induced liver injury and in those who received a liver transplant compared to survivors [190]. α-NH-butyric acid increases in serum after PHx in mice and can discriminate between survivors and non-survivors of ALF (including APAP-induced ALF) in pediatric patients as well as bilirubin and prothrombin time can [191]. Lect2 is also elevated in non-survivors of ALF (again, including APAP-induced ALF) compared to survivors [166]. Similarly, CD133/CD39 double-positive microparticles are elevated in patients with APAP-induced acute-on-chronic liver failure (ACLF), and data from rodent studies indicate that CD39 promotes liver recovery [192]. It was also recently reported that some hepatocytes adopt a senescent phenotype after injury, leading to the secretion of CXCL14, which then inhibits liver regeneration [193]. Interestingly, the authors also reported that serum CXCL14 was elevated in patients with APAP-induced ALF and could predict non-survivors. Finally, we recently discovered that some species of phosphatidic acid (PA) may be involved in liver regeneration after APAP hepatotoxicity in mice and are also elevated in the serum from APAP overdose patients with liver injury [194,195], though we have not yet tested the prognostic value of serum PA.

10. Miscellaneous Other Biomarkers

Various other biomarkers that do not fit well into the categories above have also been explored in APAP hepatotoxicity. We have repeatedly observed elevated agininosuccinate synthetase 1 (ASS1) in circulation after APAP hepatotoxicity in both mice and humans [196,197]. Furthermore, our data from mice indicate that it may be a more sensitive and specific biomarker of liver injury than ALT [196,197]. In our experiments, plasma ASS1 increased as early as 2 h post-APAP overdose, before an increase in ALT [196]. It was also elevated in models of mild liver injury but not in a model of benign ALT elevation [197]. In addition, a dose of APAP (100 mg/kg) that did not cause an increase in ALT did increase ASS1 [196]. However, more research is needed to fully evaluate the utility of ASS1. We have also shown that aldehyde dehydrogenase 1a1 (ALDH1A1), alcohol dehydrogenase 1 (ADH1), fructose-1,6-bisphophate (FBP1), and a number of other serum markers are also more specific for liver injury than ALT using the APAP model [197]. Based on that, we proposed that such markers may be useful as part of a screen-and-confirm approach to identify and diagnose idiosyncratic drug-induced liver injury in clinical trials or even clinically in which one would screen for possible injury using ALT and then confirm the injury using a more specific marker [145]. Procalcitonin, often used as a marker of bacterial infection, is also elevated in APAP overdose patients with liver injury and appears to be a result of the injury and resulting inflammation rather than an indication of infection [198,199]. Interestingly, procalcitonin elevation preceded ALT elevation by 33 h in one study [200], indicating that it may be useful as an early biomarker of liver damage to predict later ALT elevations. Unfortunately, while the latter study included a logistic regression analysis of the ability of admission procalcitonin levels to predict injury, the authors did not limit the analysis to patients who presented with normal ALT, so the prognostic value in that scenario remains unclear. Circulating fatty acid binding protein 1 (FABP1) is also elevated in liver injury [201]. It is also prognostic for death in APAP-induced ALF, especially in combination with the KCC and the ALSGPI. The serum or plasma levels of several other potential biomarkers, including C-reactive protein (CRP) [165], taurine [202], and sphingolipids [203], also change during APAP hepatotoxicity, but the clinical significance of these changes has yet to be explored.

The overall findings for all of the major biomarkers discussed above are summarized in Table 1.

Table 1. Summary of major biomarkers used or proposed for use in APAP hepatotoxicity.

Biomarker (s)/Tool (s)	Purpose	Reference (s)
* ALT, AST	Detection of ALI	[20,22,32,33]
# ALT >50 U/L at admission	Prediction of ALI (high NPV)	[41,42]
# Declining transaminases or AST/ALT <0.4	Discontinuation of NAC	[32,37]
# APAP × AT	Prediction of ALI	[50]
# LDH	Prediction of death	[39,49]
MDH1	Detection of ALI; prediction of death	[49,57,58]
* Rumack–Matthew nomogram	Prediction of ALI	[63]
# Psi parameter	Prediction of ALI	[77–80]
* APAP-protein adducts	Mechanistic: Protein alkylation; Diagnosis of APAP hepatotoxicity	[81–86]
# 95% probability intervals for APAP-protein adducts	Diagnosis of APAP hepatotoxicity	[67]
GLDH	Detection of ALI; Mechanistic: Mitochondrial damage; Prediction of ALI	[36,38,119,137]
mtDNA	Mechanistic: Mitochondrial damage	[36,38]
Nuclear DNA fragments	Mechanistic: Mitochondrial damage, DNA fragmentation	[36,38,123]
Acylcarnitines	Mechanistic: Mitochondrial damage	[120,121]
CPS1	Mechanistic: Mitochondrial damage; Prediction of death	[124,125]
Total K18	Mechanistic: Cell death mode; Prediction of ALI	[123,131,132,137]
ccK18	Mechanistic: Cell death mode	[123,131,132]
Caspase 3 activity	Mechanistic: Cell death mode	[36]
HMGB1	Mechanistic: Cell death mode; Prediction of ALI	[123,137,138]
Bile acids (e.g., glycodeoxycholic acid)	Mechanistic: Bile acid toxicity?; Prediction of death	[140,142,143]
Cytokines/chemokines	Inflammation markers	[160–163,165–167]
miR-122	Prediction of ALI	[137]
miRNA regeneration profiles	Regeneration markers	[181–184]
# AFP	Regeneration marker	[189]
# Phosphate	Regeneration marker	[190]
α-NH-butyric acid	Regeneration marker	[191]
Lect2	Regeneration marker	[166]
CXCL14	Regeneration marker	[193]
Phosphatidic acid species	Possible regeneration markers	[194,195]
ASS1	Detection of ALI	[49,196,197]
ADH1, ALDH1A1, FBP1	Detection of ALI	[197]
FABP1	Detection of ALI; Regeneration marker	[201]

* Currently used clinically. # Available clinically. Note that inclusion here does not necessarily indicate endorsement.

11. Conclusions and Future Directions in Biomarker Development

11.1. New Models for Biomarker Discovery

A challenge in identifying and validating biomarkers for APAP overdose in humans is the difficulty in obtaining serum or plasma samples from a sufficient number of APAP overdose patients, especially from non-survivors, to obtain meaningful results. Developing cell culture models may present an alternative approach. A challenge with cell culture models is that most hepatocyte cell lines, such as HepG2 cells, do not express the cytochrome P450 enzymes required to initiate APAP hepatotoxicity [204,205]. Furthermore, most hepatocyte culture systems cannot replicate the human pathophysiology to any significant degree because they lack the other cell types in the liver (Kupffer cells, stellate cells, cholangiocytes, and sinusoidal epithelial cells, for example) as well as the normal hepatic architecture. They also typically lack extrahepatic cells that may have a role in APAP-induced liver injury or repair, like neutrophils and monocytes. However, new models are emerging to overcome these challenges. HepaRG is a convenient cell line that expresses many P450s and develops APAP hepatotoxicity that mostly resembles what we see in humans and mice [94]. Meanwhile, model systems such as organ-on-chip are increasingly popular and permit the co-culture of primary hepatocytes or HepaRG cells with other hepatic cell types in structures that somewhat resemble the hepatic sinusoid [206]. Finally, multi-organ chips are also being developed that incorporate similar liver systems [207–210]. As these systems mature and become more affordable and accessible, they may be useful for the routine study of novel liver injury biomarkers which can then be validated in later clinical studies.

11.2. Understanding What Makes a Good Biomarker

Whatever methods are used to identify and validate new biomarkers, it is imperative that we come to understand what makes a good biomarker of liver injury. Aside from the usual considerations of technical and biological variations, organ specificity and specificity for liver injury are critical considerations. A challenge with ALT, for example, is that it can be elevated in the absence of liver injury [197]. Furthermore, it is not entirely specific for the liver, as it can be elevated with muscle damage, too [211]. Clinical feasibility is another key issue. For example, because fatal APAP overdose and ALF, more generally, are relatively uncommon, it may be difficult to obtain commercial interest in biomarkers to predict survival. This is an advantage of markers like LDH, which are already widely used clinically for other reasons. Another factor may be abundance within an organ. Abundance within the liver may also be an important consideration. One may ask why LDH can predict poor outcomes in APAP overdose patients while ALT cannot. It has been proposed that the molecular weight and subcellular location of a protein may be factors, the idea being that large proteins or those buried deeper into the cells—within organelles, for example—are less likely to be released. However, LDH forms a large tetramer of approximately 140 kD, and both LDH and ALT1—the dominant isoform released into serum [212–214]—are primarily cytosolic. Another possible explanation is that LDH is only released with membrane damage and leakage, reflecting true hepatocyte injury, while ALT can be released via other mechanisms that are less specific for cell death. This is plausible, but there are little data to support it at this moment. Finally, a third explanation is that LDH is either induced by APAP or is simply more abundant in the liver than ALT in the first place, such that LDH continues to increase with increased injury (and therefore with a greater probability of poor outcomes) while ALT plateaus. Indeed, our prior data indicate that LDH continues to increase for about 24 h after ALT peaks [39], though further investigation is needed to confirm that. Furthermore, we have observed far greater LDH activity than ALT activity in liver tissue homogenates, though LDH did not appear to be induced (McGill et al., unpublished observations). In any case, additional research is clearly needed to understand what physiological and biochemical properties of a biomarker are most desirable for either diagnosis or prognosis in liver injury.

11.3. Conclusions

A great deal of research has been conducted to identify circulating biomarkers for use in APAP overdose patients. ALT and the Rumack–Matthew nomogram continue to dominate clinical use, while the measurement of APAP-protein adducts is emerging as a novel diagnostic tool that may be useful when carefully interpreted. Emerging prognostic biomarkers also show promise for use in the near future. However, additional research is recommended to validate these latter markers.

Author Contributions: Conceptualization, M.R.M.; methodology, M.R.M.; software, M.R.M.; investigation, M.R.M. and S.C.C.; resources, M.R.M.; writing—original draft preparation, M.R.M.; writing—review and editing, M.R.M. and S.C.C.; visualization, M.R.M.; project administration, M.R.M.; funding acquisition, M.R.M. All authors have read and agreed to the published version of the manuscript.

Funding: M.M. was funded in part by National Institutes of Health grants UL1TR003107 and by a research grant from Haleon. The funding agencies had no role in the conceptualization, design, writing, editing or submission of this manuscript.

Institutional Review Board Statement: Not applicable.

Informed Consent Statement: Not applicable.

Data Availability Statement: Not applicable.

Acknowledgments: We thank Jack Hinson, Dean Roberts, Laura James, and Barry Rumack for their helpful discussions and correspondence. The laboratory of MRM was supported in part by the National Institutes of Health grant UL1 TR003107.

Conflicts of Interest: M.R.M. has consulted for Acetaminophen Toxicity Diagnostics, LLC, within the last ten years. He has also received research funding from GlaxoSmithKline/Haleon within the last ten years. S.C.C. has received research funding from Johnson & Johnson within the last ten years. None of these companies had a role in the conception, writing, editing, or submission of this manuscript.

References

1. Proudfoot, A.T.; Good, A.M.; Bateman, D.N. Clinical toxicology in Edinburgh, two centuries of progress. *Clin. Toxicol.* **2013**, *51*, 509–514. [CrossRef] [PubMed]
2. Davidson, D.G.; Eastham, W.N. Acute liver necrosis following overdose of paracetamol. *Br. Med. J.* **1966**, *2*, 497–499. [CrossRef] [PubMed]
3. Eder, H. Chronic Toxicity Studies on Phenacetin, N-Acetyl-p-Aminophenol (NAPA) and Acetylsalicylic Acid on Cats. *Acta Pharmacol. Toxicol.* **1964**, *21*, 197–204. [CrossRef] [PubMed]
4. Boyd, E.M.; Bereczky, G.M. Liver Necrosis from Paracetamol. *Br. J. Pharmacol. Chemother.* **1966**, *26*, 606–614. [CrossRef] [PubMed]
5. Bone, J.M. Aspirin and Gastric Bleeding. *Br. Med. J.* **1967**, *3*, 810–811. [CrossRef] [PubMed]
6. Thomson, J.S.; Prescott, L.F. Liver damage and impaired glucose tolerance after paracetamol overdosage. *Br. Med. J.* **1966**, *2*, 506–507. [CrossRef] [PubMed]
7. Toghill, P.; Williams, R.; Stephens, J.; Carroll, J. Acute Hepatic Necrosis Following an Overdose of Paracetamol. *Gastroenterology* **1969**, *56*, 773–776. [CrossRef]
8. Boyer, T.D.; Rouff, S.L. Acetaminophen-Induced Hepatic Necrosis and Renal Failure. *JAMA J. Am. Med. Assoc.* **1971**, *218*, 440–441. [CrossRef]
9. James, O.; Roberts, S.; Douglas, A.; Lesna, M.; Pulman, L.; Smith, P.; Watson, A. Liver Damage after Paracetamol Overdose. Comparison of Liver-Function Tests, Fasting Serum Bile Acids, and Liver Histology. *Lancet* **1975**, *306*, 579–581. [CrossRef]
10. McJunkin, B.; Barwick, K.W.; Little, W.C.; Winfield, J.B. Fatal Massive Hepatic Necrosis Following Acetaminophen Overdose. *JAMA* **1976**, *236*, 1874–1875. [CrossRef]
11. Barker, J.D.; de Carle, D.J.; Anuras, S. Chronic Excessive Acetaminophen Use and Liver Damage. *Ann. Intern. Med.* **1977**, *87*, 299–301. [CrossRef] [PubMed]
12. Krenzelok, E.P.; Best, L.; Manoguerra, A.S. Acetaminophen Toxity. *Am. J. Hosp. Pharm.* **1977**, *34*, 391–394. [CrossRef] [PubMed]
13. Ferguson, D.R.; Snyder, S.K.; Cameron, A.J. Hepatotoxicity in Acetaminophen Poisoning. *Mayo Clin. Proc.* **1977**, *52*, 246–248. [CrossRef] [PubMed]
14. Groarke, J.F.; Averett, J.M.; Hirschowitz, B.I. Acetaminophen and Hepatic Necrosis. *N. Engl. J. Med.* **1977**, *296*, 233. [CrossRef] [PubMed]

15. Lee, W.M. Acetaminophen Toxicity: A History of Serendipity and Unintended Consequences. *Clin. Liver Dis.* **2020**, *16*, 34–44. [CrossRef] [PubMed]
16. Manthripragada, A.D.; Zhou, E.H.; Budnitz, D.S.; Lovegrove, M.C.; Willy, M.E. Characterization of acetaminophen overdose-related emergency department visits and hospitalizations in the United States. *Pharmacoepidemiol. Drug Saf.* **2011**, *20*, 819–826. [CrossRef] [PubMed]
17. Li, C.; Martin, B.C. Trends in emergency department visits attributable to acetaminophen overdoses in the United States: 1993–2007. *Pharmacoepidemiol. Drug Saf.* **2011**, *20*, 810–818. [CrossRef] [PubMed]
18. Budnitz, D.S.; Lovegrove, M.C.; Crosby, A.E. Emergency Department Visits for Overdoses of Acetaminophen-Containing Products. *Am. J. Prev. Med.* **2011**, *40*, 585–592. [CrossRef]
19. Stravitz, R.T.; Fontana, R.J.; Karvellas, C.; Durkalski, V.; McGuire, B.; Rule, J.A.; Tujios, S.; Lee, W.M.; Acute Liver Failure Study Group. Future directions in acute liver failure. *Hepatology* **2023**, *78*, 1266–1289. [CrossRef]
20. Karmen, A.; Wróblewski, F.; LaDue, J.S. Transaminase Activity in Human Blood. *J. Clin. Investig.* **1955**, *34*, 126–133. [CrossRef]
21. Wróblewski, F.; Ladue, J.S. Serum Glutamic Pyruvic Transaminase SGP-T in Hepatic Disease: A Preliminary Report. *Ann. Intern. Med.* **1956**, *45*, 801–811. [CrossRef]
22. De Ritis, F.; Coltori, M.; Giusti, G. Transaminase Activity of Human Serum in Viral Hepatitis; Preventive Note. *Minerva Medica* **1955**, *46*, 1207–1209. [PubMed]
23. Alfred, D. Reagents and Method for Assaying Biological Samples. U.S. Patent 3,413,198, 26 November 1968.
24. Kessler, G.; Rush, R.; Leon, L.; Delea, A.; Cupiola, R. Automated 340 Nm Measurement of SGOT, SGPT and LDH. *Clin. Chem.* **1970**, *16*, 530–531.
25. Smith, A.F.; Taylor, R.H. Comparison of two-point (AutoAnalyzer II) with kinetic methods for transaminase assay. *J. Clin. Pathol.* **1973**, *26*, 42–47. [CrossRef] [PubMed]
26. McGill, M.R.; Jaeschke, H. Metabolism and Disposition of Acetaminophen: Recent Advances in Relation to Hepatotoxicity and Diagnosis. *Pharm. Res.* **2013**, *30*, 2174–2187. [CrossRef] [PubMed]
27. McGill, M.R.; Hinson, J.A. The development and hepatotoxicity of acetaminophen: Reviewing over a century of progress. *Drug Metab. Rev.* **2020**, *52*, 472–500. [CrossRef] [PubMed]
28. Jaeschke, H.; Ramachandran, A. Central mechanisms of acetaminophen hepatotoxicity: Mitochondrial dysfunction by protein adducts and oxidant stress. *Drug Metab. Dispos.* **2023**, *51*. [CrossRef]
29. Rej, R.; Keese, C.R.; Giaever, I. Direct immunological determination of aspartate aminotransferase isoenzymes. *Clin. Chem.* **1981**, *27*, 1597–1601. [CrossRef]
30. Panteghini, M.; Pagani, F.; Cuccia, C. Activity of serum aspartate aminotransferase isoenzymes in patients with acute myocardial infarction. *Clin. Chem.* **1987**, *33*, 67–71. [CrossRef]
31. Zoppini, G.; Cacciatori, V.; Negri, C.; Stoico, V.; Lippi, G.; Targher, G.; Bonora, E. The aspartate aminotransferase-to-alanine aminotransferase ratio predicts all-cause and cardiovascular mortality in patients with type 2 diabetes. *Medicine* **2016**, *95*, e4821. [CrossRef]
32. Mcgovern, A.J.; Vitkovitsky, I.V.; Jones, D.L.; Mullins, M.E. Can AST/ALT Ratio Indicate Recovery after Acute Paracetamol Poisoning? *Clin. Toxicol.* **2015**, *53*, 164–167. [CrossRef]
33. McGill, M.R. The past and present of serum aminotransferases and the future of liver injury biomarkers. *EXCLI J.* **2016**, *15*, 817–828. [CrossRef] [PubMed]
34. Maclean, D.; Peters, T.J.; Brown, R.A.; McCathie, M.; Baines, G.F.; Robertson, P.G. Treatment of Acute Paracetamol Poisoning. *Lancet* **1968**, *292*, 849–852. [CrossRef] [PubMed]
35. Singer, A.J.; Carracio, T.R.; Mofenson, H.C. The Temporal Profile of Increased Transaminase Levels in Patients with Acetaminophen-Induced Liver Dysfunction. *Ann. Emerg. Med.* **1995**, *26*, 49–53. [CrossRef] [PubMed]
36. McGill, M.R.; Sharpe, M.R.; Williams, C.D.; Taha, M.; Curry, S.C.; Jaeschke, H. The mechanism underlying acetaminophen-induced hepatotoxicity in humans and mice involves mitochondrial damage and nuclear DNA fragmentation. *J. Clin. Investig.* **2012**, *122*, 1574–1583. [CrossRef] [PubMed]
37. Curtis, R.M.; Sivilotti, M.L.A. A descriptive analysis of aspartate and alanine aminotransferase rise and fall following acetaminophen overdose. *Clin. Toxicol.* **2015**, *53*, 849–855. [CrossRef] [PubMed]
38. McGill, M.R.; Staggs, V.S.; Sharpe, M.R.; Lee, W.M.; Jaeschke, H. Serum Mitochondrial Biomarkers and Damage-Associated Molecular Patterns Are Higher in Acetaminophen Overdose Patients with Poor Outcome. *Hepatology* **2014**, *60*, 1336–1345. [CrossRef]
39. Price, J.R.; Hagrass, H.; Filip, A.B.; McGill, M.R. LDH and the MELD-LDH in Severe Acute Liver Injury and Acute Liver Failure: Preliminary Confirmation of a Novel Prognostic Score for Risk Stratification. *J. Appl. Lab. Med.* **2023**, *8*, 504–513. [CrossRef]
40. Green, T.J.; Sivilotti, M.L.; Langmann, C.; Yarema, M.; Juurlink, D.; Burns, M.J.; Johnson, D.W. When Do the Aminotransferases Rise after Acute Acetaminophen Overdose. *Clin. Toxicol.* **2010**, *48*, 787–792. [CrossRef]
41. Al-Hourani, K.; Mansi, R.; Pettie, J.; Dow, M.; Bateman, D.N.; Dear, J.W. The predictive value of hospital admission serum alanine transaminase activity in patients treated for paracetamol overdose. *QJM* **2013**, *106*, 541–546. [CrossRef]
42. Curry, S.C.; Padilla-Jones, A.; Kang, A.; Snow, J.; Heise, C. Serum ALT Activity at Commencement of N-Acetylecysteine Therapy as a Predictor of Hepatotoxocity, Hepatic Encephalopathy, and Mortality in Patients with Acetaminophen Toxicity. *J. Med. Toxicol.* **2019**, *15*, 71. [CrossRef]

43. Harrison, P.; Keays, R.; Bray, G.; Alexander, G.; Williams, R. Improved outcome of paracetamol-induced fulminant hepatic failure by late administration of acetylcysteine. *Lancet* **1990**, *335*, 1572–1573. [CrossRef] [PubMed]
44. Keays, R.; Harrison, P.M.; Wendon, J.A.; Forbes, A.; Gove, C.; Alexander, G.J.; Williams, R. Intravenous acetylcysteine in paracetamol induced fulminant hepatic failure: A prospective controlled trial. *BMJ* **1991**, *303*, 1026–1029. [CrossRef] [PubMed]
45. Mullins, M.E.; Schwarz, E. Re: Remien Etal.: Mathematical Modeling of Liver Injury and Dysfunction after Acetaminophen Overdose. *Hepatology* **2012**, *56*, 2427–2428. [CrossRef] [PubMed]
46. James, L.P.; McCullough, S.S.; Lamps, L.W.; Hinson, J.A. Effect of N-Acetylcysteine on Acetaminophen Toxicity in Mice: Relationship to Reactive Nitrogen and Cytokine Formation. *Toxicol. Sci.* **2003**, *75*, 458–467. [CrossRef] [PubMed]
47. Xie, Y.; McGill, M.R.; Dorko, K.; Kumer, S.C.; Schmitt, T.M.; Forster, J.; Jaeschke, H. Mechanisms of acetaminophen-induced cell death in primary human hepatocytes. *Toxicol. Appl. Pharmacol.* **2014**, *279*, 266–274. [CrossRef] [PubMed]
48. McGill, M.R.; Lebofsky, M.; Norris, H.-R.; Slawson, M.H.; Bajt, M.L.; Xie, Y.; Williams, C.D.; Wilkins, D.G.; Rollins, D.E.; Jaeschke, H. Plasma and liver acetaminophen-protein adduct levels in mice after acetaminophen treatment: Dose–response, mechanisms, and clinical implications. *Toxicol. Appl. Pharmacol.* **2013**, *269*, 240–249. [CrossRef]
49. Vazquez, J.H.; Kennon-McGill, S.; Byrum, S.D.; Mackintosh, S.G.; Jaeschke, H.; Williams, D.K.; Lee, W.M.; Dranoff, J.A.; McGill, M.R. Proteomics Indicates Lactate Dehydrogenase Is Prognostic in Acetaminophen-Induced Acute Liver Failure Patients and Reveals Altered Signaling Pathways. *Toxicol. Sci.* **2022**, *187*, 25–34. [CrossRef]
50. Sivilotti, M.L.A.; Green, T.J.; Langmann, C.; Yarema, M.; Juurlink, D.; Johnson, D. Multiplying the Serum Aminotransferase by the Acetaminophen Concentration to Predict Toxicity Following Overdose. *Clin. Toxicol.* **2010**, *48*, 793–799. [CrossRef]
51. Wróblewski, F.; Ladue, J.S. Lactic Dehydrogenase Activity in Blood. *Proc. Soc. Exp. Biol. Med.* **1955**, *90*, 210–213. [CrossRef]
52. Hsieh, K.M.; Blumenthal, H.T. Serum Lactic Dehydrogenase Levels in Various Disease States. *Proc. Soc. Exp. Biol. Med.* **1956**, *91*, 626–630. [CrossRef] [PubMed]
53. Hammond, K.D.; Balinsky, D. Isozyme Studies of Several Enzymes of Carbohydrate Metabolism in Human Adult and Fetal Tissues, Tumor Tissues, and Cell Cultures. *Cancer Res.* **1978**, *38*, 1323–1328. [PubMed]
54. Milne, E.; Doxey, D. Lactate dehydrogenase and its isoenzymes in the tissues and sera of clinically normal dogs. *Res. Vet. Sci.* **1987**, *43*, 222–224. [CrossRef] [PubMed]
55. Farhana, A.; Lappin, S.L. *Biochemistry, Lactate Dehydrogenase (LDH)*; StatPearls Publishing: Treasure Island, FL, USA, 2020.
56. Knezevic, C.E.; Ness, M.A.; Tsang, P.H.T.; Tenney, B.J.; Marzinke, M.A. Establishing hemolysis and lipemia acceptance thresholds for clinical chemistry tests. *Clin. Chim. Acta* **2020**, *510*, 459–465. [CrossRef] [PubMed]
57. Bing, R.J.; Castellanos, A.; Siegel, A. Diagnostic Value of Activity of Malic Dehydrogenase and Phosphohexose Isomerase; Preliminary Report of Findings in Patients with Myocardial Infarction and Liver Disease. *J. Am. Med. Assoc.* **1957**, *164*, 647–650. [CrossRef]
58. Schomaker, S.; Warner, R.; Bock, J.; Johnson, K.; Potter, D.; Van Winkle, J.; Aubrecht, J. Assessment of Emerging Biomarkers of Liver Injury in Human Subjects. *Toxicol. Sci.* **2013**, *132*, 276–283. [CrossRef]
59. Lester, D.; Greenberg, L.A. The Metabolic Fate of Acetanilid and Other Aniline Derivatives; Major Metabolites of Acetanilid Appearing in the Blood. *J. Pharmacol. Exp. Ther.* **1947**, *90*, 68–75.
60. Brodie, B.B.; Axelrod, J. The Estimation of Acetanilide and Its Metabolic Products, Aniline, n-Acetyl p-Aminophenol and p-Aminophenol (Free and Total Conjugated) in Biological Fluids and Tissues. *J. Pharmacol. Exp. Ther.* **1948**, *94*, 22–28.
61. Prescott, L.; Roscoe, P.; Wright, N.; Brown, S. Plasma-Paracetamol Half-Life and Hepatic Necrosis in Patients with Paracetamol Overdosage. *Lancet* **1971**, *297*, 519–522. [CrossRef]
62. Done, A.K. Salicylate Intoxication. Significance of Measurements of Salicylate in Blood in Cases of Acute Ingestion. *Pediatrics* **1960**, *26*, 800–807. [CrossRef]
63. Rumack, B.H.; Matthew, H. Acetaminophen Poisoning and Toxicity. *Pediatrics* **1975**, *55*, 871–876. [CrossRef] [PubMed]
64. Chiew, A.L.; Isbister, G.K.; Kirby, K.A.; Page, C.B.; Chan, B.S.H.; Buckley, N.A. Massive paracetamol overdose: An observational study of the effect of activated charcoal and increased acetylcysteine dose (ATOM-2). *Clin. Toxicol.* **2017**, *55*, 1055–1065. [CrossRef] [PubMed]
65. Chiew, A.L.; James, L.P.; Isbister, G.K.; Pickering, J.W.; McArdle, K.; Chan, B.S.; Buckley, N.A. Early acetaminophen-protein adducts predict hepatotoxicity following overdose (ATOM-5). *J. Hepatol.* **2020**, *72*, 450–462. [CrossRef] [PubMed]
66. Lewis, J.C.; Lim, M.; Lai, L.; Mendoza, E.; Albertson, T.E.; Chenoweth, J.A. Evaluation of N-acetylcysteine dose for the treatment of massive acetaminophen ingestion. *Clin. Toxicol.* **2022**, *60*, 507–513. [CrossRef] [PubMed]
67. Curry, S.C.; Padilla-Jones, A.; Ruha, A.M.; O'Connor, A.D.; Kang, A.M.; Wilkins, D.G.; Jaeschke, H.; Wilhelms, K.; Gerkin, R.D.; Graeme, K.A.; et al. The Relationship Between Circulating Acetaminophen-Protein Adduct Concentrations and Alanine Aminotransferase Activities in Patients with and Without Acetaminophen Overdose and Toxicity. *J. Med. Toxicol.* **2019**, *15*, 143–155. [CrossRef] [PubMed]
68. Kellmeyer, K.; Yates, C.; Parker, S.; Hilligoss, D. Bilirubin interference with kit determination of acetaminophen. *Clin. Chem.* **1982**, *28*, 554–555. [CrossRef] [PubMed]
69. Bertholf, R.L.; Johannsen, L.M.; Bazooband, A.; Mansouri, V. False-Positive Acetaminophen Results in a Hyperbilirubinemic Patient. *Clin. Chem.* **2003**, *49*, 695–698. [CrossRef] [PubMed]
70. Beuhler, M.; Curry, S. False Positive Acetaminophen Levels Associated with Hyperbilirubinemia. *Clin. Toxicol.* **2005**, *43*, 167–170. [CrossRef]

71. Polson, J.; Wians, F.H.; Orsulak, P.; Fuller, D.; Murray, N.G.; Koff, J.M.; Khan, A.I.; Balko, J.A.; Hynan, L.S.; Lee, W.M. False positive acetaminophen concentrations in patients with liver injury. *Clin. Chim. Acta* **2008**, *391*, 24–30. [CrossRef]
72. Chan, B.; Tsang, H.; Ng, C.W.; Ling, W.H.; Leung, D.C.; Lee, H.H.; Mak, C.M. Performance evaluation of five commercial assays for detection of acetaminophen. *J. Clin. Lab. Anal.* **2019**, *33*, e22683. [CrossRef]
73. Tyhach, R.J.; Mayer, M.; Salpeter, L. More on Interference of N-Acetylcysteine in Measurement of Acetaminophen [3] (Multiple Letters). *Clin. Chem.* **1999**, *45*, 584. [CrossRef] [PubMed]
74. Rumack, B.H.; Peterson, R.C.; Koch, G.G.; Amara, I.A. Acetaminophen Overdose: 662 Cases with Evaluation of Oral Acetylcysteine Treatment. *Arch. Intern. Med.* **1981**, *141*, 380. [CrossRef] [PubMed]
75. Smilkstein, M.J.; Knapp, G.L.; Kulig, K.W.; Rumack, B.H. Efficacy of Oral N-Acetylcysteine in the Treatment of Acetaminophen Overdose. *N. Engl. J. Med.* **1988**, *319*, 1557–1562. [CrossRef] [PubMed]
76. Makin, A.J.; Wendon, J.; Williams, R. A 7-year experience of severe acetaminophen-induced hepatotoxicity (1987–1993). *Gastroenterology* **1995**, *109*, 1907–1916. [CrossRef] [PubMed]
77. Sivilotti, M.L.A.; Good, A.M.; Yarema, M.C.; Juurlink, D.N.; Johnson, D.W. A New Predictor of Toxicity Following Acetaminophen Overdose Based on Pretreatment Exposure. *Clin. Toxicol.* **2005**, *43*, 229–234. [CrossRef]
78. Sivilotti, M.L.; Yarema, M.C.; Juurlink, D.N.; Good, A.M.; Johnson, D.W. A Risk Quantification Instrument for Acute Acetaminophen Overdose Patients Treated with N-Acetylcysteine. *Ann. Emerg. Med.* **2005**, *46*, 263–271. [CrossRef] [PubMed]
79. Chomchai, S.; Chomchai, C.; Anusornsuwan, T. Acetaminophen psi parameter: A useful tool to quantify hepatotoxicity risk in acute acetaminophen overdose. *Clin. Toxicol.* **2011**, *49*, 664–667. [CrossRef] [PubMed]
80. Chomchai, S.; Chomchai, C. Predicting acute acetaminophen hepatotoxicity with acetaminophen-aminotransferase multiplication product and the Psi parameter. *Clin. Toxicol.* **2014**, *52*, 506–511. [CrossRef]
81. James, L.P.; Chiew, A.; Abdel-Rahman, S.M.; Letzig, L.; Graudins, A.; Day, P.; Roberts, D. Acetaminophen protein adduct formation following low-dose acetaminophen exposure: Comparison of immediate-release vs extended-release formulations. *Eur. J. Clin. Pharmacol.* **2013**, *69*, 851–857. [CrossRef]
82. McGill, M.R.; James, L.P.; McCullough, S.S.; Moran, J.H.; Mathews, S.E.; Peterson, E.C.; Fleming, D.P.; Tripod, M.E.; Vazquez, J.H.; Kennon-McGill, S.; et al. Short-Term Safety of Repeated Acetaminophen Use in Patients with Compensated Cirrhosis. *Hepatol. Commun.* **2022**, *6*, 361–373. [CrossRef]
83. Davern, T.J.; James, L.P.; Hinson, J.A.; Polson, J.; Larson, A.M.; Fontana, R.J.; Lalani, E.; Munoz, S.; Shakil, A.O.; Lee, W.M. Measurement of Serum Acetaminophen–Protein Adducts in Patients with Acute Liver Failure. *Gastroenterology* **2006**, *130*, 687–694. [CrossRef] [PubMed]
84. James, L.; Capparelli, E.; Simpson, P.; Letzig, L.; Roberts, D.; Hinson, J.; Kearns, G.; Blumer, J.; Sullivan, J. Acetaminophen-Associated Hepatic Injury: Evaluation of Acetaminophen Protein Adducts in Children and Adolescents with Acetaminophen Overdose. *Clin. Pharmacol. Ther.* **2008**, *84*, 684–690. [CrossRef]
85. James, L.P.; Letzig, L.; Simpson, P.M.; Capparelli, E.; Roberts, D.W.; Hinson, J.A.; Davern, T.J.; Lee, W.M. Pharmacokinetics of Acetaminophen-Protein Adducts in Adults with Acetaminophen Overdose and Acute Liver Failure. *Drug Metab. Dispos.* **2009**, *37*, 1779–1784. [CrossRef] [PubMed]
86. Roberts, D.W.; Lee, W.M.; Hinson, J.A.; Bai, S.; Swearingen, C.J.; Stravitz, R.T.; Reuben, A.; Letzig, L.; Simpson, P.M.; Rule, J.; et al. An Immunoassay to Rapidly Measure Acetaminophen Protein Adducts Accurately Identifies Patients with Acute Liver Injury or Failure. *Clin. Gastroenterol. Hepatol.* **2017**, *15*, 555–562.e3. [CrossRef] [PubMed]
87. Mitchell, J.R.; Jollow, D.J.; Potter, W.Z.; Davis, D.C.; Gillette, J.R.; Brodie, B.B. Acetaminophen Induced Hepatic Necrosis. I. Role of Drug Metabolism. *J. Pharmacol. Exp. Ther.* **1973**, *187*, 185–194. [PubMed]
88. Jollow, D.J.; Mitchell, J.R.; Potter, W.Z.; Davis, D.C.; Gillette, J.R.; Brodie, B.B. Acetaminophen Induced Hepatic Necrosis. II. Role of Covalent Binding in Vivo. *J. Pharmacol. Exp. Ther.* **1973**, *187*, 195–202.
89. Potter, W.Z.; Davis, D.C.; Mitchell, J.R.; Jollow, D.J.; Gillette, J.R.; Brodie, B.B. Acetaminophen Induced Hepatic Necrosis. III. Cytochrome P 450 Mediated Covalent Binding in Vitro. *J. Pharmacol. Exp. Ther.* **1973**, *187*, 203–210.
90. Mitchell, J.R.; Jollow, D.J.; Potter, W.Z.; Gillette, J.R.; Brodie, B.B. Acetaminophen Induced Hepatic Necrosis. IV. Protective Role of Glutathione. *J. Pharmacol. Exp. Ther.* **1973**, *187*, 211–217.
91. Potter, W.; Thorgeirsson, S.; Jollow, D.; Mitchell, J. Acetaminophen-Induced Hepatic Necrosis V. Correlation of Hepatic Necrosis, Covalent Binding and Glutathione Depletion in Hamsters. *Pharmacology* **1974**, *12*, 129–143. [CrossRef]
92. Roberts, D.W.; Pumford, N.R.; Potter, D.W.; Benson, R.W.; Hinson, J.A. A Sensitive Immunochemical Assay for Acetaminophen-Protein Adducts. *J. Pharmacol. Exp. Ther.* **1987**, *241*, 527–533.
93. Muldrew, K.L.; James, L.P.; Coop, L.; McCullough, S.S.; Hendrickson, H.P.; Hinson, J.A.; Mayeux, P.R. Determination of Acetaminophen-Protein Adducts in Mouse Liver and Serum and Human Serum after Hepatotoxic Doses of Acetaminophen Using High-Performance Liquid Chromatography with Electrochemical Detection. *Drug Metab. Dispos.* **2002**, *30*, 446–451. [CrossRef] [PubMed]
94. McGill, M.R.; Yan, H.-M.; Ramachandran, A.; Murray, G.J.; Rollins, D.E.; Jaeschke, H. HepaRG cells: A human model to study mechanisms of acetaminophen hepatotoxicity. *Hepatology* **2011**, *53*, 974–982. [CrossRef] [PubMed]

95. Cook, S.F.; King, A.D.; Chang, Y.; Murray, G.J.; Norris, H.-R.K.; Dart, R.C.; Green, J.L.; Curry, S.C.; Rollins, D.E.; Wilkins, D.G. Quantification of a biomarker of acetaminophen protein adducts in human serum by high-performance liquid chromatography-electrospray ionization-tandem mass spectrometry: Clinical and animal model applications. *J. Chromatogr. B* **2015**, *985*, 131–141. [CrossRef] [PubMed]
96. Heard, K.J.; Green, J.L.; James, L.P.; Judge, B.S.; Zolot, L.; Rhyee, S.; Dart, R.C. Acetaminophen-cysteine adducts during therapeutic dosing and following overdose. *BMC Gastroenterol.* **2011**, *11*, 20. [CrossRef] [PubMed]
97. Kennon_McGill, S.; McGill, M. Extrahepatic toxicity of acetaminophen: Critical evaluation of the evidence and proposed mechanisms. *J. Clin. Transl. Res.* **2017**, *3*, 297–310. [CrossRef] [PubMed]
98. Curry, S.C.; Padilla-Jones, A.; O'Connor, A.D.; Ruha, A.M.; Bikin, D.S.; Wilkins, D.G.; Rollins, D.E.; Slawson, M.H.; Gerkin, R.D. Prolonged Acetaminophen-Protein Adduct Elimination During Renal Failure, Lack of Adduct Removal by Hemodiafiltration, and Urinary Adduct Concentrations After Acetaminophen Overdose. *J. Med. Toxicol.* **2015**, *11*, 169–178. [CrossRef] [PubMed]
99. Heard, K.; Green, J.L.; Anderson, V.; Bucher-Bartelson, B.; Dart, R.C. Paracetamol (acetaminophen) protein adduct concentrations during therapeutic dosing. *Br. J. Clin. Pharmacol.* **2016**, *81*, 562–568. [CrossRef] [PubMed]
100. Monte, A.A.; Sonn, B.; Saben, J.; Rumack, B.H.; Reynolds, K.M.; Dart, R.C.; Heard, K.J. The Genomics of Elevated ALT and Adducts in Therapeutic Acetaminophen Treatment: A Pilot Study. *J. Med. Toxicol.* **2020**, *17*, 160–167. [CrossRef]
101. Thomas, K.C.; Wilkins, D.G.; Curry, S.C.; Grey, T.C.; Andrenyak, D.M.; McGill, L.D.; Rollins, D.E. Detection of Acetaminophen–Protein Adducts in Decedents with Suspected Opioid–Acetaminophen Combination Product Overdose. *J. Forensic Sci.* **2016**, *61*, 1301–1306. [CrossRef]
102. Petersen, P.; Vilstrup, H. Relation between Liver Function and Hepatocyte Ultrastructure in a Case of Paracetamol Intoxication. *Digestion* **1979**, *19*, 415–419. [CrossRef]
103. Meyers, L.L.; Beierschmitt, W.P.; Khairallah, E.A.; Cohen, S.D. Acetaminophen-induced inhibition of hepatic mitochondrial respiration in mice. *Toxicol. Appl. Pharmacol.* **1988**, *93*, 378–387. [CrossRef] [PubMed]
104. Jaeschke, H. Glutathione Disulfide Formation and Oxidant Stress during Acetaminophen-Induced Hepatotoxicity in Mice in Vivo: The Protective Effect of Allopurinol. *J. Pharmacol. Exp. Ther.* **1990**, *255*, 935–941. [PubMed]
105. Kon, K.; Kim, J.-S.; Jaeschke, H.; Lemasters, J.J. Mitochondrial permeability transition in acetaminophen-induced necrosis and apoptosis of cultured mouse hepatocytes. *Hepatology* **2004**, *40*, 1170–1179. [CrossRef] [PubMed]
106. Reid, A.B.; Kurten, R.C.; McCullough, S.S.; Brock, R.W.; Hinson, J.A. Mechanisms of Acetaminophen-Induced Hepatotoxicity: Role of Oxidative Stress and Mitochondrial Permeability Transition in Freshly Isolated Mouse Hepatocytes. *J. Pharmacol. Exp. Ther.* **2005**, *312*, 509–516. [CrossRef] [PubMed]
107. Cover, C.; Mansouri, A.; Knight, T.R.; Bajt, M.L.; Lemasters, J.J.; Pessayre, D.; Jaeschke, H. Peroxynitrite-Induced Mitochondrial and Endonuclease-Mediated Nuclear DNA Damage in Acetaminophen Hepatotoxicity. *J. Pharmacol. Exp. Ther.* **2005**, *315*, 879–887. [CrossRef] [PubMed]
108. Bajt, M.L.; Cover, C.; Lemasters, J.J.; Jaeschke, H. Nuclear Translocation of Endonuclease G and Apoptosis-Inducing Factor during Acetaminophen-Induced Liver Cell Injury. *Toxicol. Sci.* **2006**, *94*, 217–225. [CrossRef] [PubMed]
109. Ramachandran, A.; Lebofsky, M.; Baines, C.P.; Lemasters, J.J.; Jaeschke, H. Cyclophilin D deficiency protects against acetaminophen-induced oxidant stress and liver injury. *Free. Radic. Res.* **2011**, *45*, 156–164. [CrossRef]
110. McGill, M.R.; Williams, C.D.; Xie, Y.; Ramachandran, A.; Jaeschke, H. Acetaminophen-induced liver injury in rats and mice: Comparison of protein adducts, mitochondrial dysfunction, and oxidative stress in the mechanism of toxicity. *Toxicol. Appl. Pharmacol.* **2012**, *264*, 387–394. [CrossRef]
111. Nguyen, N.T.; Du, K.; Akakpo, J.Y.; Umbaugh, D.S.; Jaeschke, H.; Ramachandran, A. Mitochondrial protein adduct and superoxide generation are prerequisites for early activation of c-jun N-terminal kinase within the cytosol after an acetaminophen overdose in mice. *Toxicol. Lett.* **2021**, *338*, 21–31. [CrossRef]
112. Gunawan, B.K.; Liu, Z.; Han, D.; Hanawa, N.; Gaarde, W.A.; Kaplowitz, N. c-Jun N-Terminal Kinase Plays a Major Role in Murine Acetaminophen Hepatotoxicity. *Gastroenterology* **2006**, *131*, 165–178. [CrossRef]
113. Henderson, N.C.; Pollock, K.J.; Frew, J.; Mackinnon, A.C.; Flavell, R.A.; Davis, R.J.; Sethi, T.; Simpson, K.J. Critical role of c-jun (NH2) terminal kinase in paracetamol- induced acute liver failure. *Gut* **2007**, *56*, 982–990. [CrossRef] [PubMed]
114. Win, S.; Than, T.A.; Min, R.W.M.; Aghajan, M.; Kaplowitz, N. c-Jun N-terminal kinase mediates mouse liver injury through a novel Sab (SH3BP5)-dependent pathway leading to inactivation of intramitochondrial Src. *Hepatology* **2016**, *63*, 1987–2003. [CrossRef] [PubMed]
115. Win, S.; Min, R.W.; Chen, C.Q.; Zhang, J.; Chen, Y.; Li, M.; Suzuki, A.; Abdelmalek, M.F.; Wang, Y.; Aghajan, M.; et al. Expression of mitochondrial membrane–linked SAB determines severity of sex-dependent acute liver injury. *J. Clin. Investig.* **2019**, *129*, 5278–5293. [CrossRef] [PubMed]
116. Placke, M.E.; Ginsberg, G.L.; Wyand, D.S.; Cohen, S.D. Ultrastructural Changes during Acute Acetaminophen-Induced Hepatotoxicity in the Mouse: A Time and Dose Study. *Toxicol. Pathol.* **1987**, *15*, 431–438. [CrossRef] [PubMed]
117. Wong, S.G.; Card, J.W.; Racz, W.J. The role of mitochondrial injury in bromobenzene and furosemide induced hepatotoxicity. *Toxicol. Lett.* **2000**, *116*, 171–181. [CrossRef]
118. Church, R.J.; Schomaker, S.J.; Eaddy, J.S.; Boucher, G.G.; Kreeger, J.M.; Aubrecht, J.; Watkins, P.B. Glutamate dehydrogenase as a biomarker for mitotoxicity; insights from furosemide hepatotoxicity in the mouse. *PLoS ONE* **2020**, *15*, e0240562. [CrossRef] [PubMed]

119. McGill, M.R.; Jaeschke, H. Biomarkers of Mitotoxicity after Acute Liver Injury: Further Insights into the Interpretation of Glutamate Dehydrogenase. *J. Clin. Transl. Res.* **2021**, *7*, 5. [CrossRef]
120. McGill, M.R.; Li, F.; Sharpe, M.R.; Williams, C.D.; Curry, S.C.; Ma, X.; Jaeschke, H. Circulating acylcarnitines as biomarkers of mitochondrial dysfunction after acetaminophen overdose in mice and humans. *Arch. Toxicol.* **2014**, *88*, 391–401. [CrossRef]
121. Bhattacharyya, S.; Yan, K.; Pence, L.; Simpson, P.M.; Gill, P.; Letzig, L.G.; Beger, R.D.; Sullivan, J.E.; Kearns, G.L.; Reed, M.D.; et al. Targeted liquid chromatography–mass spectrometry analysis of serum acylcarnitines in acetaminophen toxicity in children. *Biomark. Med.* **2014**, *8*, 147–159. [CrossRef]
122. Xie, Y.; McGill, M.R.; Du, K.; Dorko, K.; Kumer, S.C.; Schmitt, T.M.; Ding, W.-X.; Jaeschke, H. Mitochondrial protein adducts formation and mitochondrial dysfunction during N-acetyl-m-aminophenol (AMAP)-induced hepatotoxicity in primary human hepatocytes. *Toxicol. Appl. Pharmacol.* **2015**, *289*, 213–222. [CrossRef]
123. Craig, D.G.N.; Lee, P.; Pryde, E.A.; Masterton, G.S.; Hayes, P.C.; Simpson, K.J. Circulating apoptotic and necrotic cell death markers in patients with acute liver injury. *Liver Int.* **2011**, *31*, 1127–1136. [CrossRef] [PubMed]
124. Weerasinghe, S.V.W.; Jang, Y.-J.; Fontana, R.J.; Omary, M.B. Carbamoyl phosphate synthetase-1 is a rapid turnover biomarker in mouse and human acute liver injury. *Am. J. Physiol. Liver Physiol.* **2014**, *307*, G355–G364. [CrossRef] [PubMed]
125. Kwan, R.; Chen, L.; Park, M.-J.; Su, Z.; Weerasinghe, S.V.; Lee, W.M.; Durkalski-Mauldin, V.L.; Fontana, R.J.; Omary, M.B. The Role of Carbamoyl Phosphate Synthetase 1 as a Prognostic Biomarker in Patients with Acetaminophen-induced Acute Liver Failure. *Clin. Gastroenterol. Hepatol.* **2023**. [CrossRef] [PubMed]
126. Crouser, E.D.; Julian, M.W.; Huff, J.E.; Struck, J.; Cook, C.H. Carbamoyl phosphate synthase-1: A marker of mitochondrial damage and depletion in the liver during sepsis. *Crit. Care Med.* **2006**, *34*, 2439–2446. [CrossRef] [PubMed]
127. Leers, M.P.G.; Bergman, T.; Tribbick, G.; Persson, B.; Ramaekers, F.C.S.; Nap, M.; Schutte, B.; Kölgen, W.; Björklund, V.; Björklund, P.; et al. Immunocytochemical detection and mapping of a cytokeratin 18 neo-epitope exposed during early apoptosis. *J. Pathol.* **1999**, *187*, 567–572. [CrossRef]
128. Ueno, T.; Toi, M.; Bivén, K.; Bando, H.; Ogawa, T.; Linder, S. Measurement of an apoptotic product in the sera of breast cancer patients. *Eur. J. Cancer* **2003**, *39*, 769–774. [CrossRef] [PubMed]
129. Linder, S.; Havelka, A.M.; Ueno, T.; Shoshan, M.C. Determining tumor apoptosis and necrosis in patient serum using cytokeratin 18 as a biomarker. *Cancer Lett.* **2004**, *214*, 1–9. [CrossRef] [PubMed]
130. Rutherford, A.E.; Hynan, L.S.; Borges, C.B.; Forcione, D.G.; Blackard, J.T.; Lin, W.; Gorman, A.R.; Shaikh, O.S.; Reuben, A.; Harrison, E.; et al. Serum Apoptosis Markers in Acute Liver Failure: A Pilot Study. *Clin. Gastroenterol. Hepatol.* **2007**, *5*, 1477–1483. [CrossRef]
131. Bechmann, L.P.; Marquitan, G.; Jochum, C.; Saner, F.; Gerken, G.; Canbay, A. Apoptosis versus necrosis rate as a predictor in acute liver failure following acetaminophen intoxication compared with acute-on-chronic liver failure. *Liver Int.* **2008**, *28*, 713–716. [CrossRef]
132. Volkmann, X.; Anstaett, M.; Hadem, J.; Stiefel, P.; Bahr, M.J.; Lehner, F.; Manns, M.P.; Schulze-Osthoff, K.; Bantel, H. Caspase activation is associated with spontaneous recovery from acute liver failure. *Hepatology* **2008**, *47*, 1624–1633. [CrossRef]
133. Gujral, J.S.; Knight, T.R.; Farhood, A.; Bajt, M.L.; Jaeschke, H. Mode of Cell Death after Acetaminophen Overdose in Mice: Apoptosis or Oncotic Necrosis? *Toxicol. Sci.* **2002**, *67*, 322–328. [CrossRef] [PubMed]
134. Williams, C.D.; Koerner, M.R.; Lampe, J.N.; Farhood, A.; Jaeschke, H. Mouse strain-dependent caspase activation during acetaminophen hepatotoxicity does not result in apoptosis or modulation of inflammation. *Toxicol. Appl. Pharmacol.* **2011**, *257*, 449–458. [CrossRef] [PubMed]
135. McGregor, A.H.; More, L.J.; Simpson, K.J.; Harrison, D.J. Liver death and regeneration in paracetamol toxicity. *Hum. Exp. Toxicol.* **2003**, *22*, 221–227. [CrossRef] [PubMed]
136. Church, R.J.; Kullak-Ublick, G.A.; Aubrecht, J.; Bonkovsky, H.L.; Chalasani, N.; Fontana, R.J.; Goepfert, J.C.; Hackman, F.; King, N.M.P.; Kirby, S.; et al. Candidate biomarkers for the diagnosis and prognosis of drug-induced liver injury: An international collaborative effort. *Hepatology* **2019**, *69*, 760–773. [CrossRef] [PubMed]
137. Dear, J.W.; Clarke, J.I.; Francis, B.; Allen, L.; Wraight, J.; Shen, J.; Dargan, P.I.; Wood, D.; Cooper, J.; Thomas, S.H.L.; et al. Risk stratification after paracetamol overdose using mechanistic biomarkers: Results from two prospective cohort studies. *Lancet Gastroenterol. Hepatol.* **2018**, *3*, 104–113. [CrossRef] [PubMed]
138. Scaffidi, P.; Misteli, T.; Bianchi, M.E. Release of Chromatin Protein HMGB1 by Necrotic Cells Triggers Inflammation. *Nature* **2002**, *418*, 191–195. [CrossRef] [PubMed]
139. Basta, G.; Del Turco, S.; Navarra, T.; Lee, W.M. Circulating Levels of Soluble Receptor for Advanced Glycation End Products and Ligands of the Receptor for Advanced Glycation End Products in Patients with Acute Liver Failure. *Liver Transplant.* **2015**, *21*, 847–854. [CrossRef] [PubMed]
140. Ghallab, A.; Hassan, R.; Hofmann, U.; Friebel, A.; Hobloss, Z.; Brackhagen, L.; Begher-Tibbe, B.; Myllys, M.; Reinders, J.; Overbeck, N.; et al. Interruption of bile acid uptake by hepatocytes after acetaminophen overdose ameliorates hepatotoxicity. *J. Hepatol.* **2022**, *77*, 71–83. [CrossRef]
141. Bhushan, B.; Borude, P.; Edwards, G.; Walesky, C.; Cleveland, J.; Li, F.; Ma, X.; Apte, U. Role of Bile Acids in Liver Injury and Regeneration following Acetaminophen Overdose. *Am. J. Pathol.* **2013**, *183*, 1518–1526. [CrossRef]

142. Woolbright, B.L.; McGill, M.R.; Staggs, V.S.; Winefield, R.D.; Gholami, P.; Olyaee, M.; Sharpe, M.R.; Curry, S.C.; Lee, W.M.; Jaeschke, H.; et al. Glycodeoxycholic Acid Levels as Prognostic Biomarker in Acetaminophen-Induced Acute Liver Failure Patients. *Toxicol. Sci.* **2014**, *142*, 436–444. [CrossRef]
143. Luo, L.; Aubrecht, J.; Li, D.; Warner, R.L.; Johnson, K.J.; Kenny, J.; Colangelo, J.L. Assessment of serum bile acid profiles as biomarkers of liver injury and liver disease in humans. *PLoS ONE* **2018**, *13*, e0193824. [CrossRef] [PubMed]
144. Llewellyn, H.P.; Vaidya, V.S.; Wang, Z.; Peng, Q.; Hyde, C.; Potter, D.; Wang, J.; Zong, Q.; Arat, S.; Martin, M.; et al. Evaluating the Sensitivity and Specificity of Promising Circulating Biomarkers to Diagnose Liver Injury in Humans. *Toxicol. Sci.* **2021**, *181*, 23–34. [CrossRef] [PubMed]
145. Vazquez, J.H.; McGill, M.R. Redrawing the Map to Novel DILI Biomarkers in Circulation: Where Are We, Where Should We Go, and How Can We Get There? *Livers* **2021**, *1*, 286–293. [CrossRef]
146. Jaeschke, H.; Williams, C.D.; Ramachandran, A.; Bajt, M.L. Acetaminophen hepatotoxicity and repair: The role of sterile inflammation and innate immunity. *Liver Int.* **2012**, *32*, 8–20. [CrossRef] [PubMed]
147. Woolbright, B.L.; Jaeschke, H. Role of the inflammasome in acetaminophen-induced liver injury and acute liver failure. *J. Hepatol.* **2017**, *66*, 836–848. [CrossRef]
148. Jaeschke, H.; Ramachandran, A. Mechanisms and pathophysiological significance of sterile inflammation during acetaminophen hepatotoxicity. *Food Chem. Toxicol.* **2020**, *138*, 111240. [CrossRef] [PubMed]
149. Laskin, D.L.; Pilaro, A.M.; Ji, S. Potential role of activated macrophages in acetaminophen hepatotoxicity: II. Mechanism of macrophage accumulation and activation. *Toxicol. Appl. Pharmacol.* **1986**, *86*, 216–226. [CrossRef] [PubMed]
150. Laskin, D.L.; Pilaro, A.M. Potential role of activated macrophages in acetaminophen hepatotoxicity: I. Isolation and characterization of activated macrophages from rat liver. *Toxicol. Appl. Pharmacol.* **1986**, *86*, 204–215. [CrossRef]
151. Laskin, D.L.; Gardner, C.R.; Price, V.F.; Jollow, D.J. Modulation of macrophage functioning abrogates the acute hepatotoxicity of acetaminophen. *Hepatology* **1995**, *21*, 1045–1050. [CrossRef]
152. Ju, C.; Reilly, T.P.; Bourdi, M.; Radonovich, M.F.; Brady, J.N.; George, J.W.; Pohl, L.R. Protective Role of Kupffer Cells in Acetaminophen-Induced Hepatic Injury in Mice. *Chem. Res. Toxicol.* **2002**, *15*, 1504–1513. [CrossRef]
153. Clemens, M.M.; Vazquez, J.H.; Kennon-McGill, S.; McCullough, S.S.; James, L.P.; McGill, M.R. Pre-treatment twice with liposomal clodronate protects against acetaminophen hepatotoxicity through a pre-conditioning effect. *Liver Res.* **2020**, *4*, 145–152. [CrossRef]
154. James, L.P.; McCullough, S.S.; Knight, T.R.; Jaeschke, H.; Hinson, J.A. Acetaminophen Toxicity in Mice Lacking NADPH Oxidase Activity: Role of Peroxynitrite Formation and Mitochondrial Oxidant Stress. *Free. Radic. Res.* **2003**, *37*, 1289–1297. [CrossRef] [PubMed]
155. Holt, M.P.; Cheng, L.; Ju, C. Identification and characterization of infiltrating macrophages in acetaminophen-induced liver injury. *J. Leukoc. Biol.* **2008**, *84*, 1410–1421. [CrossRef] [PubMed]
156. Imaeda, A.B.; Watanabe, A.; Sohail, M.A.; Mahmood, S.; Mohamadnejad, M.; Sutterwala, F.S.; Flavell, R.A.; Mehal, W.Z. Acetaminophen-induced hepatotoxicity in mice is dependent on Tlr9 and the Nalp3 inflammasome. *J. Clin. Investig.* **2009**, *119*, 305–314. [CrossRef] [PubMed]
157. Williams, C.D.; Antoine, D.J.; Shaw, P.J.; Benson, C.; Farhood, A.; Williams, D.P.; Kanneganti, T.-D.; Park, B.K.; Jaeschke, H. Role of the Nalp3 inflammasome in acetaminophen-induced sterile inflammation and liver injury. *Toxicol. Appl. Pharmacol.* **2011**, *252*, 289–297. [CrossRef] [PubMed]
158. Williams, C.D.; Bajt, M.L.; Sharpe, M.R.; McGill, M.R.; Farhood, A.; Jaeschke, H. Neutrophil activation during acetaminophen hepatotoxicity and repair in mice and humans. *Toxicol. Appl. Pharmacol.* **2014**, *275*, 122–133. [CrossRef] [PubMed]
159. Nguyen, N.T.; Umbaugh, D.S.; Smith, S.; Adelusi, O.B.; Sanchez-Guerrero, G.; Ramachandran, A.; Jaeschke, H. Dose-dependent pleiotropic role of neutrophils during acetaminophen-induced liver injury in male and female mice. *Arch. Toxicol.* **2023**, *97*, 1397–1412. [CrossRef]
160. James, L.P.; Farrar, H.C.; Darville, T.L.; Sullivan, J.E.; Givens, T.G.; Kearns, G.L.; Do, G.S.W.; Simpson, P.M.; Hinson, J.A. Elevation of serum interleukin 8 levels in acetaminophen overdose in children and adolescents. *Clin. Pharmacol. Ther.* **2001**, *70*, 280–286. [CrossRef]
161. Williams, A.M.; Langley, P.G.; Osei-Hwediah, J.; Wendon, J.A.; Hughes, R.D. Hyaluronic acid and endothelial damage due to paracetamol-induced hepatotoxicity. *Liver Int.* **2003**, *23*, 110–115. [CrossRef]
162. Woolbright, B.L.; Nguyen, N.T.; McGill, M.R.; Sharpe, M.R.; Curry, S.C.; Jaeschke, H. Generation of pro-and anti-inflammatory mediators after acetaminophen overdose in surviving and non-surviving patients. *Toxicol. Lett.* **2022**, *367*, 59–66. [CrossRef]
163. James, L.P.; Simpson, P.M.; Farrar, H.C.; Kearns, G.L.; Wasserman, G.S.; Blumer, J.L.; Reed, M.D.; Sullivan, J.E.; Hinson, J.A. Cytokines and Toxicity in Acetaminophen Overdose. *J. Clin. Pharmacol.* **2005**, *45*, 1165–1171. [CrossRef] [PubMed]
164. Steuerwald, N.M.; Foureau, D.M.; Norton, H.J.; Zhou, J.; Parsons, J.C.; Chalasani, N.; Fontana, R.J.; Watkins, P.B.; Lee, W.M.; Reddy, K.R.; et al. Profiles of Serum Cytokines in Acute Drug-Induced Liver Injury and Their Prognostic Significance. *PLoS ONE* **2013**, *8*, e81974. [CrossRef] [PubMed]
165. Craig, D.G.; Lee, P.; Pryde, E.A.; Walker, S.W.; Beckett, G.J.; Hayes, P.C.; Simpson, K.J. Elevated levels of the long pentraxin 3 in paracetamol-induced human acute liver injury. *Eur. J. Gastroenterol. Hepatol.* **2013**, *25*, 359–367. [CrossRef] [PubMed]
166. Slowik, V.; the Acute Liver Failure Study Group; Borude, P.; Jaeschke, H.; Woolbright, B.L.; Lee, W.M.; Apte, U. Leukocyte cell derived chemotaxin-2 (Lect2) as a predictor of survival in adult acute liver failure. *Transl. Gastroenterol. Hepatol.* **2019**, *4*, 17. [CrossRef]

167. Craig, D.G.; Lee, P.; Pryde, E.A.; Hayes, P.C.; Simpson, K.J. Serum Neopterin and Soluble CD163 as Markers of Macrophage Activation in Paracetamol (Acetaminophen)-Induced Human Acute Liver Injury. *Aliment. Pharmacol. Ther.* **2013**, *38*, 1395–1404. [CrossRef] [PubMed]
168. Wang, K.; Zhang, S.; Marzolf, B.; Troisch, P.; Brightman, A.; Hu, Z.; Hood, L.E.; Galas, D.J. Circulating microRNAs, potential biomarkers for drug-induced liver injury. *Proc. Natl. Acad. Sci. USA* **2009**, *106*, 4402–4407. [CrossRef] [PubMed]
169. Lewis, P.J.S.; Dear, J.; Platt, V.; Simpson, K.J.; Craig, D.G.; Antoine, D.J.; French, N.S.; Dhaun, N.; Webb, D.J.; Costello, E.M.; et al. Circulating microRNAs as potential markers of human drug-induced liver injury. *Hepatology* **2011**, *54*, 1767–1776. [CrossRef] [PubMed]
170. Ward, J.; Kanchagar, C.; Veksler-Lublinsky, I.; Lee, R.C.; McGill, M.R.; Jaeschke, H.; Curry, S.C.; Ambros, V.R. Circulating microRNA profiles in human patients with acetaminophen hepatotoxicity or ischemic hepatitis. *Proc. Natl. Acad. Sci. USA* **2014**, *111*, 12169–12174. [CrossRef]
171. Krauskopf, J.; Caiment, F.; Claessen, S.M.; Johnson, K.J.; Warner, R.L.; Schomaker, S.J.; Burt, D.A.; Aubrecht, J.; Kleinjans, J.C. Application of High-Throughput Sequencing to Circulating microRNAs Reveals Novel Biomarkers for Drug-Induced Liver Injury. *Toxicol. Sci.* **2015**, *143*, 268–276. [CrossRef]
172. Yang, X.; Salminen, W.F.; Shi, Q.; Greenhaw, J.; Gill, P.S.; Bhattacharyya, S.; Beger, R.D.; Mendrick, D.L.; Mattes, W.B.; James, L.P. Potential of extracellular microRNAs as biomarkers of acetaminophen toxicity in children. *Toxicol. Appl. Pharmacol.* **2015**, *284*, 180–187. [CrossRef]
173. Krauskopf, J.; De Kok, T.M.; Schomaker, S.J.; Gosink, M.; Burt, D.A.; Chandler, P.; Warner, R.L.; Johnson, K.J.; Caiment, F.; Kleinjans, J.C.; et al. Serum microRNA signatures as "liquid biopsies" for interrogating hepatotoxic mechanisms and liver pathogenesis in human. *PLoS ONE* **2017**, *12*, e0177928. [CrossRef] [PubMed]
174. Carreiro, S.; Marvel-Coen, J.; Lee, R.; Chapman, B.; Ambros, V. Circulating microRNA Profiles in Acetaminophen Toxicity. *J. Med. Toxicol.* **2020**, *16*, 177–187. [CrossRef] [PubMed]
175. McGill, M.R.; Jaeschke, H. MicroRNAs as Signaling Mediators and Biomarkers of Drug- and Chemical-Induced Liver Injury. *J. Clin. Med.* **2015**, *4*, 1063–1078. [CrossRef] [PubMed]
176. Bernal, W. Biomarkers for risk assessment in paracetamol hepatotoxicity. *Lancet Gastroenterol. Hepatol.* **2018**, *3*, 76–77. [CrossRef] [PubMed]
177. McCrae, J.C.; Sharkey, N.; Webb, D.J.; Vliegenthart, A.D.B.; Dear, J.W. Ethanol consumption produces a small increase in circulating miR-122 in healthy individuals. *Clin. Toxicol.* **2016**, *54*, 53–55. [CrossRef] [PubMed]
178. López-Longarela, B.; Morrison, E.E.; Tranter, J.D.; Chahman-Vos, L.; Léonard, J.-F.; Gautier, J.-C.; Laurent, S.; Lartigau, A.; Boitier, E.; Sautier, L.; et al. Direct Detection of miR-122 in Hepatotoxicity Using Dynamic Chemical Labeling Overcomes Stability and isomiR Challenges. *Anal. Chem.* **2020**, *92*, 3388–3395. [CrossRef] [PubMed]
179. Kersaudy-Kerhoas, M.; Liga, A.; Roychoudhury, A.; Stamouli, M.; Grant, R.; Carrera, D.S.; Schulze, H.; Mielczarek, W.; Oosthuyzen, W.; Quintana, J.F.; et al. Microfluidic system for near-patient extraction and detection of miR-122 microRNA biomarker for drug-induced liver injury diagnostics. *Biomicrofluidics* **2022**, *16*, 024108. [CrossRef]
180. Roychoudhury, A.; Dear, J.W.; Kersaudy-Kerhoas, M.; Bachmann, T.T. Amplification-free electrochemical biosensor detection of circulating microRNA to identify drug-induced liver injury. *Biosens. Bioelectron.* **2023**, *231*, 115298. [CrossRef]
181. Tavabie, O.D.; Karvellas, C.J.; Salehi, S.; Speiser, J.L.; Rose, C.F.; Menon, K.; Prachalias, A.; Heneghan, M.A.; Agarwal, K.; Lee, W.M.; et al. A novel microRNA-based prognostic model outperforms standard prognostic models in patients with acetaminophen-induced acute liver failure. *J. Hepatol.* **2021**, *75*, 424–434. [CrossRef]
182. John, K.; Hadem, J.; Krech, T.; Wahl, K.; Manns, M.P.; Dooley, S.; Batkai, S.; Thum, T.; Schulze-Osthoff, K.; Bantel, H. MicroRNAs play a role in spontaneous recovery from acute liver failure. *Hepatology* **2014**, *60*, 1346–1355. [CrossRef]
183. Salehi, S.; Brereton, H.C.; Arno, M.J.; Darling, D.; Quaglia, A.; O'grady, J.; Heaton, N.; Aluvihare, V.R. Human Liver Regeneration Is Characterized by the Coordinated Expression of Distinct MicroRNA Governing Cell Cycle Fate. *Am. J. Transplant.* **2013**, *13*, 1282–1295. [CrossRef] [PubMed]
184. Salehi, S.; Tavabie, O.D.; Verma, S.; McPhail, M.J.W.; Farzaneh, F.; Bernal, W.; Menon, K.; Agarwal, K.; Aluvihare, V.R. Serum MicroRNA Signatures in Recovery from Acute and Chronic Liver Injury and Selection for Liver Transplantation. *Liver Transplant.* **2020**, *26*, 811–822. [CrossRef] [PubMed]
185. O'Grady, J.G.; Alexander, G.J.; Hayllar, K.M.; Williams, R. Early indicators of prognosis in fulminant hepatic failure. *Gastroenterology* **1989**, *97*, 439–445. [CrossRef] [PubMed]
186. Malinchoc, M.; Kamath, P.S.; Gordon, F.D.; Peine, C.J.; Rank, J.; ter Borg, P.C. A model to predict poor survival in patients undergoing transjugular intrahepatic portosystemic shunts. *Hepatology* **2000**, *31*, 864–871. [CrossRef]
187. Koch, D.G.; Tillman, H.; Durkalski, V.; Lee, W.M.; Reuben, A. Development of a Model to Predict Transplant-free Survival of Patients with Acute Liver Failure. *Clin. Gastroenterol. Hepatol.* **2016**, *14*, 1199–1206.e2. [CrossRef] [PubMed]
188. Walesky, C.M.; Kolb, K.E.; Winston, C.L.; Henderson, J.; Kruft, B.; Fleming, I.; Ko, S.; Monga, S.P.; Mueller, F.; Apte, U.; et al. Functional compensation precedes recovery of tissue mass following acute liver injury. *Nat. Commun.* **2020**, *11*, 5785. [CrossRef] [PubMed]
189. Schmidt, L.E.; Dalhoff, K. Alpha-fetoprotein is a predictor of outcome in acetaminophen-induced liver injury. *Hepatology* **2005**, *41*, 26–31. [CrossRef] [PubMed]

190. Schmidt, L.E.; Dalhoff, K. Serum phosphate is an early predictor of outcome in severe acetaminophen-induced hepatotoxicity. *Hepatology* **2002**, *36*, 659–665. [CrossRef]
191. Rudnick, D.A.; Dietzen, D.J.; Turmelle, Y.P.; Shepherd, R.; Zhang, S.; Belle, S.H.; Squires, R.; Karpen, S.; Dell Olio, D.; Squires, R.; et al. Serum α-NH2-Butyric Acid May Predict Spontaneous Survival in Pediatric Acute Liver Failure. *Pediatr. Transplant.* **2009**, *13*, 223–230. [CrossRef]
192. Schmelzle, M.; Splith, K.; Andersen, L.W.; Kornek, M.; Schuppan, D.; Jones-Bamman, C.; Nowak, M.; Toxavidis, V.; Salhanick, S.D.; Han, L.; et al. Increased Plasma Levels of Microparticles Expressing CD39 and CD133 in Acute Liver Injury. *Transplantation* **2013**, *95*, 63–69. [CrossRef]
193. Umbaugh, D.; Nguyen, N.; Guerrero, G.; Villaneuva, C.; Hagenbuch, B.; Ramachandran, A.; Jaeschke, H. Hepatocyte Senescence Is Initiated through a Klf6-P21 Mechanism That Mediates the Production of Cxcl14, a Novel Prognostic Biomarker of Acute Liver Failure. *Toxicologist* **2023**, *S3*, 587.
194. Lutkewitte, A.J.; Schweitzer, G.G.; Kennon-McGill, S.; Clemens, M.M.; James, L.P.; Jaeschke, H.; Finck, B.N.; McGill, M.R. Lipin deactivation after acetaminophen overdose causes phosphatidic acid accumulation in liver and plasma in mice and humans and enhances liver regeneration. *Food Chem. Toxicol.* **2018**, *115*, 273–283. [CrossRef]
195. Clemens, M.M.; Kennon-McGill, S.; Apte, U.; James, L.P.; Finck, B.N.; McGill, M.R. The inhibitor of glycerol 3-phosphate acyltransferase FSG67 blunts liver regeneration after acetaminophen overdose by altering GSK3β and Wnt/β-catenin signaling. *Food Chem. Toxicol.* **2019**, *125*, 279–288. [CrossRef] [PubMed]
196. McGill, M.R.; Cao, M.; Svetlov, A.; Sharpe, M.R.; Williams, C.D.; Curry, S.C.; Farhood, A.; Jaeschke, H.; Svetlov, S.I. Argininosuccinate synthetase as a plasma biomarker of liver injury after acetaminophen overdose in rodents and humans. *Biomarkers* **2014**, *19*, 222–230. [CrossRef] [PubMed]
197. Vazquez, J.H.; Clemens, M.M.; Allard, F.D.; Yee, E.U.; Kennon-McGill, S.; Mackintosh, S.G.; Jaeschke, H.; Hambuchen, M.D.; McGill, M.R. Identification of Serum Biomarkers to Distinguish Hazardous and Benign Aminotransferase Elevations. *Toxicol. Sci.* **2019**, *173*, 244–254. [CrossRef] [PubMed]
198. Rule, J.A.; Hynan, L.S.; Attar, N.; Sanders, C.; Korzun, W.J.; Lee, W.M.; Larson, A.M.; Liou, I.; Davern, T.; Fix, O.; et al. Procalcitonin Identifies Cell Injury, Not Bacterial Infection, in Acute Liver Failure. *PLoS ONE* **2015**, *10*, e0138566. [CrossRef] [PubMed]
199. Mallet, M.; Haq, M.; Tripon, S.; Bernard, M.; Benosman, H.; Thabut, D.; Rudler, M. Elevated procalcitonin is associated with bacterial infection during acute liver failure only when unrelated to acetaminophen intoxication. *Eur. J. Gastroenterol. Hepatol.* **2017**, *29*, 811–816. [CrossRef] [PubMed]
200. Nuzzo, A.; Salem, S.; Malissin, I.; Diallo, A.; Deye, N.; Goury, A.; Gourlain, H.; Péron, N.; Vicaut, E.; Voicu, S.; et al. Plasma procalcitonin may be an early predictor of liver injury in acetaminophen poisoning: A prospective cohort study. *United Eur. Gastroenterol. J.* **2021**, *9*, 571–580. [CrossRef]
201. Mikus, M.; Drobin, K.; Gry, M.; Bachmann, J.; Lindberg, J.; Yimer, G.; Aklillu, E.; Makonnen, E.; Aderaye, G.; Roach, J.; et al. Elevated levels of circulating CDH5 and FABP1 in association with human drug-induced liver injury. *Liver Int.* **2017**, *37*, 132–140. [CrossRef]
202. Ghandforoush-Sattari, M.; Mashayekhi, S. Evaluation of taurine as a biomarker of liver damage in paracetamol poisoning. *Eur. J. Pharmacol.* **2008**, *581*, 171–176. [CrossRef]
203. Gai, Z.; Samodelov, S.L.; Alecu, I.; Hornemann, T.; Grove, J.I.; Aithal, G.P.; Visentin, M.; Kullak-Ublick, G.A. Plasma Sphingoid Base Profiles of Patients Diagnosed with Intrinsic or Idiosyncratic Drug-induced Liver Injury. *Int. J. Mol. Sci.* **2023**, *24*, 3013. [CrossRef] [PubMed]
204. Westerink, W.M.; Schoonen, W.G. Cytochrome P450 enzyme levels in HepG2 cells and cryopreserved primary human hepatocytes and their induction in HepG2 cells. *Toxicol. Vitr.* **2007**, *21*, 1581–1591. [CrossRef] [PubMed]
205. Hart, S.N.; Li, Y.; Nakamoto, K.; Subileau, E.-A.; Steen, D.; Zhong, X.-B. A Comparison of Whole Genome Gene Expression Profiles of HepaRG Cells and HepG2 Cells to Primary Human Hepatocytes and Human Liver Tissues. *Drug Metab. Dispos.* **2010**, *38*, 988–994. [CrossRef] [PubMed]
206. Ewart, L.; Apostolou, A.; Briggs, S.A.; Carman, C.V.; Chaff, J.T.; Heng, A.R.; Jadalannagari, S.; Janardhanan, J.; Jang, K.-J.; Joshipura, S.R.; et al. Performance assessment and economic analysis of a human Liver-Chip for predictive toxicology. *Commun. Med.* **2022**, *2*, 154. [CrossRef] [PubMed]
207. Maschmeyer, I.; Hasenberg, T.; Jaenicke, A.; Lindner, M.; Lorenz, A.K.; Zech, J.; Garbe, L.-A.; Sonntag, F.; Hayden, P.; Ayehunie, S.; et al. Chip-based human liver–intestine and liver–skin co-cultures—A first step toward systemic repeated dose substance testing in vitro. *Eur. J. Pharm. Biopharm.* **2015**, *95*, 77–87. [CrossRef] [PubMed]
208. Lin, N.; Zhou, X.; Geng, X.; Drewell, C.; Hübner, J.; Li, Z.; Zhang, Y.; Xue, M.; Marx, U.; Li, B. Repeated dose multi-drug testing using a microfluidic chip-based coculture of human liver and kidney proximal tubules equivalents. *Sci. Rep.* **2020**, *10*, 8879. [CrossRef] [PubMed]
209. Novak, R.; Ingram, M.; Marquez, S.; Das, D.; Delahanty, A.; Herland, A.; Maoz, B.M.; Jeanty, S.S.F.; Somayaji, M.R.; Burt, M.; et al. Robotic fluidic coupling and interrogation of multiple vascularized organ chips. *Nat. Biomed. Eng.* **2020**, *4*, 407–420. [CrossRef]
210. Ronaldson-Bouchard, K.; Teles, D.; Yeager, K.; Tavakol, D.N.; Zhao, Y.; Chramiec, A.; Tagore, S.; Summers, M.; Stylianos, S.; Tamargo, M.; et al. A multi-organ chip with matured tissue niches linked by vascular flow. *Nat. Biomed. Eng.* **2022**, *6*, 351–371. [CrossRef]

211. Schomaker, S.; Potter, D.; Warner, R.; Larkindale, J.; King, N.; Porter, A.C.; Owens, J.; Tomlinson, L.; Sauer, J.-M.; Johnson, K.; et al. Serum glutamate dehydrogenase activity enables early detection of liver injury in subjects with underlying muscle impairments. *PLoS ONE* **2020**, *15*, e0229753. [CrossRef]
212. Miyazaki, M.; Rosenblum, J.S.; Kasahara, Y.; Nakagawa, I.; Patricelli, M.P. Determination of enzymatic source of alanine aminotransferase activity in serum from dogs with liver injury. *J. Pharmacol. Toxicol. Methods* **2009**, *60*, 307–315. [CrossRef]
213. Yang, R.-Z.; Park, S.; Reagan, W.J.; Goldstein, R.; Zhong, S.; Lawton, M.; Rajamohan, F.; Qian, K.; Liu, L.; Gong, D.-W. Alanine aminotransferase isoenzymes: Molecular cloning and quantitative analysis of tissue expression in rats and serum elevation in liver toxicity. *Hepatology* **2009**, *49*, 598–607. [CrossRef]
214. Rafter, I.; Gråberg, T.; Kotronen, A.; Strömmer, L.; Mattson, C.M.; Kim, R.W.; Ehrenborg, E.; Andersson, H.B.; Yki-Järvinen, H.; Schuppe-Koistinen, I.; et al. Isoform-specific alanine aminotransferase measurement can distinguish hepatic from extrahepatic injury in humans. *Int. J. Mol. Med.* **2012**, *30*, 1241–1249. [CrossRef]

livers

MDPI

Review

High-Dose Acetaminophen as a Treatment for Cancer

Jeffrey Wu [1], Bradley Maller [2,3], Rujul Kaul [2], Andrea Galabow [2], Allyn Bryan [2] and Alexander Neuwelt [2,*]

1 Department of Neurology, School of Medicine, Oregon Health and Sciences University, 3181 Sam Jackson Park Rd., Portland, OR 97239, USA; wujeff@yahoo.com
2 Department of Veterans Affairs, 1201 Broad Rock Blvd, Richmond, VA 23249, USA; bradly.maller@vcuhealth.org (B.M.); rujul.kaul@va.gov (R.K.); shellie.galabow@va.gov (A.G.)
3 Department of Internal Medicine, School of Medicine, Virginia Commonwealth University, 1201 E Marshall St., Richmond, VA 23298, USA
* Correspondence: alexander.neuwelt@va.gov

Abstract: The use of high-dose acetaminophen (AAP) with n-acetylcysteine (NAC) rescue was studied as an anti-cancer treatment in phase I trials with promising signals of anti-tumor efficacy. Correlative analysis suggested that AAP has a free-radical-independent mechanism of anti-tumor activity—in contrast to the well-established mechanism of AAP hepatotoxicity. Subsequent "reverse translational" studies in the pre-clinical setting have identified novel mechanisms of action of high-dose AAP, including modulation of JAK-STAT signaling in both the tumor cell and the tumor immune microenvironment. Importantly, these effects are free-radical-independent and not reversed by concurrent administration of the established AAP rescue agents fomepizole and NAC. By administering high-dose AAP concurrently with fomepizole and NAC, 100-fold higher AAP levels than those of standard dosing can be achieved in mice without detected toxicity and with substantial anti-tumor efficacy against commonly used mouse models of lung and breast cancer that are resistant to standard first-line anti-cancer therapies. With these recent advances, additional clinical trials of high-dose AAP with concurrent NAC and fomepizole-based rescue are warranted.

Keywords: acetaminophen; N-acetylcysteine; fomepizole; cancer

1. AAP Is Hepatotoxic in Overdose

Acetaminophen (AAP) is a commonly used drug throughout the world, standardly taken as an anti-nociceptive and fever-reducing agent. AAP is metabolized by a variety of pathways, including glucuronidation, sulfation, and fatty acid amide hydrolase (FAAH)-mediated conversion to N-arachidonoylphenolamine (AM404); AM404 is thought to be an active metabolite that contributes to the anti-nociceptive properties of AAP [1]. Additionally, CYP2E1-mediated conversion of AAP into N-acetyl-p-benzoquinone imine (NAPQI) is a minor metabolic pathway, comprising about 5–10% of AAP metabolism [2]. NAPQI is a reactive intermediate that under normal conditions is rapidly bound and detoxified by intracellular glutathione (GSH). However, upon AAP overdose, intracellular GSH becomes depleted and NAPQI binds cellular proteins, predominantly within the liver, resulting in toxicity [3]. Of note, NAPQI bound to cellular proteins, termed protein adducts, can be measured using mass spectrometry and is a relatively specific measure of AAP toxicity [4]. Key evidence for the mechanisms of AAP liver toxicity come from studies demonstrating substantially improved tolerability of high doses of AAP in CYP2E1 KO mice [5].

2. Strategies to Prevent AAP Toxicity

The FDA-approved antidote for AAP toxicity is n-acetylcysteine (NAC), which can be administered either orally or intravenously. NAC functions both as a GSH precursor and also as a potent thiol anti-oxidant that binds and detoxifies NAPQI, thus mitigating AAP hepatotoxicity. Clinically, when NAC is administered within 6–8 h of AAP overdose, outcomes are positive the vast majority of the time with a relatively minimal risk of mortality [3,6,7]. Of note, as outlined in a Cochrane database review, the data supporting the use of NAC as a clinical antidote to AAP toxicity are largely based on single-arm, non-randomized studies [8]. Thus, the extent to which patients that overdose on AAP may spontaneously recover is not completely understood.

Fomepizole (4-methylpyrazole, 4-MP) is a potent CYP2E1 inhibitor that is increasingly being utilized as an adjunctive therapy in the management of AAP overdose [9,10]. Fomepizole is FDA-approved for the treatment of ethylene glycol and methanol toxicity and has a relatively well-established safety profile with few significant toxicities [11]. Fomepizole inhibits CYP2E1-mediated NAPQI formation and subsequent free-radical-mediated stress response in the mitochondria upon AAP overdose via inhibition of N-terminal JNK phosphorylation [12]. Fomepizole rescue prevents the formation of oxidative metabolites, such as APAP-Cys, while not affecting other metabolic pathways such as glucuronidation [12].

Numerous other antidotes to AAP toxicity have been evaluated pre-clinically, including 25-hydroxycholesterol-3-sulfate [13] and heparan sulfates [14]. However, these drugs have not been evaluated in human patients for protection against AAP toxicity; fomepizole and NAC are the drugs with the most clinical data supporting their use.

3. Early Pre-Clinical Studies of High-Dose AAP for the Treatment of Cancer

The initial pre-clinical studies using high-dose AAP as a treatment for cancer utilized hepatoma cell lines HEPG2 and PLC/PRF/5 [15]. These studies were based on the presumption that n-acetylcysteine functions as an "antagonist" to AAP, i.e., neutralizing both the toxicity and efficacy of AAP. Wu et al. designed experiments with the goal of allowing NAC to selectively rescue normal hepatocytes but not malignant hepatoma cells from high-dose AAP treatment. The experiments took advantage of the presence of receptors for galactose-terminal (asialo-)glycoproteins on normal hepatocytes. A conjugate was created by coupling NAC to galactose-terminal (asialo-)fetuin. It was demonstrated that HEPG2 cells (capable of taking up galactose-terminal (asialo-)fetuin) were effectively rescued by the modified NAC; however, PLC/PRF/5 cells could not take up the galactose-terminal (asialo-)fetuin-bound NAC and thus were not rescued.

4. Clinical Trials of High-Dose AAP as a Treatment of Cancer

Clinical trials evaluating high-dose AAP as a treatment for cancer were conceived based on relatively vague principles that AAP may have differential effects on neoplastic cells relative to normal cells, thus permitting selective rescue of normal cells using NAC-based rescue approaches. For instance, the clinical trials cited studies that utilized NAC to blunt the toxicity of alkylating agents and radiation to normal cells without preventing tumoricidal activity [16]. In reality, these clinical trials were designed based on relatively scant pre-clinical rationale and in the absence of in vitro or in vivo mouse studies directly evaluating the anti-tumor properties of high-dose AAP with delayed NAC rescue—the treatment regimen used in the studies [17].

Kobrinsky et al. enrolled 19 patients onto their trial of high-dose AAP from 1990 to 1991 [17]. The patients had a wide range of malignancies, including pancreatic cancer, prostate cancer, and esophageal cancer, among others. The majority of patients had solid tumors, while one patient had acute leukemia. AAP was administered orally as a concentrated slurry. NAC was administered starting 8 h after the AAP treatment using a 16-hour infusion (NAC dosing was similar to what is used in the management of AAP overdose). Delayed NAC rescue was used based on the concern that NAC functions as an "antagonist" of AAP and concurrent administration would therefore neutralize its efficacy. However, no rationale was provided for why delayed NAC would rescue the normal liver but not the cancer.

Treatment with high-dose AAP was performed weekly for 4 weeks and continued until disease progression or unacceptable toxicity. AAP was started at 6 g/m^2 and escalated up to a maximum of 20 g/m^2. A total of 78 courses of high-dose AAP were administered.

Out of 14 patients assessed for response, 3 had a partial response (responding patients had esophageal cancer, pancreatic cancer, and small-cell lung cancer), 3 were "improved," and 3 patients had a mixed response. Thus, the overall response rate among assessable patients was 3/14 or 21%. Interestingly, 8 of the patients with chronic pain reported complete analgesic control for 12–24 h after the injection. No dose-limiting liver toxicities were observed. The most common adverse events were nausea (associated with swallowing the large volume of AAP slurry) and drowsiness that usually resolved around the time the NAC infusion was started. In pharmacological analysis, AAP was noted to have a half-life of 3.6 h with mean serum AAP concentration at 4 h of 245 µg/mL (range 95–473 µg/mL).

While the published manuscript was a clinical trial, in the Discussion section it was revealed that "Corden and Bartlett-Heubus have demonstrated a reproducible antiproliferative effect of HDAC on L1210 leukemia cells in vitro despite no demonstrable decrease in intracellular glutathione [17]". This observation was the first to suggest a possible free-radical-independent mechanism of anti-tumor activity in high-dose AAP.

A subsequent phase I clinical trial of high-dose AAP was performed by Wolchok et al. in patients with advanced melanoma at Memorial Sloan Kettering Cancer Center [18]. The trial evaluated a combination of AAP and carmustine (BCNU). The authors hypothesized that AAP would deplete tumoral GSH, a molecule known to be involved in chemotherapy resistance, and thus sensitize tumors to BCNU. However, a GSH-mediated mechanism of synergy between AAP and chemotherapy had not yet been tested in animal models.

Wolchok et al. designed the study to sequentially dose-escalate AAP and BCNU. The starting dose of AAP was 10 g/m^2 every 3 weeks; BCNU was started at 10 mg/m^2. AAP was escalated by 5 g/m^2 in cohorts until the DLT (dose-limiting toxicity) was reached. Once the DLT of AAP was reached, BCNU dosing was subsequently elevated using a 3 + 3 design. AAP was again given as a slurry; however, due to nausea and unpleasant taste, some patients required placement of an NG tube. NAC rescue was started 6–8 h after AAP treatment.

Two patients experienced grade IV liver toxicity at 20 g/m^2 AAP and thus 15 g/m^2 was identified as the maximum tolerated dose; 150 mg/m^2 was identified as the MTD of BCNU. Mean peak AAP levels in the 15 g/m^2 AAP cohort was 267 µg/mL. As a correlative biomarker, GSH levels were measured in peripheral blood mononuclear cells (PBMCs) pre- and post-AAP treatment. Interestingly, AAP was shown not to deplete GSH levels in PBMCs—likely because of low CYP2E1 expression in immune cells [19].

Out of the 27 enrolled patients, 2 experienced a partial response (7.4%). The relatively low response rate observed in this phase I trial of AAP could be secondary to the inability to dose-escalate to adequate levels of AAP (1/3 patients in the 20 g/m^2 cohort experienced a partial response). Thus, with improved rescue regimens, higher AAP doses may be achieved, resulting in improved response rates. Alternatively, AAP may have limited efficacy against melanoma, a tumor that responds to distinct therapies relative to other solid tumors (for instance, melanoma is generally resistant to chemotherapy) [18].

The final clinical case of AAP being used to treat cancer was published in 2005 by Kobrinsky et al. [20]. A 30-month-old child was diagnosed with advanced hepatoblastoma. The patient was initially treated with doxorubicin, but unfortunately progressed. As a second-line therapy, the patient was given 90 mg/m^2 cisplatin, 1.5 mg/m^2 vincristine, and 600 mg/m^2 5-flurouracil. However, the patient's tumor proved refractory to this therapy. Finally, the patient was treated with 30 g/m^2 AAP along with delayed NAC rescue and concurrent cisplatin 90 mg/m^2. The patient experienced a profound response, with AFP falling from 6700 ng/mL at the start of therapy to 430 ng/mL after the fourth treatment cycle. The patient had his remaining disease surgically resected and only a 5 mm area of viable tumor was present on pathology. At the time of publication, the patient was 8 years out from surgery and disease-free [20] (Table 1).

Table 1. Clinical experience of high-dose acetaminophen in cancer patients.

Citation	Intervention	Duration	Patients Enrolled (*n*)	Outcomes
Kobrinsky, 1996 [17]	Oral AAP with dose escalation and delayed NAC rescue for diverse malignancies.	Until disease progression or unacceptable toxicity	19	Toxicity: No dose-limiting toxicities at doses of up to 20 g/m^2 AAP. Efficacy: Three out of fourteen evaluated patients (21%) had a partial response.
Wolchok, 2003 [18]	Carmustine dose escalation, oral AAP dose escalation, and delayed NAC rescue for advanced malignant melanoma.	Until disease progression or unacceptable toxicity	27	Toxicity: Two patients experienced grade IV liver toxicity at 20 g/m^2 AAP, so 15 g/m^2 was the maximum tolerated dose (in combination with carmustine). Efficacy: Two patients had a partial response.
Kobrinksy, 2005 [20]	Case report of treatment of progressive hepatoblastoma with high-dose (30 g/m^2) AAP, NAC, and cisplatin.	Four cycles, then surgical resection of tumor	1	Toxicity: No toxicities noted. Efficacy: Near-complete response followed by resection of residual necrotic tumor. Patient disease-free for 8 years at time of publication.

5. Unanswered Questions from Clinical Trials of High-Dose AAP

The clinical trials of high-dose AAP were performed on the basis of theoretical, if unproven, concepts and generally in the absence of pre-clinical data. The goal of the clinical trials was to selectively rescue the toxicity of high-dose AAP using NAC while not reversing AAP's tumoricidal effects. However, there was no firm pre-clinical basis—beyond theoretical concepts and extrapolations from unrelated data sets—suggesting how this could be accomplished.

Furthermore, the mechanistic rationale cited in the clinical trials for potential AAP efficacy, i.e., that AAP would lead to intra-tumoral GSH depletion and subsequent free radical injury, had not been shown in any pre-clinical models outside of the liver. Indeed, as discussed above, Kobrinsky et al. noted in vitro evidence of anti-leukemic activity of AAP in the absence of GSH depletion [17], and Wolchok et al. found that AAP did not cause GSH depletion in the PBMCs of treated patients, again suggesting an alternative mechanism of the anti-tumor activity of high-dose AAP [18].

In brief, the three key unanswered questions from the clinical trials can be summarized as follows:

(1) Does AAP have tumoricidal activity via GSH depletion, i.e., analogous to the mechanism of toxicity in the liver, and if not, what is the mechanism?
(2) Is it possible to selectively rescue the normal liver without rescuing the tumoricidal effects of high-dose AAP?
(3) What is the optimal rescue regimen that would allow for safe dose escalation of AAP to levels needed for anti-tumor efficacy? Is NAC alone truly the optimal rescue strategy, or are other drugs/combinations of drugs more effective?

As a result of the above unanswered questions, additional clinical trials of high-dose AAP have not been performed despite the promising results of the phase I trials outlined above. Over the last several years, our group has aimed to perform "reverse translational" studies, i.e., perform in vitro and in vivo data laboratory experiments to help explain the promising yet mechanistically nebulous clinical observations.

6. High-Dose AAP Selectively Depletes Glutathione in the Liver but Not the Tumor in Pre-Clinical Models

We evaluated the pre-clinical efficacy of high-dose AAP with delayed NAC rescue using hepatocarcinoma and hepatoblastoma models. In these studies, we demonstrated GSH depletion in liver tumor cells in vitro; however, high doses of AAP (5–20 mM) and a relatively long duration of AAP treatment (up to 18 h in cell culture, despite AAP having a half-life of 2–4 h) were used. Our in vitro studies additionally demonstrated synergism between AAP and cisplatin. NAC reversed AAP cytotoxicity towards tumor cells when administered concurrently but demonstrated decreased tumor protection when administered at delayed timepoints in vitro [21].

We subsequently evaluated the efficacy of AAP in a pre-clinical model of ovarian cancer [22,23]. AAP demonstrated increased cytotoxic activity when given with paclitaxel and cisplatin in vitro using the human SKOV3 ovarian cancer cell line. AAP in combination with cisplatin or paclitaxel led to profound loss of mitochondrial membrane potential in treated tumor cells, suggesting that the observed synergy may be mediated by toxicity towards tumor cell mitochondria.

In evaluating the pharmacology of high-dose AAP, we observed that AAP levels were similar in the brain, liver, tumor, and serum of rats treated with high-dose AAP. However, GSH levels were depleted only in the liver but not the tumor, brain, or serum of AAP-treated rats. The finding of selective GSH depletion in the liver but not the tumor was highly novel and directly undermined the proposed mechanism of anti-tumor activity of high-dose AAP, i.e., that it has anti-tumor activity via GSH depletion [23].

Further, our finding that AAP depletes GSH in the liver but not the tumor, subsequently validated in other models [24], suggests a mechanism for selective rescue of normal liver using NAC. NAC functions as a GSH precursor and anti-oxidant; if AAP leads to GSH depletion only in the liver, then NAC can be administered concurrently with high-dose AAP and no tumor protection would be expected. The selective depletion of GSH in the liver upon treatment with high-dose AAP is due to selective expression of CYP2E1 in the liver relative to other organs [19] (Figure 1). If NAC selectively rescues the liver but not the tumor from high-dose AAP treatment, then this raises the possibility of concurrent administration of the two drugs. The potential for AAP administration with concurrent NAC-based rescue could enhance treatment tolerability considering the known improved clinical outcomes when NAC is administered promptly after AAP overdose [3].

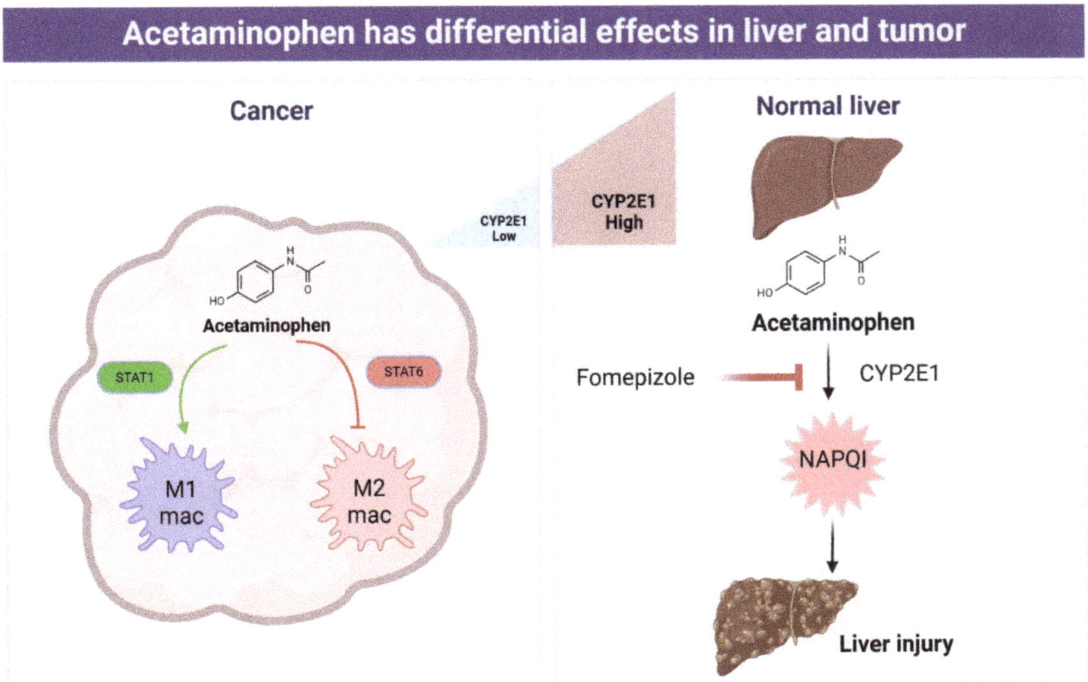

Figure 1. High-dose acetaminophen inhibits M2 polarization of tumor-associated macrophages, leading to anti-tumor immune response. Within the liver, the CYP2E1 inhibitor fomepizole prevents NAPQI formation and resultant toxicity. Differential rescue of liver but not tumor from acetaminophen by fomepizole is a result of selective expression of CYP2E1 in the liver.

7. Identification of Free-Radical-Independent Mechanisms of Anti-Tumor Activity of High-Dose AAP

If high-dose AAP does not have anti-cancer activity via GSH depletion and associated free radical injury, then an alternative mechanism must exist. We demonstrated that AAP has anti-cancer stem cell (CSC) activity in multiple pre-clinical models of cancer, an effect that was not reversed by concurrent administration of NAC. Mechanistically, AAP inhibits STAT3 phosphorylation, a protein that is central to the activity and proliferation of CSCs, via direct binding. In STAT3 knockdown lung cancer cells, the anti-CSC effects of AAP are lost, underscoring the physiological relevance of our findings. These data provide additional credence to the concept that NAC may be administered concurrently with AAP for selective rescue from toxicity without compromising anti-tumor activity [24].

JAK-STAT signaling plays a central role in many facets of the anti-tumor immune response. Given our finding that AAP modulates JAK-STAT signaling in tumor cells, we next evaluated the effect of AAP on the adaptive immune system. We observed that AAP inhibits STAT6—involved in pro-tumorigenic M2 polarization of macrophages—but not STAT1—involved in pro-inflammatory anti-tumor M1 macrophage polarization. In vitro and in vivo, high-dose AAP decreased expression of M2 markers in tumor-associated macrophages (such as arginase and CD206) at both the RNA and protein levels. M1 markers, such as iNOS, MHC I, and CD80, were relatively unaffected. Using the mouse syngeneic 4T1 triple negative breast cancer model, it was found that high-dose AAP had profound anti-cancer activity that was lost in macrophage-depleted mice treated with F4/80 antibodies, underscoring the central role of the innate immune system in mediating AAP anti-tumor activity in vivo [25] (Figure 1).

8. Optimization of High-Dose AAP Rescue Cocktail

As discussed above, the data supporting NAC as the standard rescue agent for AAP overdose are based largely on single-arm non-randomized trials [8]. Furthermore, there is a paucity of data comparing the efficacy of NAC to alternative rescue agents that have demonstrated pre-clinical promise, such as heparan sulfates [14], 25-hydroxycholesterol-3-sulfate [13], and the CYP2E1 inhibitor fomepizole [26]. Our lab directly compared the most established antidotes to AAP toxicity, NAC and fomepizole, in pre-clinical mouse models. At doses of up to 650 mg/kg, AAP concurrent treatment with fomepizole completely prevented hepatotoxicity. On the other hand, NAC (100 mg/kg IP) provided no significant protection. The lack of observed hepato-protection of NAC in these pre-clinical models is surprising, yet has similarly been observed in other studies [13,27]. Higher doses of NAC (500–1200 mg/kg) have demonstrated improved efficacy in preventing AAP toxicity in mouse models [28,29], but are well beyond the maximal safe dose in humans [30].

CYP2E1 mediates a minor AAP metabolic pathway (about 5–10% of AAP metabolism) that creates a transient reactive intermediate NAPQI that locally binds cellular proteins in the liver, leading to hepatotoxicity. The active AAP metabolite AM404 is generated in a CYP2E1-independent manner (Figure 2) [31]. While fomepizole prevents AAP hepatotoxicity in vivo, fomepizole did not reverse the anti-tumor effects of AAP in vitro or in vivo [32]—likely because CYP2E1 is expressed selectively in the liver (Figure 1) [19]. In fact, using fomepizole-based rescue, we were able to safely dose-escalate AAP to the levels needed for profound anti-tumor activity, 100-fold higher than standard AAP dosing, in commonly used mouse cancer models (LLC lung cancer and 4T1 breast cancer) without any detected toxicity [32].

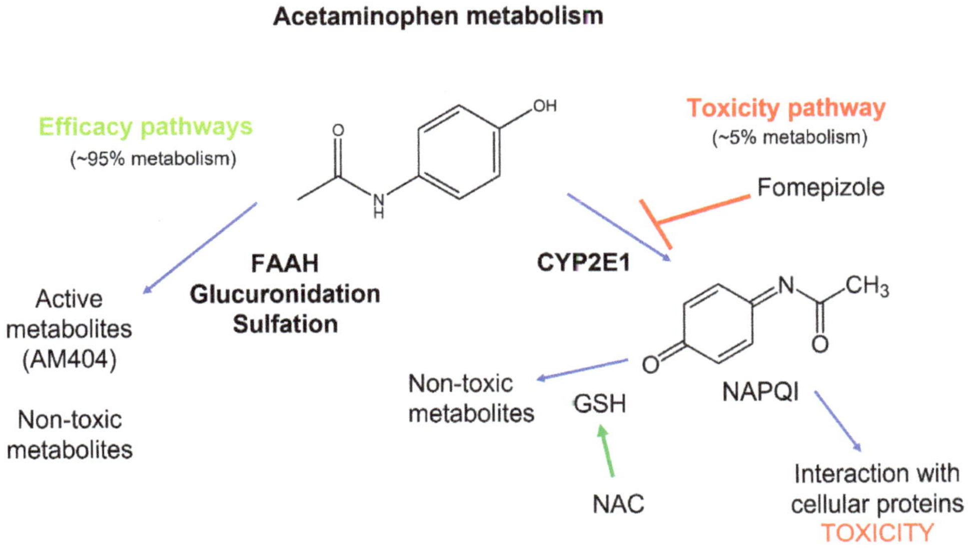

Figure 2. Acetaminophen metabolic pathways. CYP2E1-mediated metabolism is a minor metabolic pathway that leads to toxicity and can be blocked with CYP2E1 inhibitors such as fomepizole to prevent toxicity and preserve anti-tumor efficacy.

9. Future Directions—AAP as Anti-Cancer Therapeutic

While the precise anti-tumor mechanisms of high-dose AAP are better understood now relative to when the initial clinical trials were conducted in the 1990s [17], much remains to be learned. Animal studies suggest that high-dose AAP has anti-tumor properties through disruption of the JAK-STAT signaling pathway, both in the tumor cell and in tumor-associated macrophages [24,25]. Given the complexity and interconnectedness of the tumor immune microenvironment, it is suspected that other immune cells play important roles in mediating AAP's anti-tumor immune response. The JAK-STAT signaling pathway, for example, is known to play a role in the maturation of dendritic cells and the activation of helper T cells [33]. Currently, our lab is comprehensively evaluating changes in the tumor immune microenvironment induced by high-dose AAP using such methodologies as single-cell RNA sequencing and multiplex flow cytometry. With improved understanding of the specific molecular interactions at play, patient selection for clinical trials may be optimized, and rationally designed synergistic combinations with other active drugs may be evaluated. Ultimately, improved understanding of high-dose AAP mechanism of action may inform the design of subsequent-generation drugs with improved target specificity and potency.

Additional safety data of high-dose AAP in human patients are needed. In the study by Kobrinsky et al., 19 patients with diverse tumor histologies were treated with high-dose AAP followed by delayed NAC rescue. Dose-limiting liver toxicity was not seen in this study [17]. Subsequently, however, Wolchok et al. observed grade IV liver toxicity in two patients treated with 20 g/m^2 AAP [18]; the maximum tolerated dose was set at 15 g/m^2 AAP. In our pre-clinical mouse models, higher doses of AAP could be tolerated without hepatotoxicity when administered with fomepizole-based rescue strategies [32] relative to the NAC regimens used in the initial clinical trials. Human trials are needed to comprehensively evaluate the safety profile, pharmacokinetics, and pharmacodynamics of high-dose AAP with fomepizole-based rescue across a range of doses in patients with advanced cancer.

Early pre-clinical data suggest the efficacy of AAP in diverse cancer models, including hepatic cancer, breast cancer, lung cancer, ovarian cancer, and even atypical teratoid rhabdoid tumor models [21–24]; the use of AAP in brain tumors is particularly compelling, considering that AAP readily crosses the blood–brain barrier. However, the relative efficacy of AAP in various tumor histologies—including solid tumors versus hematologic malignancies—remains to be comprehensively elucidated. Ultimately, large clinical datasets may be needed to assess the clinical efficacy of AAP in diverse malignancies—both alone and in rational combinations with existing anti-tumor agents. Additionally, robust correlative studies from clinical trials will be needed to evaluate the role of JAK-STAT signaling and the immune system in mediating the anti-tumor activity of high-dose AAP.

10. Future Directions—Analgesic Potential of AAP/Fomepizole

Patients with advanced cancer often have debilitating pain syndromes associated with their disease, requiring high doses of narcotic pain medicines. Traditional chemotherapy regimens are associated with substantial symptomatic toxicities, including nausea, fatigue, and weakness, that may directly or indirectly exacerbate chronic pain syndromes. The potential of high-dose AAP to not only have anti-cancer activity but also contribute potent analgesic control may be a compelling added benefit of our approach. Kobrinsky et al. noted complete analgesia for 12–24 h in eight patients with chronic pain syndrome receiving high-dose AAP [17] for the treatment of advanced cancer. As described above (Figure 2), AM404 is an active analgesic metabolite of AAP that is created in a CYP2E1-independent fashion via deacetylation of AAP to para-aminophenol followed by fatty acid amide hydrolase (FAAH)-catalyzed conjugation with arachidonic acid [34]. Thus, the CYP2E1 inhibitor fomepizole is unlikely to mitigate the analgesic effects of AAP, and high-dose AAP with fomepizole rescue may be a potent analgesic cocktail that spares the toxicities of narcotics, such as constipation, respiratory depression and ultimately dependance. Further research studying the analgesic benefits of high-dose AAP with fomepizole-based rescue will require detailed evaluation in both animal and human studies.

11. Conclusions

High-dose AAP has demonstrated promise in phase I clinical trials for the treatment of patients with advanced malignancy. Lack of understanding of therapeutic mechanisms has limited the subsequent development of AAP as an anti-cancer drug. More recently, "reverse translational" pre-clinical studies have provided substantial mechanistic insights that may facilitate future clinical trials of high-dose AAP in patients with cancer. Most importantly, recently published data provide evidence that AAP may be administered concurrently with highly effective antidotes such as fomepizole to prevent toxicity without compromising therapeutic anti-tumor efficacy. With these recent advances, we believe it is imperative that high-dose AAP with fomepizole-based rescue be evaluated in clinical trials for patients with advanced cancer.

Author Contributions: Conceptualization, A.N.; writing—original draft preparation, A.N.; writing—review and editing, J.W., A.G., B.M., A.B., R.K. and A.N. All authors have read and agreed to the published version of the manuscript.

Funding: This research was funded by the Department of Veterans Affairs, grant number 5IK2BX004914-03.

Institutional Review Board Statement: Not applicable.

Informed Consent Statement: Not applicable.

Data Availability Statement: Data is contained within the article.

Conflicts of Interest: The Department of Veterans Affairs (AN and AB) has submitted provisional IP on the concurrent use of CYP2E1 inhibitors with acetaminophen.

References

1. Saliba, S.W.; Marcotegui, A.R.; Fortwangler, E.; Ditrich, J.; Perazzo, J.C.; Munoz, E.; de Oliveira, A.C.P.; Fiebich, B.L. AM404, paracetamol metabolite, prevents prostaglandin synthesis in activated microglia by inhibiting COX activity. *J. Neuroinflammation* **2017**, *14*, 246. [CrossRef] [PubMed]
2. Yoon, E.; Babar, A.; Choudhary, M.; Kutner, M.; Pyrsopoulos, N. Acetaminophen-Induced Hepatotoxicity: A Comprehensive Update. *J. Clin. Transl. Hepatol.* **2016**, *4*, 131–142. [CrossRef] [PubMed]
3. Heard, K.J. Acetylcysteine for acetaminophen poisoning. *N. Engl. J. Med.* **2008**, *359*, 285–292. [CrossRef] [PubMed]
4. Davern, T.J., 2nd; James, L.P.; Hinson, J.A.; Polson, J.; Larson, A.M.; Fontana, R.J.; Lalani, E.; Munoz, S.; Shakil, A.O.; Lee, W.M.; et al. Measurement of serum acetaminophen-protein adducts in patients with acute liver failure. *Gastroenterology* **2006**, *130*, 687–694. [CrossRef] [PubMed]
5. Lee, S.S.; Buters, J.T.; Pineau, T.; Fernandez-Salguero, P.; Gonzalez, F.J. Role of CYP2E1 in the hepatotoxicity of acetaminophen. *J. Biol. Chem.* **1996**, *271*, 12063–12067. [CrossRef] [PubMed]
6. Yip, L.; Dart, R.C. A 20-hour treatment for acute acetaminophen overdose *N. Engl. J. Med.* **2003**, *348*, 2471–2472. [CrossRef] [PubMed]
7. Smilkstein, M.J.; Knapp, G.L.; Kulig, K.W.; Rumack, B.H. Efficacy of oral N-acetylcysteine in the treatment of acetaminophen overdose. Analysis of the national multicenter study (1976 to 1985). *N. Engl. J. Med.* **1988**, *319*, 1557–1562. [CrossRef] [PubMed]
8. Brok, J.; Buckley, N.; Gluud, C. Interventions for paracetamol (acetaminophen) overdose. *Cochrane Database Syst. Rev.* **2006**, CD003328. [CrossRef]
9. Filip, A.B.; Berg, S.E.; Mullins, M.E.; Schwarz, E.S.; Toxicology Investigators, C. Fomepizole as an adjunctive therapy for acetaminophen poisoning: Cases reported to the toxicology investigators consortium (ToxIC) database 2015–2020. *Clin. Toxicol.* **2022**, *60*, 1006–1011. [CrossRef]
10. Pepin, L.; Matsler, N.; Fontes, A.; Heard, K.; Flaherty, B.F.; Monte, A.A. Fomepizole Therapy for Acetaminophen-Induced Liver Failure in an Infant. *Pediatrics* **2023**, *152*, e2022061033. [CrossRef]
11. Rasamison, R.; Besson, H.; Berleur, M.P.; Schicchi, A.; Megarbane, B. Analysis of fomepizole safety based on a 16-year post-marketing experience in France. *Clin. Toxicol.* **2020**, *58*, 742–747. [CrossRef] [PubMed]
12. Akakpo, J.Y.; Ramachandran, A.; Kandel, S.E.; Ni, H.M.; Kumer, S.C.; Rumack, B.H.; Jaeschke, H. 4-Methylpyrazole protects against acetaminophen hepatotoxicity in mice and in primary human hepatocytes. *Hum. Exp. Toxicol.* **2018**, *37*, 1310–1322. [CrossRef] [PubMed]
13. Wang, Y.; Pandak, W.M.; Lesnefsky, E.J.; Hylemon, P.B.; Ren, S. 25-Hydroxycholesterol 3-Sulfate Recovers Acetaminophen Induced Acute Liver Injury via Stabilizing Mitochondria in Mouse Models. *Cells* **2021**, *10*, 3027. [CrossRef]
14. Arnold, K.; Xu, Y.; Sparkenbaugh, E.M.; Li, M.; Han, X.; Zhang, X.; Xia, K.; Piegore, M.; Zhang, F.; Zhang, X.; et al. Design of anti-inflammatory heparan sulfate to protect against acetaminophen-induced acute liver failure. *Sci. Transl. Med.* **2020**, *12*, eaav8075. [CrossRef] [PubMed]
15. Wu, G.Y.; Wu, C.H.; Rubin, M.I. Acetaminophen hepatotoxicity and targeted rescue: A model for specific chemotherapy of hepatocellular carcinoma. *Hepatology* **1985**, *5*, 709–713. [CrossRef] [PubMed]
16. Wanamarta, A.H.; van Rijn, J.; Blank, L.E.; Haveman, J.; van Zandwijk, N.; Joenje, H. Effect of N-acetylcysteine on the antiproliferative action of X-rays or bleomycin in cultured human lung tumor cells. *J. Cancer Res. Clin. Oncol.* **1989**, *115*, 340–344. [CrossRef]
17. Kobrinsky, N.L.; Hartfield, D.; Horner, H.; Maksymiuk, A.; Minuk, G.Y.; White, D.F.; Feldstein, T.J. Treatment of advanced malignancies with high-dose acetaminophen and N-acetylcysteine rescue. *Cancer Investig.* **1996**, *14*, 202–210. [CrossRef] [PubMed]
18. Wolchok, J.D.; Williams, L.; Pinto, J.T.; Fleisher, M.; Krown, S.E.; Hwu, W.J.; Livingston, P.O.; Chang, C.; Chapman, P.B. Phase I trial of high dose paracetamol and carmustine in patients with metastatic melanoma. *Melanoma Res.* **2003**, *13*, 189–196. [CrossRef]
19. Bieche, I.; Narjoz, C.; Asselah, T.; Vacher, S.; Marcellin, P.; Lidereau, R.; Beaune, P.; de Waziers, I. Reverse transcriptase-PCR quantification of mRNA levels from cytochrome (CYP)1, CYP2 and CYP3 families in 22 different human tissues. *Pharmacogenet Genom.* **2007**, *17*, 731–742. [CrossRef]
20. Kobrinsky, N.L.; Sjolander, D.E.; Goldenberg, J.A.; Ortmeier, T.C. Successful treatment of doxorubicin and cisplatin resistant hepatoblastoma in a child with Beckwith-Wiedemann syndrome with high dose acetaminophen and N-acetylcysteine rescue. *Pediatr. Blood Cancer* **2005**, *45*, 222–225. [CrossRef]
21. Neuwelt, A.J.; Wu, Y.J.; Knap, N.; Losin, M.; Neuwelt, E.A.; Pagel, M.A.; Warmann, S.; Fuchs, J.; Czauderna, P.; Wozniak, M. Using acetaminophen's toxicity mechanism to enhance cisplatin efficacy in hepatocarcinoma and hepatoblastoma cell lines. *Neoplasia* **2009**, *11*, 1003–1011. [CrossRef] [PubMed]
22. Neuwelt, A.J.; Nguyen, T.; Wu, Y.J.; Donson, A.M.; Vibhakar, R.; Venkatamaran, S.; Amani, V.; Neuwelt, E.A.; Rapkin, L.B.; Foreman, N.K. Preclinical high-dose acetaminophen with N-acetylcysteine rescue enhances the efficacy of cisplatin chemotherapy in atypical teratoid rhabdoid tumors. *Pediatr. Blood Cancer* **2014**, *61*, 120–127. [CrossRef]
23. Wu, Y.J.; Neuwelt, A.J.; Muldoon, L.L.; Neuwelt, E.A. Acetaminophen enhances cisplatin- and paclitaxel-mediated cytotoxicity to SKOV3 human ovarian carcinoma. *Anticancer Res.* **2013**, *33*, 2391–2400. [PubMed]
24. Pingali, P.; Wu, Y.J.; Boothello, R.; Sharon, C.; Li, H.; Sistla, S.; Sankaranarayanan, N.V.; Desai, U.R.; Le, A.T.; Doebele, R.C.; et al. High dose acetaminophen inhibits STAT3 and has free radical independent anti-cancer stem cell activity. *Neoplasia* **2021**, *23*, 348–359. [CrossRef] [PubMed]

25. Bryan, A.; Pingali, P.; Joslyn, M.; Li, H.; Bernas, T.; Koblinski, J.; Landry, J.; Lee, W.S.; Patel, B.; Neuwelt, A. High-Dose Acetaminophen with N-acetylcysteine Rescue Inhibits M2 Polarization of Tumor-Associated Macrophages. *Cancers* **2023**, *15*, 4770. [CrossRef] [PubMed]
26. Akakpo, J.Y.; Ramachandran, A.; Curry, S.C.; Rumack, B.H.; Jaeschke, H. Comparing N-acetylcysteine and 4-methylpyrazole as antidotes for acetaminophen overdose. *Arch. Toxicol.* **2022**, *96*, 453–465. [CrossRef] [PubMed]
27. Khayyat, A.; Tobwala, S.; Hart, M.; Ercal, N. N-acetylcysteine amide, a promising antidote for acetaminophen toxicity. *Toxicol. Lett.* **2016**, *241*, 133–142. [CrossRef]
28. Akakpo, J.Y.; Ramachandran, A.; Duan, L.; Schaich, M.A.; Jaeschke, M.W.; Freudenthal, B.D.; Ding, W.X.; Rumack, B.H.; Jaeschke, H. Delayed Treatment With 4-Methylpyrazole Protects Against Acetaminophen Hepatotoxicity in Mice by Inhibition of c-Jun n-Terminal Kinase. *Toxicol. Sci.* **2019**, *170*, 57–68. [CrossRef] [PubMed]
29. James, L.P.; McCullough, S.S.; Lamps, L.W.; Hinson, J.A. Effect of N-acetylcysteine on acetaminophen toxicity in mice: Relationship to reactive nitrogen and cytokine formation. *Toxicol. Sci.* **2003**, *75*, 458–467. [CrossRef]
30. Dosa, E.; Heltai, K.; Radovits, T.; Molnar, G.; Kapocsi, J.; Merkely, B.; Fu, R.; Doolittle, N.D.; Toth, G.B.; Urdang, Z.; et al. Dose escalation study of intravenous and intra-arterial N-acetylcysteine for the prevention of oto- and nephrotoxicity of cisplatin with a contrast-induced nephropathy model in patients with renal insufficiency. *Fluids Barriers CNS* **2017**, *14*, 26. [CrossRef]
31. Muramatsu, S.; Shiraishi, S.; Miyano, K.; Sudo, Y.; Toda, A.; Mogi, M.; Hara, M.; Yokoyama, A.; Kawasaki, Y.; Taniguchi, M.; et al. Metabolism of AM404 From Acetaminophen at Human Therapeutic Dosages in the Rat Brain. *Anesth. Pain. Med.* **2016**, *6*, e32873. [CrossRef]
32. Bryan, A.; Pingali, P.; Faber, A.; Landry, J.; Akakpo, J.; Jaeschke, H.; Li, H.; Lee, W.; May, L.; Patel, B.; et al. High dose acetaminophen with concurrent CYP2E1 inhibition has profound anti-cancer activity without liver toxicity. *J. Pharmacol. Exp. Ther.* **2023**, *388*, 209–217. [CrossRef]
33. Villarino, A.V.; Kanno, Y.; Ferdinand, J.R.; O'Shea, J.J. Mechanisms of Jak/STAT signaling in immunity and disease. *J. Immunol.* **2015**, *194*, 21–27. [CrossRef]
34. Hogestatt, E.D.; Jonsson, B.A.; Ermund, A.; Andersson, D.A.; Bjork, H.; Alexander, J.P.; Cravatt, B.F.; Basbaum, A.I.; Zygmunt, P.M. Conversion of acetaminophen to the bioactive N-acylphenolamine AM404 via fatty acid amide hydrolase-dependent arachidonic acid conjugation in the nervous system. *J. Biol. Chem.* **2005**, *280*, 31405–31412. [CrossRef]

livers

MDPI

Review

Role of Mitochondrial Iron Uptake in Acetaminophen Hepatotoxicity †

Jiangting Hu [1,2], Anna-Liisa Nieminen [1,2,3], Zhi Zhong [1,2] and John J. Lemasters [1,2,3,4,*]

1 Center for Cell Death, Injury & Regeneration, Medical University of South Carolina, Charleston, SC 29425, USA; huj@musc.edu (J.H.); nieminen@musc.edu (A.-L.N.); zhong@musc.edu (Z.Z.)
2 Department of Drug Discovery & Biomedical Sciences, Medical University of South Carolina, Charleston, SC 29425, USA
3 Hollings Cancer Center, Medical University of South Carolina, Charleston, SC 29425, USA
4 Department of Biochemistry & Molecular Biology, Medical University of South Carolina, Charleston, SC 29425, USA
* Correspondence: jjlemasters@musc.edu; Fax: +1-843-876-2353

† Portions of this paper were adapted from the PhD dissertation of J.H. supervised by J.J.L.

Abstract: Overdose of acetaminophen (APAP) produces fulminant hepatic necrosis. The underlying mechanism of APAP hepatotoxicity involves mitochondrial dysfunction, including mitochondrial oxidant stress and the onset of mitochondrial permeability transition (MPT). Reactive oxygen species (ROS) play an important role in APAP-induced hepatotoxicity, and iron is a critical catalyst for ROS formation. This review summarizes the role of mitochondrial ROS formation in APAP hepatotoxicity and further focuses on the role of iron. Normally, hepatocytes take up Fe^{3+}-transferrin bound to transferrin receptors via endocytosis. Concentrated into lysosomes, the controlled release of iron is required for the mitochondrial biosynthesis of heme and non-heme iron-sulfur clusters. After APAP overdose, the toxic metabolite, NAPQI, damages lysosomes, causing excess iron release and the mitochondrial uptake of Fe^{2+} by the mitochondrial calcium uniporter (MCU). NAPQI also inhibits mitochondrial respiration to promote ROS formation, including H_2O_2, with which Fe^{2+} reacts to form highly reactive •OH through the Fenton reaction. •OH, in turn, causes lipid peroxidation, the formation of toxic aldehydes, induction of the MPT, and ultimately, cell death. Fe^{2+} also facilitates protein nitration. Targeting pathways of mitochondrial iron movement and consequent iron-dependent mitochondrial ROS formation is a promising strategy to intervene against APAP hepatotoxicity in a clinical setting.

Keywords: acetaminophen; iron; mitochondria; NAPQI; •OH; oxidative stress

1. Introduction

1.1. Epidemiology of Acetaminophen Hepatotoxicity

Acetaminophen (also known as Tylenol®, paracetamol, and N-acetyl-para-aminophenol and commonly abbreviated for the latter as APAP) is one of the most used antipyretic and analgesic medications and is often combined with cough-and-cold remedies and narcotic pain relievers. APAP is generally very safe in therapeutic doses. However, an overdose of APAP causes severe liver injury, leading to elevations of serum transaminases (ALT and AST), hepatic necrosis, and even acute liver failure requiring liver transplantation [1]. APAP hepatotoxicity is the leading cause of acute liver failure in the United States, and up to 50% of cases are unintentional [2]. The currently recommended maximal therapeutic dose is 4 g/day. However, it is estimated that 6% of adults in the USA are taking over 4 g/day due to APAP combination medications [3].

1.2. Metabolism of APAP

At therapeutic doses in humans, 85–90% of APAP becomes conjugated with sulfate and glucuronide and is excreted in urine. Only a small portion of APAP is metabolically activated by cytochrome P450 enzymes (mainly CYP2E1) to the toxic and reactive metabolite, *N*-acetyl-*p*-benzoquinoneimine (NAPQI). Under normal conditions, NAPQI is efficiently detoxified by conjugation with glutathione (GSH) [4]. After an overdose of APAP, the sulfate and glucuronide pathways become saturated, and CYP450 produces relatively more NAPQI. Subsequently, GSH becomes depleted by conjugation with NAPQI, and additional NAPQI can no longer be detoxified, which then leads to liver damage [5,6].

1.3. Risk Factors of APAP Hepatotoxicity

APAP toxicity shows a threshold dose dependence such that therapeutic doses are completely non-toxic, but the threshold dose causing liver damage varies between individuals. Not all individuals with APAP overdose progress to acute liver failure. Moreover, even at a therapeutic dose, APAP hepatotoxicity can occur under certain conditions. Accordingly, the safe upper limit of APAP for therapeutic indications remains controversial [7–9]. Genetic variation within the CYP450 system can cause differing sensitivity to APAP hepatotoxicity, as well as to other risk factors [10,11].

Malnutrition, fasting, and chronic liver disease may increase the risk of APAP hepatotoxicity by decreasing hepatic levels of GSH. A 6 h fast depletes hepatic GSH levels in mice by 44% [12]. Patients with already low GSH stores as a result of fasting or malnutrition can develop severe hepatotoxicity at recommended doses of APAP [13]. Infants and adults who are alcoholic or who take certain CYP450-inducing drugs may also be more prone to liver injury from APAP [14–16]. Commonly used upregulating CYP450 drugs include rifampin, isoniazid, and phenobarbital. Chronic alcohol use also causes CYP450 enzyme induction with the increased toxic metabolism of APAP to NAPQI and enhanced hepatotoxicity, even at therapeutic doses. Fibrates, nonsteroidal anti-inflammatory drugs (NSAIDs), and alcohol are associated with a higher incidence of death in patients with APAP-associated liver injury [17]. Nonalcoholic fatty liver disease (NAFLD), recently renamed metabolic dysfunction-associated steatotic liver disease (MASLD) [18], is also associated with increased CYP2E1 activity and is accompanied by an increased risk of APAP-induced hepatotoxicity [19].

1.4. Treatment for APAP Hepatotoxicity

Early diagnosis means early intervention, which is crucial to prevent APAP-induced acute liver failure (ALF). *N*-acetylcysteine (NAC) is the preferred antidote for APAP toxicity. NAC prevents hepatotoxicity by replenishing GSH stores, binding with NAPQI, and enhancing sulfate conjugation [20]. NAC may further limit APAP toxicity through antioxidant and anti-inflammatory effects. For maximal protection against liver injury, NAC should be given within 8 h after an APAP overdose in patients whose plasma APAP levels are above the "possible hepatic toxicity" line of the Rumack–Matthew nomogram [21,22]. NAC can be given intravenously or by mouth with similar efficacy for improving outcomes in APAP overdoses [23]. However, the indications and dosage for NAC are debated. Other treatments include activated charcoal and liver transplantation. Activated charcoal can be used within 4 h after taking APAP to limit the gastrointestinal absorption of APAP [24]. However, this treatment is ineffective in most cases because of the rapid absorption of APAP. Liver transplantation is the ultimate treatment for patients with ALF [25].

2. Role of Mitochondria in Pathogenesis of APAP Hepatotoxicity

The toxic metabolite NAPQI, rather than APAP itself, causes hepatotoxicity [26]. The main mechanism causing liver injury is thought to be covalent NAPQI protein adduct formation, which leads to mitochondrial dysfunction, oxidative stress due to GSH depletion by conjugation with NAPQI, and cell death [27].

2.1. Mitochondrial Permeability Transition in APAP Hepatotoxicity

Mitochondria are a primary target of NAPQI. The expression of some CYP2E1 in the mitochondrial inner membrane rather than the endoplasmic reticulum may account, at least in part, for mitochondrial NAPQI protein adduct formation [28–30]. Mitochondrial protein adduct formation with NAPQI causes oxidative stress, which leads to various mitochondrial dysfunctions, including respiratory inhibition, decreased hepatic ATP, decreased mitochondrial membrane potential ($\Delta\Psi$), and the onset of the mitochondrial permeability transition (MPT) [31,32]. Interestingly, low-dose APAP, which does not cause necrosis in vivo, can still produce MPT-dependent mitochondrial depolarization, which is reversible [33,34].

The MPT is an abrupt increase in the permeability of the mitochondrial inner membrane to molecules of less than about 1500 Daltons in molecular weight [35,36]. Ca^{2+} activates MPT onset, whereas cyclosporin A (CsA) and non-immunosuppressive analogs like NIM811 inhibit permeability transition (PT) pore opening [37,38]. In one model, PT pores are formed by the voltage-dependent anion channel (VDAC) in the outer membrane, the adenine nucleotide translocator (ANT) in the inner membrane, and cyclophilin D (CypD) in the matrix. However, the genetic deletion of ANT1/ANT2 and VDAC does not prevent the onset of the MPT [39–41], although more recent studies in triple ANT1, 2, and 4 and CypD-deficient mice and cell lines indicate that the MPT requires ANT and CsA-binding CypD [42,43]. Other studies suggest that dimers or oligomers of the mitochondrial F_1F_O-ATP synthase or the c-rings of the F_O subunit of the synthase form PT pores [44–46], but other studies show that Ca^{2+}-induced PT pore-opening persists after genetic interventions that prevent assembly ATP synthase monomers, dimers, or oligomers [47–49]. Another recent study concludes that the ATP synthase is a negative rather than a positive regulator of PT pores [50]. In addition, regulated and unregulated conductance modes for PT pores have been described: one activated by Ca^{2+} and inhibited by CsA and the other not requiring Ca^{2+} for activation and not inhibited by CsA [51]. Consistent with regulated and unregulated pore opening, a different model of pore formation and gating proposes that PT pores are created by misfolded integral membrane proteins damaged by oxidants and other stresses. These misfolded proteins aggregate at exposed hydrophilic surfaces within the membrane bilayer to form aqueous channels. Chaperone-like proteins, including CypD, a peptidyl-prolyl cis-trans isomerase or foldase, initially block conductance through these misfolded protein clusters. However, increased Ca^{2+} acting on CypD opens these regulated PT pores, which is an effect blocked by CsA. When protein clusters exceed chaperones available to block conductance, unregulated pore opening occurs [51,52]. Thus, in this proposal, PT pores comprise multiple different molecular species, which is a conclusion increasingly made in experimental studies [42,53–55]. Nonetheless, the precise molecular composition of the PT pore or pores remains controversial.

CsA specifically blocks the MPT by binding to CypD [56]. NIM811 (N-methyl-4-isoleucine cyclosporin) is a non-immunosuppressive derivative of CsA that inhibits the MPT equivalently to CsA in isolated mitochondria [33,57]. NIM811 is protective to cultured hepatocytes and livers in vivo after a variety of injurious stresses, including ischemia/reperfusion injury, transplantation, massive hepatectomy, and cholestatic injury [58–61]. CsA and NIM811 also inhibit the MPT and attenuate APAP hepatotoxicity both in vivo and in vitro [31,33,62,63]. As discussed above, PT pores have two open conductance modes—a Ca^{2+}-activated and CsA-sensitive regulated mode associated with early PT pore opening and an unregulated mode occurring later, which does not require Ca^{2+} and is not inhibited by CsA [51]. In cultured mouse hepatocytes, CsA and NIM811 delay but do not prevent APAP-induced mitochondrial depolarization, indicating that APAP initially induces a regulated MPT that is later superseded by an unregulated MPT [31]. Ultimately, the release of proapoptotic mitochondrial proteins, together with the cessation of ATP production, leads to cell death [31,64,65].

2.2. Apoptosis and Necrosis in APAP Hepatotoxicity

Whether apoptosis or necrosis is the major mode of cell death in APAP hepatotoxicity has been a controversial topic. The MPT plays an important role in the development of both necrotic and apoptotic cell death [66]. Specifically, the uncoupling of oxidative phosphorylation after the MPT causes ATP depletion, which leads to necrotic cell killing, whereas the mitochondrial outer membrane rupture after MPT-induced mitochondrial swelling causes cytochrome *c* release and apoptosis. In vitro, APAP mainly induces necrosis in cultured mouse hepatocytes. However, apoptosis increases when necrotic cell death is blocked [67]. Animal studies suggest that APAP-induced hepatic damage is predominantly oncotic necrosis rather than apoptosis [68]. Although modest caspase activation resulting from the release of mitochondrial proteins may occur after APAP, it is insufficient to actually cause significant apoptotic cell death [69]. Nonetheless, a human study reported increased serum apoptotic markers in patients with APAP-induced acute liver failure and suggested the predictive role of apoptotic markers in the progression of acute liver failure after APAP overdose [70].

2.3. c-Jun N-Terminal Protein Kinase Activation in APAP Hepatotoxicity

In mice and cultured mouse hepatocytes after APAP exposure, c-Jun N-terminal protein kinase (JNK), a mitogen-activated protein kinase (MAPK), becomes phosphorylated, signifying activation [71]. Phospho-JNK (p-JNK) then translocates to mitochondria by binding and phosphorylating the outer membrane protein SAB, an abbreviation for the SH3 domain-binding protein that preferentially associates with Bruton's tyrosine kinase [72,73]. The subsequent release of protein tyrosine phosphatase nonreceptor type 6 (PTPN6) from SAB in the intermembrane space leads to the dephosphorylation of mitochondrial tyrosine-protein kinase c-SRC [74]. Decreased phospho-c-SRC leads to the inhibition of the respiratory chain, which enhances the generation of reactive oxygen species (ROS) [73,75]. The amplified oxidant stress then causes sustained JNK activation and promotes an APAP-induced MPT [32,76]. Platanosides, a botanical drug combination, decrease liver injury from APAP overdose in mice, possibly by preventing sustained JNK activation [77]. After low-dose APAP is given to mice, reversible hepatic mitochondrial dysfunction occurs associated with transient JNK activation [33].

3. Role of Oxidative Stress in APAP Hepatotoxicity

Oxidative stress is a principal mediator of toxicity and has been suggested as an important mechanism in APAP-induced hepatotoxicity. ROS formation increases after APAP exposure and agents that augment antioxidant defenses and scavenge ROS protect against APAP toxicity in vitro and in vivo [78]. The formation of ROS like $O_2\bullet^-$ occurs selectively in mitochondria after the initial metabolism of APAP and originates at least in part from Complex III of the respiratory chain [79–82].

The Fenton or iron-catalyzed Haber–Weiss reaction is critical following oxidative stress during APAP toxicity [83]. Initially, superoxide ($O_2\bullet^-$) may be formed by activated NADPH oxidase, loosely coupled CYP2E1, and the NAPQI-dependent disruption of the mitochondrial respiratory chain. Dismutation catalyzed by superoxide dismutase (SOD) converts $O_2\bullet^-$ to H_2O_2. After an APAP overdose, H_2O_2 cannot be completely detoxified by glutathione peroxidase since its cofactor, GSH, becomes depleted by NAPQI. $O_2\bullet^-$ also reduces ferric iron (Fe^{3+}) to ferrous iron (Fe^{2+}). Fe^{2+}, thus, formed reacts rapidly with H_2O_2 to form the highly reactive hydroxyl radical ($\bullet$OH) [27,81,83]. $\bullet$OH, in turn, damages protein and DNA, as well as causing lipid peroxidation and the breakdown of membranes. However, the most critical effect of this oxidative stress is the induction of the MPT, which produces bioenergetic failure and, ultimately, cell death [31,63].

4. Iron Metabolism

Iron is essential in the catalysis of many, if not most, enzymatic reactions that involve electron transfer and play a critical role in cellular survival. However, free iron is toxic due to its ability to generate free radicals via the Fenton reaction and to catalyze lipid peroxidation chain reactions [83,84]. Thus, the control of this necessary but potentially toxic metal is important for human health and disease. Iron homeostasis is tightly controlled by the regulation of its cellular import, storage, and intracellular movement [85,86].

4.1. Cellular Iron Metabolism

In animal cells, non-heme iron is transported into cells through two main pathways: transferrin (Tf)-bound iron uptake and non-Tf-bound iron (NTBI) uptake. NTBI uptake occurs when the body absorbs dietary iron from the intestinal lumen, or when Tf becomes saturated with iron because of iron overload. Although the exact NTBI uptake pathway is unclear, it is proposed that reductases, such as duodenal cytochrome *b* (Dcytb), reduce Fe^{3+} to Fe^{2+}, which is then imported into cells via divalent metal transporter 1 (DMT1) or ZRT/IRT-like proteins (ZIPs) [87–89].

Under physiological conditions, almost all serum iron is bound to Tf. The uptake of Tf-bound iron through Tf receptor-1 (TfR1) is the major pathway for the delivery of iron into cells [85,86]. Tf-dependent iron delivery begins with the binding of diferric Tf to TfR1 on the cell surface, followed by the endocytosis of the Tf-TfR1 complex. As pH decreases during endosome maturation and fusion with lysosomes, Fe^{3+} dissociates from Tf, and both Tf and TfR1 recycle to the cell surface for another round of iron uptake. A ferrireductase (Steap3) then reduces dissociated Fe^{3+} to Fe^{2+} within the endosomal/lysosomal compartment. Fe^{2+} subsequently exits the endosomal/lysosomal compartment into the cytosol via DMT1 or ZIP14 [90,91]. The release of Fe^{2+} from endosomal/lysosomal membranes appears to involve an Fe^{2+}/H^+ exchange mechanism [92]. Iron released to the cytosol is in a soluble, chelatable state, which constitutes the labile iron pool (LIP). From this pool, iron can be stored in ferritin, utilized for metabolism (*e.g.*, imported into mitochondria for the synthesis of heme and Fe-S clusters), used to generate ROS, or exported from the cell by ferroportin 1 (FPN1) [85,86]. Notably, lysosomes are additionally involved in intracellular iron recycling because of the degradation of many macromolecules containing iron inside the lysosomal lumen [93].

4.2. Mitochondrial Iron Metabolism

Mitochondria utilize iron for the synthesis of heme and Fe-S clusters [94–97]. Iron moves into mitochondria using the following hypothesized mechanisms: (i) Iron-loaded endosomes/lysosomes interact directly with mitochondria by a "kiss-and-run" mechanism, leading to mitochondrial iron uptake [98]. (ii) Iron from ferritin transfers into mitochondria after ferritin complex degradation [99–101]. These mechanisms remain incompletely understood and need further study.

Two transporters, the mitochondrial calcium uniporter (MCU) and the two isoforms of mitoferrin (Mfrn1/2), play essential roles in transporting iron across the inner membrane. MCU catalyzes the electrogenic mitochondrial uptake of both Ca^{2+} and Fe^{2+} driven by the negative inside mitochondrial $\Delta\Psi$, which is blocked by the specific MCU inhibitor, Ru360 [81,102–104]. Mfrn1 and its paralog Mfrn2 also mediate mitochondrial iron uptake in erythroid and non-erythroid cells, respectively [105,106]. Because mitochondrial iron uptake is needed for heme synthesis, the deletion of Mfrn1 in hematopoietic tissues leads to anemia [106]. Some evidence indicates that Mfrn2 physically interacts with MCU, possibly as a component and/or regulator of the MCU complex [107].

Once imported into mitochondria, iron is utilized for the synthesis of heme and Fe-S clusters, which are incorporated into respiratory and other enzymes inside the mitochondria or exported to the cytosol to become prosthetic groups for cytosolic enzymes. Mitochondrial iron is also stored in mitochondrial ferritin (FTMT) [108].

4.3. Role of Iron in Common Models of Acute Liver Injury

However, when mitochondrial iron uptake results in iron overload and simultaneously H_2O_2 is generated by mitochondrial respiration that cannot be detoxified by antioxidant systems, Fe^{2+} and H_2O_2 react to form •OH, leading to lipid peroxidation, mitochondrial dysfunction, DNA damage, and a form of necrotic cell death now called ferroptosis [83,104,109,110]. Iron chelators like desferal and starch-desferal decrease mitochondrial ROS formation, MPT opening, and cell killing in cultured rat hepatocyte models of hypoxia/ischemia [104]. Desferal also protects against lethal injury to cultured hepatocytes from *tert*-butyl hydroperoxide, as does the lipid radical scavenger, N,N-diphenyl-p-phenylenediamine (DPPD) [111,112]. Another iron chelator, deferasirox, protects against concanavalin A-induced hepatic injury and fibrosis in rats [113]. Cytoprotection by iron chelators against hypoxia/ischemia, oxidative stress, and APAP hepatotoxicity infers a critical role for iron in the pathogenesis of injury, most likely by catalyzing •OH formation and subsequent lipid peroxidation [104,111,114–117].

5. Iron and Acetaminophen Hepatotoxicity

5.1. Evidence for Mitochondrial Iron Uptake in Acetaminophen Hepatotoxicity

After APAP overdose, the mitochondrial generation of ROS is a critical factor triggering the MPT, and iron promotes this oxidative stress [81]. Iron chelators and antioxidants that scavenge ROS protect against APAP toxicity in vitro and in vivo [114,118–121]. Treatment with the iron chelator, desferal (also called deferoxamine or desferrioxamine), increases the time required for APAP to induce ROS and mitochondrial dysfunction in cultured mouse hepatocytes [122]. After iron chelation with desferal, the addition of iron to the culture medium restores the sensitivity of hepatocytes to APAP toxicity in vitro [114,120]. Moreover, the treatment of mouse hepatocytes with the iron donor 3,5,5-trimethyl-hexanoyl ferrocene (TMHF) causes APAP-induced ROS formation and mitochondrial dysfunction to occur at earlier time points than APAP treatment alone, which is partially prevented by desferal [122].

Several fluorescent probes can visualize intracellular iron movement between organelles. The exogenously added calcein-acetoxymethylester (AM) is de-esterified in the cytosol to release calcein-free acid, whose fluorescence is quenched by chelatable Fe^{2+} [92,104,123]. Mitoferrofluor (MFF) is another iron indicator that accumulates electrophoretically into mitochondria in response to $\Delta\Psi$ and then binds covalently to mitochondrial proteins. Like green-fluorescing calcein, red-fluorescing MFF is quenched by chelatable Fe^{2+} [124]. Calcein and MFF can be used together or in combination with fluorescent indicators of mitochondrial $\Delta\Psi$, such as red-fluorescing tetramethylrhodamine methylester (TMRM) and green-fluorescing rhodamine 123 (Rh123) [81,124]. To visualize lysosomes, cells can be pre-loaded with red-fluorescing rhodamine-dextran, which is taken up via endocytosis and delivered to the lysosomes [116].

In cultured mouse hepatocytes, APAP causes lysosomes to rupture and release rhodamine-dextran into the cytosol within 4 h (Figure 1, top row). The mechanism underlying APAP-induced lysosomal rupture is not known. The APAP metabolite, NAPQI, may react covalently with lysosomal membrane components to cause the rupture. In parallel, cytosolic calcein fluorescence becomes quenched, though this is not the case for the fluorescence of calcein-free acid added to the extracellular medium, indicating an increase in cytosolic Fe^{2+} due to its release from lysosomes (Figure 1, bottom row) [81]. Starch-desferal suppresses the increase in cytosolic and mitochondrial Fe^{2+} after APAP [81]. Since membrane-impermeant starch-desferal is taken up via endocytosis into the lysosomal/endosomal compartment like rhodamine-dextran, the prevention of APAP-induced increases in cytosolic and mitochondrial Fe^{2+} by starch-desferal confirms that endosomes/lysosomes are the source of mobilizable chelatable iron entering the cytosol and mitochondria during APAP hepatotoxicity. Other sources of iron may promote the Fenton reaction in mitochondria. For example, ROS promote heme oxygenase 1 (HO-1) translocation to mitochondria in cardiomyocytes, leading to iron release from heme [125]. Further study is needed to determine whether HO-1 is involved in APAP hepatotoxicity.

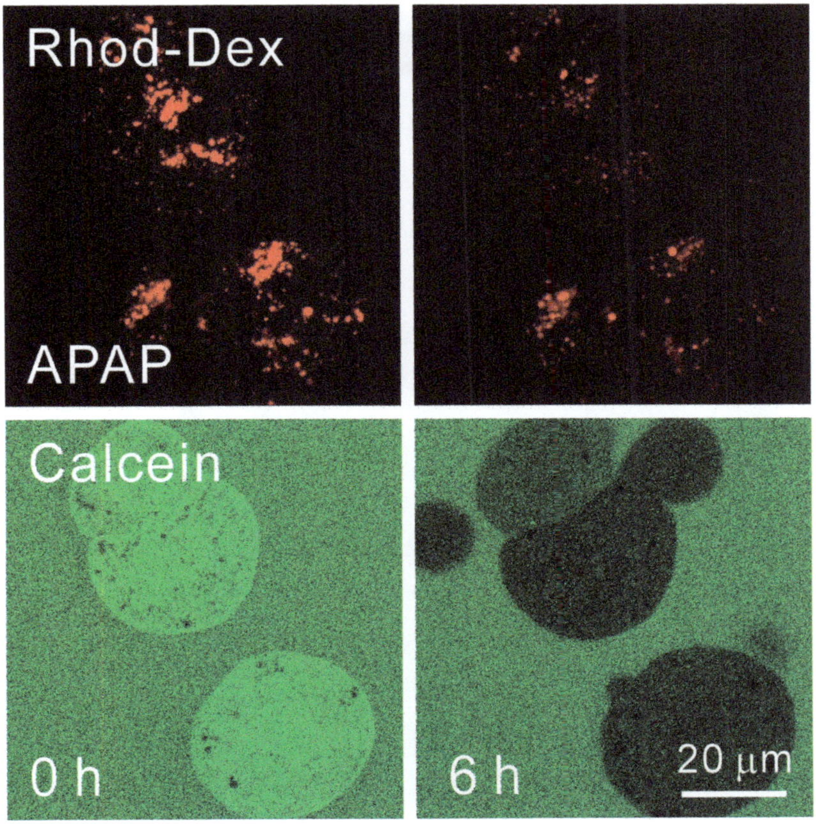

Figure 1. Acetaminophen-dependent lysosomal permeabilization and release of Fe^{2+} into the cytosol. Wildtype mouse hepatocytes were isolated from mice injected with 70 kDa rhodamine-dextran and then loaded with 1 µM calcein-AM. Rhodamine-dextran labeled lysosomes, whereas calcein-AM was de-esterified to release calcein-free acid into the cytosol. In the presence of 20 mM of fructose plus 5 mM of glycine to prevent cell death after APAP-induced disruption of mitochondrial metabolism, hepatocytes were then exposed to acetaminophen (APAP, 10 mM). Before APAP (0 h), rhodamine-dextran-labeled lysosomes were intact, and cytosolic calcein fluorescence was bright in comparison to the fluorescence of 300 µM of calcein-free acid placed in the extracelluar medium. At 4 h after APAP, many rhodamine-dextran–labeled lysosomes disappeared in parallel with the quenching of calcein fluorescence. This calcein quenching signified increased cytosolic chelatable Fe^{2+}. As lysosomes disappeared, diffuse red fluorescence appeared in the cytosol, signifying that acetaminophen permeabilized many lysosomes. After [116].

5.2. Role of the Mitochondrial Calcium Uniporter in Mitochondrial Iron Uptake during Acetaminophen Hepatotoxicity

Movement into the mitochondria of Fe^{2+} released from ruptured lysosomes is mediated by MCU, an electrogenic Ca^{2+} transporter that also conducts Fe^{2+}, since the MCU inhibitors, Ru360 and minocycline, block MFF quenching but not calcein quenching after APAP [81]. Further support for this role of MCU is provided by studies using mice with a hepatocyte-specific MCU (hsMCU) deficiency. In wildtype hepatocytes, mitochondrial MFF fluorescence is bright but subsequently progressively decreases after APAP exposure, beginning within 4 h and becoming virtually complete after 12 h (Figure 2A, bottom row). In parallel, mitochondrial depolarization (the loss of Rh123 fluorescence), signifying the onset of the MPT, begins to occur within 8 h and is complete within 12 h (Figure 2A, top row). By contrast, in hsMCU KO hepatocytes that are deficient in MCU, mitochondrial MFF quenching and mitochondrial depolarization are suppressed after APAP (Figure 2B). Nonetheless, cytosolic calcein fluorescence is just as strongly quenched after APAP in MCU-deficient hepatocytes as in wildtype hepatocytes showing that lysosomes still release Fe^{2+} (Figures 1 and 3). Both in vitro and in vivo, lysosomal iron chelation with starch-desferal and the inhibition of MCU-mediated mitochondrial iron uptake protect against APAP-induced hepatotoxicity [81,116,117,126]. Notably, both the global- and hepatocyte-specific deficiency of MCU decreases APAP hepatotoxicity in vivo as assessed by ALT release and necrosis by histology without altering hepatic APAP metabolism [126]. In addition, the co-treatment of APAP with $FeSO_4$ dramatically increases APAP-induced hepatotoxicity, which is prevented by desferal [27].

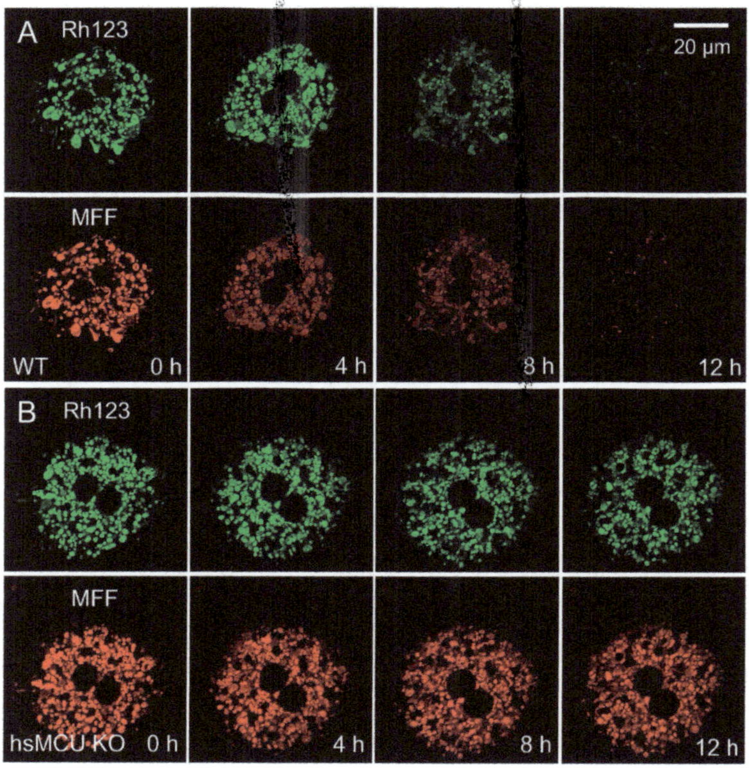

Figure 2. Suppression of mitochondrial iron uptake and depolarization after acetaminophen treatment of hepatocytes deficient in the mitochondrial calcium uniporter. Wildtype and hsMCU KO hepatocytes were loaded with 300 nM of Rh123 plus 1 μM of MFF and exposed to 10 mM APAP in the presence of 20 mM of fructose plus 5 mM of glycine. Rh123 is a green-fluorescing indicator of mitochondrial ΔΨ. Mitoferrofluor (MFF) accumulates electrophoretically into mitochondria, binds covalently, and becomes quenched as mitochondrial Fe^{2+} increases. (**A**) In wildtype (WT) hepatocytes, red mitochondrial MFF fluorescence was bright at 0 h but subsequently quenched progressively, beginning within 4 h and becoming virtually complete after 12 h (bottom row). Mitochondrial depolarization (loss of green Rh123 fluorescence) began to occur at 8 h and was complete after 12 h (top row). (**B**) In hsMCU KO hepatocytes, mitochondrial MFF quenching and mitochondrial depolarization were suppressed after APAP. After [126].

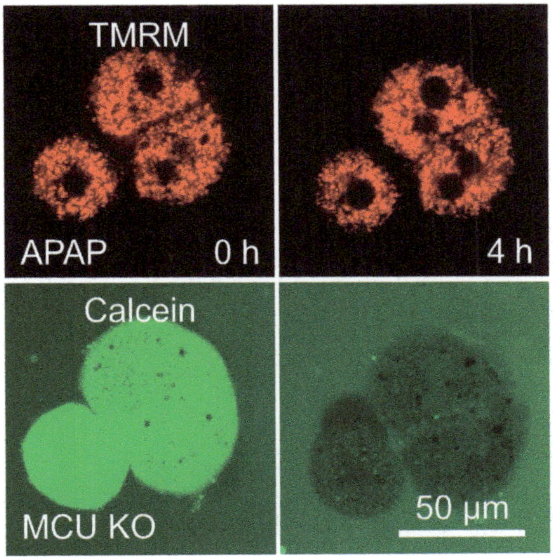

Figure 3. Increased cytosolic Fe^{2+} in MCU-deficient hepatocytes after acetaminophen. Hepatocytes were loaded with 300 nM of TMRM plus 1 µM of calcein-AM and incubated with 300 µM of calcein-free before exposure to 10 mM APAP in the presence of 20 mM fructose plus 5 mM glycine. TMRM is a red-fluorescing indicator of mitochondrial $\Delta\Psi$. When MCU-deficient hepatocytes were exposed to 10 mM APAP, mitochondrial depolarization (loss of TMRM fluorescence) was suppressed. However, the green cytosolic calcein fluorescence decreased substantially similarly to wildtype hepatocytes, signifying increased cytosolic chelatable Fe^{2+}. After [126].

5.3. Possible Roles of Kupffer Cells and JNK in Iron-Dependency of Acetaminophen Hepatotoxicity

Kupffer cells are liver-resident macrophages that are involved in the phagocytosis of senescent red blood cells and the recycling of iron [127]. Kupffer cells are also a potential source of oxidant stress promoting cell death [128]. Human and mouse studies indicate that Kupffer cells and infiltrating monocyte-derived macrophages have both injury-promoting and injury-repair functions after APAP overdose [129–133]. Although MCU deficiency in hepatocytes decreases liver necrosis and ALT release after APAP in mice, MCU deficiency in Kupffer cells does not alter APAP hepatotoxicity [126].

JNK activation in the cytosol and translocation of p-JNK to mitochondria are important early events promoting the MPT and cell death in APAP hepatotoxicity [32]. Recent in vivo studies in mice show that neither desferal nor Fe^{2+} treatment affects JNK activation and its translocation to mitochondria after APAP overdose [27]. These findings suggest that the effect of iron is not at the early stages of the response to APAP but specifically at later events within mitochondria.

5.4. "Two Hit" Hypothesis

Overall, these results support a "two hit" hypothesis for the role of oxidative stress and iron in APAP hepatotoxicity (Figure 4) [81] (see also [104]). In the first hit, CYP2E1 metabolizes APAP to NAPQI, which induces mitochondrial protein adduct formation, the disruption of mitochondrial respiration, and consequent generation of $O_2^{\bullet-}$ and H_2O_2. These ROS also activate JNK, which translocates to mitochondria to further inhibit respiration with the feed-forward effect of enhancing mitochondrial ROS generation even more. In the second hit, toxic NAPQI causes lysosomal breakdown and the release of chelatable Fe^{2+} into the cytosol. Fe^{2+} is then taken up into mitochondria via MCU. In the presence of $O_2^{\bullet-}$ and H_2O_2, such mitochondrial Fe^{2+} loading induces •OH formation via the Fenton reaction, which in turn causes MPT onset, mitochondria depolarization, bioenergetic failure, and cell death. Iron imported into mitochondria also facilitates protein nitration by peroxynitrite ($ONOO^-$), which is formed from the reaction of $O_2^{\bullet-}$ with nitric oxide (NO) [27].

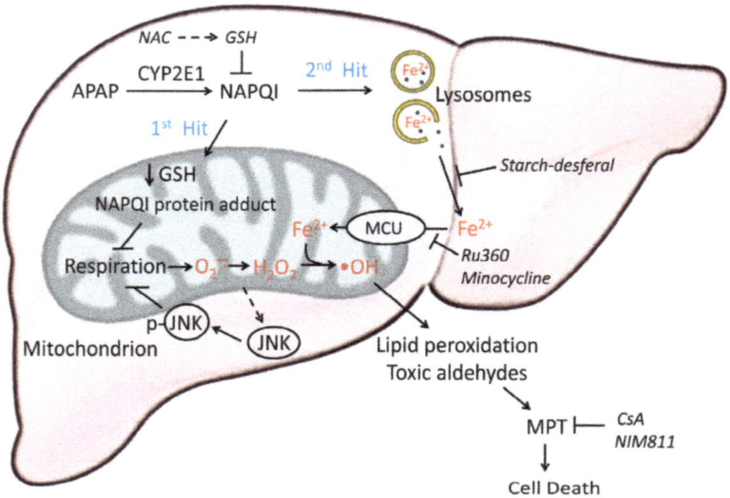

Figure 4. Two-hit model of APAP hepatotoxicity. After an overdose of APAP, the first hit occurs when APAP causes GSH depletion, NAPQI protein adduct formation, and the inhibition of mitochondrial respiration, which induces $O_2^{\bullet-}$ and H_2O_2 formation. ROS-induced JNK phosphorylation and activation further enhance respiratory inhibition and mitochondrial ROS formation. The second hit occurs when NAPQI damages lysosomes and releases Fe^{2+} into the cytosol, which is then taken up into mitochondria via the electrogenic MCU to promote intramitochondrial •OH formation by the Fenton reaction. •OH, in turn, induces lipid peroxidation, the formation of toxic aldehydes, MPT onset, and mitochondrial bioenergetic failure, leading to the loss of cell viability. Starch-desferal chelates lysosomal iron to prevent the release of chelatable iron after lysosomal disruption and subsequent uptake into mitochondria to promote •OH formation. Ru360 and minocycline block mitochondrial iron uptake via MCU to also suppress iron-catalyzed •OH formation in the mitochondrial matrix. CsA and NIM811 inhibit MPT. Blocking either hit protects against APAP-induced hepatic injury.

5.5. Ferroptosis during Acetaminophen Hepatotoxicity

Iron has long been known to promote lipid peroxidation and cell death in various models of cell injury (see [112,115,120,134,135]). During APAP toxicity to cultured hepatocytes, DPPD, a scavenger of lipid radicals, prevents both lipid peroxidation and cell death [111,136]. Similarly, ferrostatin-1, a scavenger of alkoxyl radicals that propagate lipid peroxidation chain reactions, protects against APAP-induced hepatotoxicity in mice [137]. Non-apoptotic iron-dependent cell death involving lipid peroxidation and mitochondrial iron-loading has more recently been named ferroptosis [110,138]. A novel ferroptosis inhibitor, mifepristone, prevents APAP-induced hepatotoxicity in vitro and in mice in vivo [139], and growth arrest-specific 1 (GAS1) overexpression promotes ferroptosis and aggravates APAP-induced hepatocellular injury both in vitro and in vivo [140].

5.6. Role of Peroxynitrite and Protein Nitration in Acetaminophen Hepatotoxicity

Protein nitration is an important pathophysiological event in APAP hepatotoxicity [141,142]. During APAP overdose, respiratory chain dysfunction leads to the generation of $O_2\bullet^-$, which reacts with NO to form reactive and toxic $ONOO^-$ in the mitochondrial matrix [27,143]. The mitochondrial uptake of iron released from lysosomes then promotes $ONOO^-$-dependent nitration of protein tyrosine residues to form nitrotyrosine protein adducts [27,144]. This stress further induces the MPT in APAP toxicity (Figure 5). Consistent with this mechanism in vivo after APAP overdose, desferal and the MCU blocker, minocycline, attenuate immunostaining for nitrotyrosine protein adducts and the release of the mitochondrial intermembrane protein, cytochrome *c*, which is a consequence of mitochondrial swelling after MPT onset [27]. The co-treatment of APAP with $FeSO_4$ in mice further increases nitrotyrosine staining and the release of cytochrome *c*, as well as causing lipid peroxidation, which desferal inhibits [27]. Moreover, the mitochondria-specific SOD mimetic, mito-TEMPO, protects against APAP-induced liver injury and nitrotyrosine protein adduct formation in mice [145].

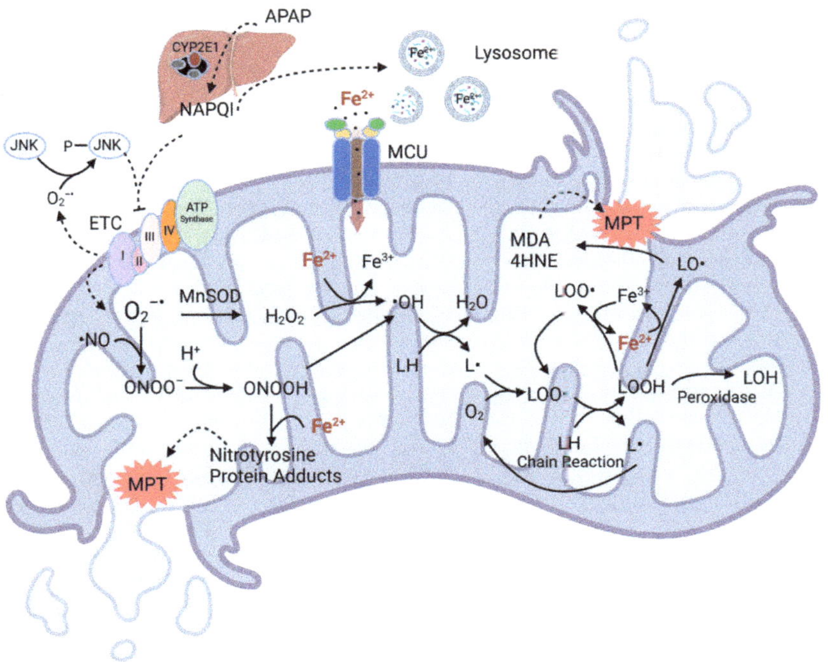

Figure 5. Role of iron in oxidative stress in APAP-induced mitochondrial damage. After an overdose of APAP, NAPQI binds to mitochondrial proteins to inhibit mitochondrial respiration. Respiratory inhibition leads to increased levels of flavin semiquinones and ubisemiquinone, which react with oxygen to form $O_2\bullet^-$. Such respiratory inhibition and ROS generation are further amplified through ROS-driven JNK activation. $O_2\bullet^-$ reacts rapidly with NO to form $ONOO^-$. The iron influx into mitochondria facilitates the reaction of $ONOO^-$ with proteins to produce nitrotyrosine adducts, ultimately promoting the MPT. SOD2 in mitochondria also converts $O_2\bullet^-$ to H_2O_2. Fe^{2+}, which is released from damaged lysosomes, is taken up into mitochondria via MCU and reacts with H_2O_2 to form the toxic •OH, which induces L• formation. L• then initiates an oxygen-dependent chain reaction generating peroxyl radicals (LOO•) and lipid peroxides (LOOHs). In the presence of Fe^{2+}, LOOH produces LO•. The beta scission of LO• then leads to the formation of reactive aldehydes like MDA and 4HNE, which also promote MPT onset. This figure was created with BioRender.com.

5.7. *Aldehydes as Drivers of Acetaminophen Hepatotoxicity*

•OH from Fenton chemistry reacts with unsaturated lipids to initiate a lipid peroxidation chain reaction with the formation of lipid radicals (L•), lipid peroxides (LOOH), and peroxyl radicals (LOO•). Iron is an important catalyst to then promote a subsequent alkoxyl radical (LO•) and more LOO• formation. Notably, the spontaneous non-enzymatic beta-scission of LO• generates a variety of aldehydes, including malondialdehyde (MDA) and 4-hydroxynonenal (4-HNE), which are often used as biomarkers for lipid peroxidation. However, MDA, 4-HNE, and other aldehydes formed downstream of lipid peroxidation are toxic, reactive, and mutagenic, with MDA reported to be the most mutagenic and 4-HNE the most toxic [146–148].

Lipid peroxidation in APAP hepatotoxicity was initially indicated by the appearance of exhalated hydrocarbons in mice in vivo and by MDA formation in liver homogenates in vitro that inducers and inhibitors of P450 enzymes, respectively, up and down modulate [149,150]. However, these studies were performed with mice fed a vitamin E-deficient diet high in polyunsaturated fatty acids that made the animals sensitive to lipid peroxidation induced by APAP [150,151]. A follow-up study with mice fed a regular diet showed minimal evidence for lipid peroxidation after APAP [152]. Furthermore, mice fed a diet high in vitamin E diet do not show decreased APAP hepatotoxicity, suggesting that endogenous defense mechanisms are normally sufficient to prevent excessive lipid peroxidation after APAP [152]. Additionally, the co-treatment of Fe^{2+} with APAP increases lipid peroxidation in vivo in mice, which desferal almost completely prevents [27,153]. Nonetheless, other reports show that APAP stimulates lipid peroxidation in isolated mouse and rat hepatocytes in vitro [154,155], and mass spectroscopy reveals lipid peroxides derived from n-6 fatty acids, mainly from arachidonic acid, after APAP overdose [137]. Moreover, 4-HNE adduct formation increases after APAP in mice fed normal chow [156].

N-(1,3-benzodioxol-5-ylmethyl)-2,6-dichlorobenzamide (Alda-1) is an activator of mitochondrial aldehyde dehydrogenase-2 (ALDH2) and is responsible for detoxifying aldehyde oxidation to fatty acids [157]. After APAP in vivo, Alda-1 decreases 4-HNE adduct formation, APAP-induced liver injury, and mitochondrial dysfunction, indicating that lipid peroxidation-derived aldehydes are important mediators of APAP hepatotoxicity. Lipid peroxidation may occur relatively selectively in mitochondria that are the source of •OH from Fenton chemistry and whose membranes are enriched in arachidonic acid.

6. Summary and Conclusions

Iron-catalyzed free radical generation in mitochondria plays an important role in APAP toxicity (Figure 5). Initially, the toxic APAP metabolite, NAPQI, binds to mitochondrial proteins to inhibit mitochondrial respiration. Inhibited respiration leads to increased levels of ubisemiquinone and flavin semiquinone, which transfer their unpaired electrons to oxygen to form $O_2\bullet^-$. Respiratory inhibition is further amplified through JNK activation, leading to greater $O_2\bullet^-$ generation. $O_2\bullet^-$ reacts with nitric oxide to produce peroxynitrite or is converted to H_2O_2 by SOD. Since NAPQI depletes GSH after APAP overdose, GSH is no longer available to detoxify peroxynitrite and H_2O_2, as would occur normally. NAPQI also damages lysosomes, causing Fe^{2+} release into the cytosol and subsequent uptake into mitochondria via the MCU. Mitochondrial loading with Fe^{2+} facilitates nitrotyrosine protein adduct formation and Fenton chemistry with H_2O_2 to produce the highly reactive •OH. •OH, in turn, causes lipid peroxidation, the formation of toxic aldehydes, and induction of the MPT, ultimately leading to cell death. Accordingly, blocking pathways of iron movement into mitochondria via MCU, preventing iron-related mitochondrial •OH and $ONOO^-$ formation, and accelerating aldehyde metabolism are potential novel strategies to intervene against APAP hepatotoxicity in a clinical setting.

Author Contributions: J.H. wrote the first draft of the manuscript. A.-L.N., Z.Z. and J.J.L. contributed sections and edited the manuscript. All authors have read and agreed to the published version of the manuscript.

Funding: Work in the authors' laboratory was supported, in part, by grants AA021191, AA025379, AA022815, DK073336, DK119523, DK102142, ES031335, and UL1 TR001450 from the National Institutes of Health, United States. Imaging and spectroscopy facilities were supported, in part, by P20 GM130457, P30 CA138313, P30 DK123704, P30 GM140964, P30 GM118247, and 1 S10 OD018113.

Institutional Review Board Statement: Not applicable.

Informed Consent Statement: Not applicable.

Data Availability Statement: No new data were created or analyzed. Data sharing is not applicable to this article.

Conflicts of Interest: The authors declare no conflicts of interest.

Abbreviations

•OH, hydroxyl radical; ΔΨ, membrane potential; Alda-1, N-(1,3-benzodioxol-5-ylmethyl)-2,6-dichlorobenzamide; ALDH2, mitochondrial aldehyde dehydrogenase-2; ALF, acute liver failure; AM, acetoxymethylester; ANT, adenine nucleotide translocator; APAP, N-acetyl-para-aminophenol, acetaminophen; CsA, cyclosporin A; CypD, cyclophilin D; DMT1, divalent metal transporter 1; DPD, dipyridyl; DPPD′ N,N′-diphenyl-p-phenylenediamine; FPN1, ferroportin 1; FTMT, mitochondrial ferritin; GAS1, growth arrest-specific 1; GSH, glutathione; HDM, hormonally defined medium; 4-HNE, 4-hydroxynonenal; HO-1, heme oxygenase 1; JNK, c-Jun N-terminal protein kinase; LIP, labile iron pool; L•, lipid radicals; LOO•, peroxyl radical; LOOH, lipid peroxide; MAPK, mitogen-activated protein kinase; MASLD, metabolic dysfunction-associated steatotic liver disease; MCU, mitochondrial calcium uniporter; MDA, malondialdehyde; MFF, mitoferrofluor; Mfrn, mitoferrin; MPT, mitochondrial permeability transition; NAC, N-acetylcysteine; NAPQI, N-acetyl-p-benzoquinone imine; NO, nitric oxide; NTBI, non- transferrin-bound iron; $ONOO^-$, peroxynitrite; p-JNK, phospho-JNK; PI, propidium iodide; PT, permeability transition; PTPN6, protein tyrosine phosphatase nonreceptor type 6; Rh123, rhodamine 123; ROS, reactive oxygen species; SAB, SH3 domain-binding protein that preferentially associates with Bruton's tyrosine kinase; SOD, superoxide dismutase; Tf, transferrin; TfR1, Tf receptor-1; TMHF, 3,5,5-trimethyl-hexanoyl ferrocene; TMRM, tetramethylrhodamine methylester; VDAC, voltage-dependent anion channels; ZIPs, ZRT/IRT-like proteins.

References

1. Fisher, E.S.; Curry, S.C. Evaluation and treatment of acetaminophen toxicity. *Adv. Pharmacol.* **2019**, *85*, 263–272. [CrossRef]
2. Michna, E.; Duh, M.S.; Korves, C.; Dahl, J.L. Removal of opioid/acetaminophen combination prescription pain medications: Assessing the evidence for hepatotoxicity and consequences of removal of these medications. *Pain Med.* **2010**, *11*, 369–378. [CrossRef]
3. Blieden, M.; Paramore, L.C.; Shah, D.; Ben-Joseph, R. A perspective on the epidemiology of acetaminophen exposure and toxicity in the United States. *Expert Rev. Clin. Pharmacol.* **2014**, *7*, 341–348. [CrossRef]
4. Mitchell, J.R.; Jollow, D.J.; Potter, W.Z.; Gillette, J.R.; Brodie, B.B. Acetaminophen-induced hepatic necrosis. IV. Protective role of glutathione. *J. Pharmacol. Exp. Ther.* **1973**, *187*, 211–217.
5. McGill, M.R.; Jaeschke, H. Metabolism and disposition of acetaminophen: Recent advances in relation to hepatotoxicity and diagnosis. *Pharm. Res.* **2013**, *30*, 2174–2187. [CrossRef] [PubMed]
6. Ramachandran, A.; Jaeschke, H. Mitochondria in Acetaminophen-Induced Liver Injury and Recovery: A Concise Review. *Livers* **2023**, *3*, 219–231. [CrossRef] [PubMed]
7. Goyal, R.K.; Rajan, S.S.; Essien, E.J.; Sansgiry, S.S. Effectiveness of FDA's new over-the-counter acetaminophen warning label in improving consumer risk perception of liver damage. *J. Clin. Pharm. Ther.* **2012**, *37*, 681–685. [CrossRef]
8. Schilling, A.; Corey, R.; Leonard, M.; Eghtesad, B. Acetaminophen: Old drug, new warnings. *Cleve Clin. J. Med.* **2010**, *77*, 19–27. [CrossRef] [PubMed]
9. McGill, M.R.; James, L.P.; McCullough, S.S.; Moran, J.H.; Mathews, S.E.; Peterson, E.C.; Fleming, D.P.; Tripod, M.E.; Vazquez, J.H.; Kennon-McGill, S.; et al. Short-Term Safety of Repeated Acetaminophen Use in Patients with Compensated Cirrhosis. *Hepatol. Commun.* **2022**, *6*, 361–373. [CrossRef]
10. Myers, R.P.; Shaheen, A.A.; Li, B.; Dean, S.; Quan, H. Impact of liver disease, alcohol abuse, and unintentional ingestions on the outcomes of acetaminophen overdose. *Clin. Gastroenterol. Hepatol.* **2008**, *6*, 918–925, quiz 837. [CrossRef]
11. Bacle, A.; Pronier, C.; Gilardi, H.; Polard, E.; Potin, S.; Scailteux, L.M. Hepatotoxicity risk factors and acetaminophen dose adjustment, do prescribers give this issue adequate consideration? A French university hospital study. *Eur. J. Clin. Pharmacol.* **2019**, *75*, 1143–1151. [CrossRef] [PubMed]
12. Vogt, B.L.; Richie, J.P., Jr. Fasting-induced depletion of glutathione in the aging mouse. *Biochem. Pharmacol.* **1993**, *46*, 257–263. [CrossRef] [PubMed]
13. Kurtovic, J.; Riordan, S.M. Paracetamol-induced hepatotoxicity at recommended dosage. *J. Intern. Med.* **2003**, *253*, 240–243. [CrossRef] [PubMed]
14. Zimmerman, H.J.; Maddrey, W.C. Acetaminophen (paracetamol) hepatotoxicity with regular intake of alcohol: Analysis of instances of therapeutic misadventure. *Hepatology* **1995**, *22*, 767–773. [CrossRef] [PubMed]

15. James, L.P.; Alonso, E.M.; Hynan, L.S.; Hinson, J.A.; Davern, T.J.; Lee, W.M.; Squires, R.H.; Pediatric Acute Liver Failure Study, G. Detection of acetaminophen protein adducts in children with acute liver failure of indeterminate cause. *Pediatrics* **2006**, *118*, e676–e681. [CrossRef] [PubMed]
16. Chidiac, A.S.; Buckley, N.A.; Noghrehchi, F.; Cairns, R. Paracetamol (acetaminophen) overdose and hepatotoxicity: Mechanism, treatment, prevention measures, and estimates of burden of disease. *Expert Opin. Drug Metab. Toxicol.* **2023**, *19*, 297–317. [CrossRef]
17. Suzuki, A.; Yuen, N.; Walsh, J.; Papay, J.; Hunt, C.M.; Diehl, A.M. Co-medications that modulate liver injury and repair influence clinical outcome of acetaminophen-associated liver injury. *Clin. Gastroenterol. Hepatol.* **2009**, *7*, 882–888. [CrossRef] [PubMed]
18. Rinella, M.E.; Lazarus, J.V.; Ratziu, V.; Francque, S.M.; Sanyal, A.J.; Kanwal, F.; Romero, D.; Abdelmalek, M.F.; Anstee, Q.M.; Arab, J.P.; et al. A multisociety Delphi consensus statement on new fatty liver disease nomenclature. *Hepatology* **2023**, *78*, 1966–1986. [CrossRef] [PubMed]
19. Michaut, A.; Moreau, C.; Robin, M.A.; Fromenty, B. Acetaminophen-induced liver injury in obesity and nonalcoholic fatty liver disease. *Liver Int.* **2014**, *34*, e171–e179. [CrossRef] [PubMed]
20. Larson, A.M. Acetaminophen hepatotoxicity. *Clin. Liver Dis.* **2007**, *11*, 525–548. [CrossRef] [PubMed]
21. Bunchorntavakul, C.; Reddy, K.R. Acetaminophen-related hepatotoxicity. *Clin. Liver Dis.* **2013**, *17*, 587–607. [CrossRef] [PubMed]
22. Rumack, B.H.; Peterson, R.C.; Koch, G.G.; Amara, I.A. Acetaminophen overdose. 662 cases with evaluation of oral acetylcysteine treatment. *Arch. Intern. Med.* **1981**, *141*, 380–385. [CrossRef] [PubMed]
23. Perry, H.E.; Shannon, M.W. Efficacy of oral versus intravenous N-acetylcysteine in acetaminophen overdose: Results of an open-label, clinical trial. *J. Pediatr.* **1998**, *132*, 149–152. [CrossRef] [PubMed]
24. Yeates, P.J.; Thomas, S.H. Effectiveness of delayed activated charcoal administration in simulated paracetamol (acetaminophen) overdose. *Br. J. Clin. Pharmacol.* **2000**, *49*, 11–14. [CrossRef] [PubMed]
25. Russo, M.W.; Galanko, J.A.; Shrestha, R.; Fried, M.W.; Watkins, P. Liver transplantation for acute liver failure from drug induced liver injury in the United States. *Liver Transpl.* **2004**, *10*, 1018–1023. [CrossRef] [PubMed]
26. Athersuch, T.J.; Antoine, D.J.; Boobis, A.R.; Coen, M.; Daly, A.K.; Possamai, L.; Nicholson, J.K.; Wilson, I.D. Paracetamol metabolism, hepatotoxicity, biomarkers and therapeutic interventions: A perspective. *Toxicol. Res.* **2018**, *7*, 347–357. [CrossRef] [PubMed]
27. Adelusi, O.B.; Ramachandran, A.; Lemasters, J.J.; Jaeschke, H. The role of Iron in lipid peroxidation and protein nitration during acetaminophen-induced liver injury in mice. *Toxicol. Appl. Pharmacol.* **2022**, *445*, 116043. [CrossRef] [PubMed]
28. Anandatheerthavarada, H.K.; Addya, S.; Dwivedi, R.S.; Biswas, G.; Mullick, J.; Avadhani, N.G. Localization of multiple forms of inducible cytochromes P450 in rat liver mitochondria: Immunological characteristics and patterns of xenobiotic substrate metabolism. *Arch. Biochem. Biophys.* **1997**, *339*, 136–150. [CrossRef] [PubMed]
29. Robin, M.A.; Anandatheerthavarada, H.K.; Fang, J.K.; Cudic, M.; Otvos, L.; Avadhani, N.G. Mitochondrial targeted cytochrome P450 2E1 (P450 MT5) contains an intact N terminus and requires mitochondrial specific electron transfer proteins for activity. *J. Biol. Chem.* **2001**, *276*, 24680–24689. [CrossRef]
30. Massart, J.; Begriche, K.; Hartman, J.H.; Fromenty, B. Role of Mitochondrial Cytochrome P450 2E1 in Healthy and Diseased Liver. *Cells* **2022**, *11*, 288. [CrossRef]
31. Kon, K.; Kim, J.S.; Jaeschke, H.; Lemasters, J.J. Mitochondrial permeability transition in acetaminophen-induced necrosis and apoptosis of cultured mouse hepatocytes. *Hepatology* **2004**, *40*, 1170–1179. [CrossRef] [PubMed]
32. Hanawa, N.; Shinohara, M.; Saberi, B.; Gaarde, W.A.; Han, D.; Kaplowitz, N. Role of JNK translocation to mitochondria leading to inhibition of mitochondria bioenergetics in acetaminophen-induced liver injury. *J. Biol. Chem.* **2008**, *283*, 13565–13577. [CrossRef] [PubMed]
33. Hu, J.; Ramshesh, V.K.; McGill, M.R.; Jaeschke, H.; Lemasters, J.J. Low Dose Acetaminophen Induces Reversible Mitochondrial Dysfunction Associated with Transient c-Jun N-Terminal Kinase Activation in Mouse Liver. *Toxicol. Sci.* **2016**, *150*, 204–215. [CrossRef]
34. Dunn, K.W.; Martinez, M.M.; Wang, Z.; Mang, H.E.; Clendenon, S.G.; Sluka, J.P.; Glazier, J.A.; Klaunig, J.E. Mitochondrial depolarization and repolarization in the early stages of acetaminophen hepatotoxicity in mice. *Toxicology* **2020**, *439*, 152464. [CrossRef] [PubMed]
35. Zoratti, M.; Szabo, I. The mitochondrial permeability transition. *Biochim. Biophys. Acta* **1995**, *1241*, 139–176. [CrossRef]
36. Antoniel, M.; Giorgio, V.; Fogolari, F.; Glick, G.D.; Bernardi, P.; Lippe, G. The oligomycin-sensitivity conferring protein of mitochondrial ATP synthase: Emerging new roles in mitochondrial pathophysiology. *Int. J. Mol. Sci.* **2014**, *15*, 7513–7536. [CrossRef] [PubMed]
37. Crompton, M.; Ellinger, H.; Costi, A. Inhibition by cyclosporin A of a Ca2+-dependent pore in heart mitochondria activated by inorganic phosphate and oxidative stress. *Biochem. J.* **1988**, *255*, 357–360. [PubMed]
38. Waldmeier, P.C.; Feldtrauer, J.J.; Qian, T.; Lemasters, J.J. Inhibition of the mitochondrial permeability transition by the nonimmunosuppressive cyclosporin derivative NIM811. *Mol. Pharmacol.* **2002**, *62*, 22–29. [CrossRef] [PubMed]
39. Krauskopf, A.; Eriksson, O.; Craigen, W.J.; Forte, M.A.; Bernardi, P. Properties of the permeability transition in VDAC1(-/-) mitochondria. *Biochim. Biophys. Acta* **2006**, *1757*, 590–595. [CrossRef] [PubMed]
40. Baines, C.P.; Kaiser, R.A.; Sheiko, T.; Craigen, W.J.; Molkentin, J.D. Voltage-dependent anion channels are dispensable for mitochondrial-dependent cell death. *Nat. Cell Biol.* **2007**, *9*, 550–555. [CrossRef] [PubMed]

41. Kokoszka, J.E.; Waymire, K.G.; Levy, S.E.; Sligh, J.E.; Cai, J.; Jones, D.P.; MacGregor, G.R.; Wallace, D.C. The ADP/ATP translocator is not essential for the mitochondrial permeability transition pore. *Nature* **2004**, *427*, 461–465. [CrossRef] [PubMed]
42. Karch, J.; Bround, M.J.; Khalil, H.; Sargent, M.A.; Latchman, N.; Terada, N.; Peixoto, P.M.; Molkentin, J.D. Inhibition of mitochondrial permeability transition by deletion of the ANT family and CypD. *Sci. Adv.* **2019**, *5*, eaaw4597. [CrossRef] [PubMed]
43. Bround, M.J.; Havens, J.R.; York, A.J.; Sargent, M.A.; Karch, J.; Molkentin, J.D. ANT-dependent MPTP underlies necrotic myofiber death in muscular dystrophy. *Sci. Adv.* **2023**, *9*, eadi2767. [CrossRef] [PubMed]
44. Giorgio, V.; von Stockum, S.; Antoniel, M.; Fabbro, A.; Fogolari, F.; Forte, M.; Glick, G.D.; Petronilli, V.; Zoratti, M.; Szabo, I.; et al. Dimers of mitochondrial ATP synthase form the permeability transition pore. *Proc. Natl. Acad. Sci. USA* **2013**, *110*, 5887–5892. [CrossRef] [PubMed]
45. Carraro, M.; Giorgio, V.; Šileikytė, J.; Sartori, G.; Forte, M.; Lippe, G.; Zoratti, M.; Szabò, I.; Bernardi, P. Channel formation by yeast F-ATP synthase and the role of dimerization in the mitochondrial permeability transition. *J. Biol. Chem.* **2014**, *289*, 15980–15985. [CrossRef] [PubMed]
46. Alavian, K.N.; Beutner, G.; Lazrove, E.; Sacchetti, S.; Park, H.A.; Licznerski, P.; Li, H.; Nabili, P.; Hockensmith, K.; Graham, M.; et al. An uncoupling channel within the c-subunit ring of the F1FO ATP synthase is the mitochondrial permeability transition pore. *Proc. Natl. Acad. Sci. USA* **2014**, *111*, 10580–10585. [CrossRef]
47. He, J.; Carroll, J.; Ding, S.; Fearnley, I.M.; Walker, J.E. Permeability transition in human mitochondria persists in the absence of peripheral stalk subunits of ATP synthase. *Proc. Natl. Acad. Sci. USA* **2017**, *114*, 9086–9091. [CrossRef] [PubMed]
48. He, J.; Ford, H.C.; Carroll, J.; Ding, S.; Fearnley, I.M.; Walker, J.E. Persistence of the mitochondrial permeability transition in the absence of subunit c of human ATP synthase. *Proc. Natl. Acad. Sci. USA* **2017**, *114*, 3409–3414. [CrossRef]
49. Carroll, J.; He, J.; Ding, S.; Fearnley, I.M.; Walker, J.E. Persistence of the permeability transition pore in human mitochondria devoid of an assembled ATP synthase. *Proc. Natl. Acad. Sci. USA* **2019**, *116*, 12816–12821. [CrossRef] [PubMed]
50. Pekson, R.; Liang, F.G.; Axelrod, J.L.; Lee, J.; Qin, D.; Wittig, A.J.H.; Paulino, V.M.; Zheng, M.; Peixoto, P.M.; Kitsis, R.N. The mitochondrial ATP synthase is a negative regulator of the mitochondrial permeability transition pore. *Proc. Natl. Acad. Sci. USA* **2023**, *120*, e2303713120. [CrossRef] [PubMed]
51. He, L.; Lemasters, J.J. Regulated and unregulated mitochondrial permeability transition pores: A new paradigm of pore structure and function? *FEBS Lett.* **2002**, *512*, 1–7. [CrossRef] [PubMed]
52. He, L.; Lemasters, J.J. Heat shock suppresses the permeability transition in rat liver mitochondria. *J. Biol. Chem.* **2003**, *278*, 16755–16760. [CrossRef] [PubMed]
53. Neginskaya, M.A.; Solesio, M.E.; Berezhnaya, E.V.; Amodeo, G.F.; Mnatsakanyan, N.; Jonas, E.A.; Pavlov, E.V. ATP Synthase C-Subunit-Deficient Mitochondria Have a Small Cyclosporine A-Sensitive Channel, but Lack the Permeability Transition Pore. *Cell Rep.* **2019**, *26*, 11–17.e12. [CrossRef]
54. Neginskaya, M.A.; Morris, S.E.; Pavlov, E.V. Both ANT and ATPase are essential for mitochondrial permeability transition but not depolarization. *iScience* **2022**, *25*, 105447. [CrossRef] [PubMed]
55. Carrer, A.; Tommasin, L.; Šileikytė, J.; Ciscato, F.; Filadi, R.; Urbani, A.; Forte, M.; Rasola, A.; Szabò, I.; Carraro, M.; et al. Defining the molecular mechanisms of the mitochondrial permeability transition through genetic manipulation of F-ATP synthase. *Nat. Commun.* **2021**, *12*, 4835. [CrossRef] [PubMed]
56. Connern, C.P.; Halestrap, A.P. Recruitment of mitochondrial cyclophilin to the mitochondrial inner membrane under conditions of oxidative stress that enhance the opening of a calcium-sensitive non-specific channel. *Biochem. J.* **1994**, *302 Pt 2*, 321–324. [CrossRef] [PubMed]
57. Waldmeier, P.C.; Zimmermann, K.; Qian, T.; Tintelnot-Blomley, M.; Lemasters, J.J. Cyclophilin D as a drug target. *Curr. Med. Chem* **2003**, *10*, 1485–1506. [CrossRef] [PubMed]
58. Rehman, H.; Ramshesh, V.K.; Theruvath, T.P.; Kim, I.; Currin, R.T.; Giri, S.; Lemasters, J.J.; Zhong, Z. NIM811 (N-methyl-4-isoleucine cyclosporine), a mitochondrial permeability transition inhibitor, attenuates cholestatic liver injury but not fibrosis in mice. *J. Pharmacol. Exp. Ther.* **2008**, *327*, 699–706. [CrossRef] [PubMed]
59. Theruvath, T.P.; Zhong, Z.; Pediaditakis, P.; Ramshesh, V.K.; Currin, R.T.; Tikunov, A.; Holmuhamedov, E.; Lemasters, J.J. Minocycline and N-methyl-4-isoleucine cyclosporin (NIM811) mitigate storage/reperfusion injury after rat liver transplantation through suppression of the mitochondrial permeability transition. *Hepatology* **2008**, *47*, 236–246. [CrossRef] [PubMed]
60. Rehman, H.; Sun, J.; Shi, Y.; Ramshesh, V.K.; Liu, Q.; Currin, R.T.; Lemasters, J.J.; Zhong, Z. NIM811 prevents mitochondrial dysfunction, attenuates liver injury, and stimulates liver regeneration after massive hepatectomy. *Transplantation* **2011**, *91*, 406–412. [CrossRef] [PubMed]
61. Zhong, Z.; Theruvath, T.P.; Currin, R.T.; Waldmeier, P.C.; Lemasters, J.J. NIM811, a mitochondrial permeability transition inhibitor, prevents mitochondrial depolarization in small-for-size rat liver grafts. *Am. J. Transplant.* **2007**, *7*, 1103–1111. [CrossRef] [PubMed]
62. Masubuchi, Y.; Suda, C.; Horie, T. Involvement of mitochondrial permeability transition in acetaminophen-induced liver injury in mice. *J. Hepatol.* **2005**, *42*, 110–116. [CrossRef] [PubMed]
63. Reid, A.B.; Kurten, R.C.; McCullough, S.S.; Brock, R.W.; Hinson, J.A. Mechanisms of acetaminophen-induced hepatotoxicity: Role of oxidative stress and mitochondrial permeability transition in freshly isolated mouse hepatocytes. *J. Pharmacol. Exp. Ther.* **2005**, *312*, 509–516. [CrossRef] [PubMed]
64. Lemasters, J.J. Dying a Thousand Deaths: Redundant Pathways From Different Organelles to Apoptosis and Necrosis. *Gastroenterology* **2005**, *129*, 351–360. [CrossRef]

65. Kon, K.; Ikejima, K.; Okumura, K.; Aoyama, T.; Arai, K.; Takei, Y.; Lemasters, J.J.; Sato, N. Role of apoptosis in acetaminophen hepatotoxicity 19. *J. Gastroenterol. Hepatol.* **2007**, *22* (Suppl. S1), S49–S52. [CrossRef] [PubMed]
66. Kim, J.S.; Qian, T.; Lemasters, J.J. Mitochondrial permeability transition in the switch from necrotic to apoptotic cell death in ischemic rat hepatocytes. *Gastroenterology* **2003**, *124*, 494–503. [CrossRef] [PubMed]
67. Lemasters, J.J.; Nieminen, A.L.; Qian, T.; Trost, L.C.; Elmore, S.P.; Nishimura, Y.; Crowe, R.A.; Cascio, W.E.; Bradham, C.A.; Brenner, D.A.; et al. The mitochondrial permeability transition in cell death: A common mechanism in necrosis, apoptosis and autophagy. *Biochim. Biophys. Acta* **1998**, *1366*, 177–196. [CrossRef] [PubMed]
68. Gujral, J.S.; Knight, T.R.; Farhood, A.; Bajt, M.L.; Jaeschke, H. Mode of cell death after acetaminophen overdose in mice: Apoptosis or oncotic necrosis? *Toxicol. Sci.* **2002**, *67*, 322–328. [CrossRef] [PubMed]
69. Jaeschke, H.; Williams, C.D.; Farhood, A. No evidence for caspase-dependent apoptosis in acetaminophen hepatotoxicity. *Hepatology* **2011**, *53*, 718–719. [CrossRef]
70. Possamai, L.A.; McPhail, M.J.; Quaglia, A.; Zingarelli, V.; Abeles, R.D.; Tidswell, R.; Puthucheary, Z.; Rawal, J.; Karvellas, C.J.; Leslie, E.M.; et al. Character and temporal evolution of apoptosis in acetaminophen-induced acute liver failure*. *Crit. Care Med.* **2013**, *41*, 2543–2550. [CrossRef] [PubMed]
71. Gunawan, B.K.; Liu, Z.X.; Han, D.; Hanawa, N.; Gaarde, W.A.; Kaplowitz, N. c-Jun N-terminal kinase plays a major role in murine acetaminophen hepatotoxicity. *Gastroenterology* **2006**, *131*, 165–178. [CrossRef] [PubMed]
72. Win, S.; Than, T.A.; Han, D.; Petrovic, L.M.; Kaplowitz, N. c-Jun N-terminal kinase (JNK)-dependent acute liver injury from acetaminophen or tumor necrosis factor (TNF) requires mitochondrial Sab protein expression in mice. *J. Biol. Chem.* **2011**, *286*, 35071–35078. [CrossRef] [PubMed]
73. Win, S.; Than, T.A.; Kaplowitz, N. Mitochondrial P-JNK target, SAB (SH3BP5), in regulation of cell death. *Front. Cell Dev. Biol.* **2024**, *12*, 1359152. [CrossRef]
74. Win, S.; Than, T.A.; Min, R.W.; Aghajan, M.; Kaplowitz, N. c-Jun N-terminal kinase mediates mouse liver injury through a novel Sab (SH3BP5)-dependent pathway leading to inactivation of intramitochondrial Src. *Hepatology* **2016**, *63*, 1987–2003. [CrossRef] [PubMed]
75. Win, S.; Than, T.A.; Fernandez-Checa, J.C.; Kaplowitz, N. JNK interaction with Sab mediates ER stress induced inhibition of mitochondrial respiration and cell death. *Cell Death Dis.* **2014**, *5*, e989. [CrossRef] [PubMed]
76. Win, S.; Than, T.A.; Zhang, J.; Oo, C.; Min, R.W.M.; Kaplowitz, N. New insights into the role and mechanism of c-Jun-N-terminal kinase signaling in the pathobiology of liver diseases. *Hepatology* **2018**, *67*, 2013–2024. [CrossRef] [PubMed]
77. Samuvel, D.J.; Nguyen, N.T.; Jaeschke, H.; Lemasters, J.J.; Wang, X.; Choo, Y.M.; Hamann, M.T.; Zhong, Z. Platanosides, a Potential Botanical Drug Combination, Decrease Liver Injury Caused by Acetaminophen Overdose in Mice. *J. Nat. Prod.* **2022**, *85*, 1779–1788. [CrossRef] [PubMed]
78. Jaeschke, H.; Bajt, M.L. Intracellular signaling mechanisms of acetaminophen-induced liver cell death. *Toxicol. Sci.* **2006**, *89*, 31–41. [CrossRef] [PubMed]
79. Bajt, M.L.; Knight, T.R.; Lemasters, J.J.; Jaeschke, H. Acetaminophen-induced oxidant stress and cell injury in cultured mouse hepatocytes: Protection by N-acetyl cysteine. *Toxicol. Sci.* **2004**, *80*, 343–349. [CrossRef] [PubMed]
80. Jaeschke, H. Glutathione disulfide formation and oxidant stress during acetaminophen-induced hepatotoxicity in mice in vivo: The protective effect of allopurinol. *J. Pharmacol. Exp. Ther.* **1990**, *255*, 935–941. [PubMed]
81. Hu, J.; Kholmukhamedov, A.; Lindsey, C.C.; Beeson, C.C.; Jaeschke, H.; Lemasters, J.J. Translocation of iron from lysosomes to mitochondria during acetaminophen-induced hepatocellular injury: Protection by starch-desferal and minocycline. *Free Radic. Biol. Med.* **2016**, *97*, 418–426. [CrossRef] [PubMed]
82. Nguyen, N.T.; Du, K.; Akakpo, J.Y.; Umbaugh, D.S.; Jaeschke, H.; Ramachandran, A. Mitochondrial protein adduct and superoxide generation are prerequisites for early activation of c-jun N-terminal kinase within the cytosol after an acetaminophen overdose in mice. *Toxicol. Lett.* **2021**, *338*, 21–31. [CrossRef] [PubMed]
83. Kehrer, J.P.; Klotz, L.O. Free radicals and related reactive species as mediators of tissue injury and disease: Implications for Health. *Crit. Rev. Toxicol.* **2015**, *45*, 765–798. [CrossRef] [PubMed]
84. Minotti, G.; Aust, S.D. Redox cycling of iron and lipid peroxidation. *Lipids* **1992**, *27*, 219–226. [CrossRef] [PubMed]
85. Galy, B.; Conrad, M.; Muckenthaler, M. Mechanisms controlling cellular and systemic iron homeostasis. *Nat. Rev. Mol. Cell Biol.* **2024**, *25*, 133–155. [CrossRef] [PubMed]
86. Lane, D.J.; Merlot, A.M.; Huang, M.L.; Bae, D.H.; Jansson, P.J.; Sahni, S.; Kalinowski, D.S.; Richardson, D.R. Cellular iron uptake, trafficking and metabolism: Key molecules and mechanisms and their roles in disease. *Biochim. Biophys. Acta* **2015**, *1853*, 1130–1144. [CrossRef] [PubMed]
87. McKie, A.T.; Barrow, D.; Latunde-Dada, G.O.; Rolfs, A.; Sager, G.; Mudaly, E.; Mudaly, M.; Richardson, C.; Barlow, D.; Bomford, A.; et al. An iron-regulated ferric reductase associated with the absorption of dietary iron. *Science* **2001**, *291*, 1755–1759. [CrossRef] [PubMed]
88. Gunshin, H.; Mackenzie, B.; Berger, U.V.; Gunshin, Y.; Romero, M.F.; Boron, W.F.; Nussberger, S.; Gollan, J.L.; Hediger, M.A. Cloning and characterization of a mammalian proton-coupled metal-ion transporter. *Nature* **1997**, *388*, 482–488. [CrossRef] [PubMed]
89. Jenkitkasemwong, S.; Wang, C.Y.; Mackenzie, B.; Knutson, M.D. Physiologic implications of metal-ion transport by ZIP14 and ZIP8. *Biometals* **2012**, *25*, 643–655. [CrossRef] [PubMed]

90. Ohgami, R.S.; Campagna, D.R.; Greer, E.L.; Antiochos, B.; McDonald, A.; Chen, J.; Sharp, J.J.; Fujiwara, Y.; Barker, J.E.; Fleming, M.D. Identification of a ferrireductase required for efficient transferrin-dependent iron uptake in erythroid cells. *Nat. Genet.* **2005**, *37*, 1264–1269. [CrossRef] [PubMed]
91. Ohgami, R.S.; Campagna, D.R.; McDonald, A.; Fleming, M.D. The Steap proteins are metalloreductases. *Blood* **2006**, *108*, 1388–1394. [CrossRef] [PubMed]
92. Uchiyama, A.; Kim, J.S.; Kon, K.; Jaeschke, H.; Ikejima, K.; Watanabe, S.; Lemasters, J.J. Translocation of iron from lysosomes into mitochondria is a key event during oxidative stress-induced hepatocellular injury. *Hepatology* **2008**, *48*, 1644–1654. [CrossRef] [PubMed]
93. Kurz, T.; Terman, A.; Gustafsson, B.; Brunk, U.T. Lysosomes in iron metabolism, ageing and apoptosis. *Histochem. Cell Biol.* **2008**, *129*, 389–406. [CrossRef]
94. Lill, R. Function and biogenesis of iron-sulphur proteins. *Nature* **2009**, *460*, 831–838. [CrossRef] [PubMed]
95. Lill, R.; Hoffmann, B.; Molik, S.; Pierik, A.J.; Rietzschel, N.; Stehling, O.; Uzarska, M.A.; Webert, H.; Wilbrecht, C.; Muhlenhoff, U. The role of mitochondria in cellular iron-sulfur protein biogenesis and iron metabolism. *Biochim. Biophys. Acta* **2012**, *1823*, 1491–1508. [CrossRef] [PubMed]
96. Braymer, J.J.; Freibert, S.A.; Rakwalska-Bange, M.; Lill, R. Mechanistic concepts of iron-sulfur protein biogenesis in Biology. *Biochim. Biophys. Acta Mol. Cell Res.* **2021**, *1868*, 118863. [CrossRef] [PubMed]
97. Kořený, L.; Oborník, M.; Horáková, E.; Waller, R.F.; Lukeš, J. The convoluted history of haem biosynthesis. *Biol. Rev. Camb. Philos. Soc.* **2022**, *97*, 141–162. [CrossRef] [PubMed]
98. Sheftel, A.D.; Zhang, A.S.; Brown, C.; Shirihai, O.S.; Ponka, P. Direct interorganellar transfer of iron from endosome to mitochondrion. *Blood* **2007**, *110*, 125–132. [CrossRef] [PubMed]
99. Asano, T.; Komatsu, M.; Yamaguchi-Iwai, Y.; Ishikawa, F.; Mizushima, N.; Iwai, K. Distinct mechanisms of ferritin delivery to lysosomes in iron-depleted and iron-replete cells. *Mol. Cell Biol.* **2011**, *31*, 2040–2052. [CrossRef]
100. De Domenico, I.; Vaughn, M.B.; Li, L.; Bagley, D.; Musci, G.; Ward, D.M.; Kaplan, J. Ferroportin-mediated mobilization of ferritin iron precedes ferritin degradation by the proteasome. *EMBO J.* **2006**, *25*, 5396–5404. [CrossRef] [PubMed]
101. De Domenico, I.; Ward, D.M.; Kaplan, J. Specific iron chelators determine the route of ferritin degradation. *Blood* **2009**, *114*, 4546–4551. [CrossRef] [PubMed]
102. Flatmark, T.; Romslo, I. Energy-dependent accumulation of iron by isolated rat liver mitochondria. Requirement of reducing equivalents and evidence for a unidirectional flux of Fe(II) across the inner membrane. *J. Biol. Chem.* **1975**, *250*, 6433–6438. [CrossRef] [PubMed]
103. Matlib, M.A.; Zhou, Z.; Knight, S.; Ahmed, S.; Choi, K.M.; Krause-Bauer, J.; Phillips, R.; Altschuld, R.; Katsube, Y.; Sperelakis, N.; et al. Oxygen-bridged dinuclear ruthenium amine complex specifically inhibits Ca2+ uptake into mitochondria in vitro and in situ in single cardiac myocytes. *J. Biol. Chem.* **1998**, *273*, 10223–10231. [CrossRef] [PubMed]
104. Zhang, X.; Lemasters, J.J. Translocation of iron from lysosomes to mitochondria during ischemia predisposes to injury after reperfusion in rat hepatocytes. *Free Radic. Biol. Med.* **2013**, *63*, 243–253. [CrossRef] [PubMed]
105. Shaw, G.C.; Cope, J.J.; Li, L.; Corson, K.; Hersey, C.; Ackermann, G.E.; Gwynn, B.; Lambert, A.J.; Wingert, R.A.; Traver, D.; et al. Mitoferrin is essential for erythroid iron assimilation. *Nature* **2006**, *440*, 96–100. [CrossRef] [PubMed]
106. Troadec, M.B.; Warner, D.; Wallace, J.; Thomas, K.; Spangrude, G.J.; Phillips, J.; Khalimonchuk, O.; Paw, B.H.; Ward, D.M.; Kaplan, J. Targeted deletion of the mouse Mitoferrin1 gene: From anemia to protoporphyria. *Blood* **2011**, *117*, 5494–5502. [CrossRef] [PubMed]
107. Nieminen, A.L.; Schwartz, J.; Hung, H.I.; Blocker, E.R.; Gooz, M.; Lemasters, J.J. Mitoferrin-2 (Mfrn2) regulates the electrogenic mitochondrial calcium uniporter and inter-acts physically with MCU. *Biophys. J.* **2014**, *106*, 581a–582a. [CrossRef]
108. Dietz, J.V.; Fox, J.L.; Khalimonchuk, O. Down the Iron Path: Mitochondrial Iron Homeostasis and Beyond. *Cells* **2021**, *10*, 2198. [CrossRef] [PubMed]
109. Aust, S.D.; Morehouse, L.A.; Thomas, C.E. Role of metals in oxygen radical reactions. *J. Free Radic. Biol. Med.* **1985**, *1*, 3–25. [CrossRef]
110. Dixon, S.J.; Lemberg, K.M.; Lamprecht, M.R.; Skouta, R.; Zaitsev, E.M.; Gleason, C.E.; Patel, D.N.; Bauer, A.J.; Cantley, A.M.; Yang, W.S.; et al. Ferroptosis: An iron-dependent form of nonapoptotic cell death. *Cell* **2012**, *149*, 1060–1072. [CrossRef] [PubMed]
111. Masaki, N.; Kyle, M.E.; Farber, J.L. tert-Butyl hydroperoxide kills cultured hepatocytes by peroxidizing membrane lipids. *Arch. Biochem. Biophys.* **1989**, *269*, 390–399. [CrossRef] [PubMed]
112. Nieminen, A.L.; Byrne, A.M.; Herman, B.; Lemasters, J.J. Mitochondrial permeability transition in hepatocytes induced by t-BuOOH: NAD(P)H and reactive oxygen species. *Am. J. Physiol.* **1997**, *272*, C1286–C1294. [CrossRef] [PubMed]
113. Adel, N.; Mantawy, E.M.; El-Sherbiny, D.A.; El-Demerdash, E. Iron chelation by deferasirox confers protection against concanavalin A-induced liver fibrosis: A mechanistic approach. *Toxicol. Appl. Pharmacol.* **2019**, *382*, 114748. [CrossRef] [PubMed]
114. Gerson, R.J.; Casini, A.; Gilfor, D.; Serroni, A.; Farber, J.L. Oxygen-mediated cell injury in the killing of cultured hepatocytes by acetaminophen. *Biochem. Biophys. Res. Commun.* **1985**, *126*, 1129–1137. [CrossRef] [PubMed]
115. Byrne, A.M.; Lemasters, J.J.; Nieminen, A.L. Contribution of increased mitochondrial free Ca^{2+} to the mitochondrial permeability transition induced by tert-butylhydroperoxide in rat hepatocytes. *Hepatology* **1999**, *29*, 1523–1531. [CrossRef] [PubMed]

116. Kon, K.; Kim, J.S.; Uchiyama, A.; Jaeschke, H.; Lemasters, J.J. Lysosomal iron mobilization and induction of the mitochondrial permeability transition in acetaminophen-induced toxicity to mouse hepatocytes. *Toxicol. Sci.* **2010**, *117*, 101–108. [CrossRef] [PubMed]
117. Hu, J.; Lemasters, J.J. Suppression of iron mobilization from lysosomes to mitochondria attenuates liver injury after acetaminophen overdose in vivo in mice: Protection by minocycline. *Toxicol. Appl. Pharmacol.* **2020**, *392*, 114930. [CrossRef] [PubMed]
118. Adamson, G.M.; Harman, A.W. Oxidative stress in cultured hepatocytes exposed to acetaminophen. *Biochem. Pharmacol.* **1993**, *45*, 2289–2294. [CrossRef] [PubMed]
119. Schnellmann, J.G.; Pumford, N.R.; Kusewitt, D.F.; Bucci, T.J.; Hinson, J.A. Deferoxamine delays the development of the hepatotoxicity of acetaminophen in mice. *Toxicol. Lett.* **1999**, *106*, 79–88. [CrossRef]
120. Kyle, M.E.; Miccadei, S.; Nakae, D.; Farber, J.L. Superoxide dismutase and catalase protect cultured hepatocytes from the cytotoxicity of acetaminophen. *Biochem. Biophys. Res. Commun.* **1987**, *149*, 889–896. [CrossRef] [PubMed]
121. Kyle, M.E.; Nakae, D.; Serroni, A.; Farber, J.L. 1,3-(2-Chloroethyl)-1-nitrosourea potentiates the toxicity of acetaminophen both in the phenobarbital-induced rat and in hepatocytes cultured from such animals. *Mol. Pharmacol.* **1988**, *34*, 584–589. [PubMed]
122. Moon, M.S.; Richie, J.P.; Isom, H.C. Iron potentiates acetaminophen-induced oxidative stress and mitochondrial dysfunction in cultured mouse hepatocytes. *Toxicol. Sci.* **2010**, *118*, 119–127. [CrossRef] [PubMed]
123. Epsztejn, S.; Kakhlon, O.; Glickstein, H.; Breuer, W.; Cabantchik, I. Fluorescence analysis of the labile iron pool of mammalian cells. *Anal. Biochem.* **1997**, *248*, 31–40. [CrossRef] [PubMed]
124. Kholmukhamedov, A.; Li, L.; Lindsey, C.C.; Hu, J.; Nieminen, A.L.; Takemoto, K.; Beeson, G.C.; Beneker, C.M.; McInnes, C.; Beeson, C.C.; et al. A new fluorescent sensor mitoferrofluor indicates the presence of chelatable iron in polarized and depolarized mitochondria. *J. Biol. Chem.* **2022**, *298*, 102336. [CrossRef] [PubMed]
125. Chen, Y.; Guo, X.; Zeng, Y.; Mo, X.; Hong, S.; He, H.; Li, J.; Fatima, S.; Liu, Q. Oxidative stress induces mitochondrial iron overload and ferroptotic cell death. *Sci. Rep.* **2023**, *13*, 15515. [CrossRef] [PubMed]
126. Hu, J.; Nieminen, A.L.; Weemhoff, J.L.; Jaeschke, H.; Murphy, L.G.; Dent, J.A.; Lemasters, J.J. The mitochondrial calcium uniporter mediates mitochondrial Fe^{2+} uptake and hepatotoxicity after acetaminophen. *Toxicol. Appl. Pharmacol.* **2023**, *479*, 116722. [CrossRef] [PubMed]
127. Sukhbaatar, N.; Weichhart, T. Iron Regulation: Macrophages in Control. *Pharmaceuticals* **2018**, *11*, 137. [CrossRef] [PubMed]
128. Jaeschke, H.; Farhood, A. Neutrophil and Kupffer cell-induced oxidant stress and ischemia-reperfusion injury in rat liver. *Am. J. Physiol.* **1991**, *260*, G355–G362. [CrossRef] [PubMed]
129. Michael, S.L.; Pumford, N.R.; Mayeux, P.R.; Niesman, M.R.; Hinson, J.A. Pretreatment of mice with macrophage inactivators decreases acetaminophen hepatotoxicity and the formation of reactive oxygen and nitrogen species. *Hepatology* **1999**, *30*, 186–195. [CrossRef] [PubMed]
130. Ju, C.; Reilly, T.P.; Bourdi, M.; Radonovich, M.F.; Brady, J.N.; George, J.W.; Pohl, L.R. Protective role of Kupffer cells in acetaminophen-induced hepatic injury in mice. *Chem. Res. Toxicol.* **2002**, *15*, 1504–1513. [CrossRef] [PubMed]
131. Triantafyllou, E.; Pop, O.T.; Possamai, L.A.; Wilhelm, A.; Liaskou, E.; Singanayagam, A.; Bernsmeier, C.; Khamri, W.; Petts, G.; Dargue, R.; et al. MerTK expressing hepatic macrophages promote the resolution of inflammation in acute liver failure. *Gut* **2018**, *67*, 333–347. [CrossRef] [PubMed]
132. Qiu, K.; Pan, Y.; Huang, W.; Li, M.; Yan, X.; Zhou, Z.; Qi, J. CXCL5 Promotes Acetaminophen-Induced Hepatotoxicity by Activating Kupffer Cells. *Int. J. Mol. Sci.* **2023**, *24*, 12180. [CrossRef] [PubMed]
133. Nguyen, N.T.; Umbaugh, D.S.; Sanchez-Guerrero, G.; Ramachandran, A.; Jaeschke, H. Kupffer cells regulate liver recovery through induction of chemokine receptor CXCR2 on hepatocytes after acetaminophen overdose in mice. *Arch. Toxicol.* **2022**, *96*, 305–320. [CrossRef] [PubMed]
134. Starke, P.E.; Farber, J.L. Ferric iron and superoxide ions are required for the killing of cultured hepatocytes by hydrogen peroxide. Evidence for the participation of hydroxyl radicals formed by an iron-catalyzed Haber-Weiss reaction. *J. Biol. Chem.* **1985**, *260*, 10099–10104. [CrossRef] [PubMed]
135. Gores, G.J.; Flarsheim, C.E.; Dawson, T.L.; Nieminen, A.L.; Herman, B.; Lemasters, J.J. Swelling, reductive stress, and cell death during chemical hypoxia in hepatocytes. *Am. J. Physiol.* **1989**, *257*, C347–C354. [CrossRef] [PubMed]
136. Farber, J.L.; Leonard, T.B.; Kyle, M.E.; Nakae, D.; Serroni, A.; Rogers, S.A. Peroxidation-dependent and peroxidation-independent mechanisms by which acetaminophen kills cultured rat hepatocytes. *Arch. Biochem. Biophys.* **1988**, *267*, 640–650. [CrossRef] [PubMed]
137. Yamada, N.; Karasawa, T.; Kimura, H.; Watanabe, S.; Komada, T.; Kamata, R.; Sampilvanjil, A.; Ito, J.; Nakagawa, K.; Kuwata, H.; et al. Ferroptosis driven by radical oxidation of n-6 polyunsaturated fatty acids mediates acetaminophen-induced acute liver failure. *Cell Death Dis.* **2020**, *11*, 144. [CrossRef] [PubMed]
138. Stockwell, B.R.; Friedmann Angeli, J.P.; Bayir, H.; Bush, A.I.; Conrad, M.; Dixon, S.J.; Fulda, S.; Gascon, S.; Hatzios, S.K.; Kagan, V.E.; et al. Ferroptosis: A regulated cell death nexus linking metabolism, redox biology, and disease. *Cell* **2017**, *171*, 273–285. [CrossRef] [PubMed]
139. Shi, Y.; Xu, N.; Liu, B.; Ma, Y.; Fu, X.; Shang, Y.; Huang, Q.; Yao, Q.; Chen, J.; Li, H. Mifepristone protects acetaminophen induced liver injury through NRF2/GSH/GST mediated ferroptosis suppression. *Free Radic. Biol. Med.* **2024**, *222*, 229–243. [CrossRef]
140. Tao, J.; Xue, C.; Wang, X.; Chen, H.; Liu, Q.; Jiang, C.; Zhang, W. GAS1 Promotes Ferroptosis of Liver Cells in Acetaminophen-Induced Acute Liver Failure. *Int. J. Med. Sci.* **2023**, *20*, 1616–1630. [CrossRef] [PubMed]

141. Hinson, J.A.; Pike, S.L.; Pumford, N.R.; Mayeux, P.R. Nitrotyrosine-protein adducts in hepatic centrilobular areas following toxic doses of acetaminophen in mice. *Chem. Res. Toxicol.* **1998**, *11*, 604–607. [CrossRef] [PubMed]
142. Knight, T.R.; Kurtz, A.; Bajt, M.L.; Hinson, J.A.; Jaeschke, H. Vascular and hepatocellular peroxynitrite formation during acetaminophen toxicity: Role of mitochondrial oxidant stress. *Toxicol. Sci.* **2001**, *62*, 212–220. [CrossRef] [PubMed]
143. Cover, C.; Mansouri, A.; Knight, T.R.; Bajt, M.L.; Lemasters, J.J.; Pessayre, D.; Jaeschke, H. Peroxynitrite-induced mitochondrial and endonuclease-mediated nuclear DNA damage in acetaminophen hepatotoxicity. *J. Pharmacol. Exp. Ther.* **2005**, *315*, 879–887. [CrossRef] [PubMed]
144. Campolo, N.; Bartesaghi, S.; Radi, R. Metal-catalyzed protein tyrosine nitration in biological systems. *Redox Rep.* **2014**, *19*, 221–231. [CrossRef] [PubMed]
145. Du, K.; Farhood, A.; Jaeschke, H. Mitochondria-targeted antioxidant Mito-Tempo protects against acetaminophen hepatotoxicity. *Arch. Toxicol.* **2017**, *91*, 761–773. [CrossRef] [PubMed]
146. Esterbauer, H.; Eckl, P.; Ortner, A. Possible mutagens derived from lipids and lipid precursors. *Mutat. Res.* **1990**, *238*, 223–233. [CrossRef] [PubMed]
147. Esterbauer, H.; Cheeseman, K.H. Determination of aldehydic lipid peroxidation products: Malonaldehyde and 4-hydroxynonenal. *Methods Enzymol.* **1990**, *186*, 407–421. [CrossRef] [PubMed]
148. Esterbauer, H.; Schaur, R.J.; Zollner, H. Chemistry and biochemistry of 4-hydroxynonenal, malonaldehyde and related aldehydes. *Free Radic. Biol. Med.* **1991**, *11*, 81–128. [CrossRef] [PubMed]
149. Wendel, A.; Feuerstein, S.; Konz, K.H. Acute paracetamol intoxication of starved mice leads to lipid peroxidation in vivo. *Biochem. Pharmacol.* **1979**, *28*, 2051–2055. [CrossRef] [PubMed]
150. Wendel, A.; Feuerstein, S. Drug-induced lipid peroxidation in mice--I. Modulation by monooxygenase activity, glutathione and selenium status. *Biochem. Pharmacol.* **1981**, *30*, 2513–2520. [CrossRef] [PubMed]
151. Wendel, A.; Jaeschke, H.; Gloger, M. Drug-induced lipid peroxidation in mice--II. Protection against paracetamol-induced liver necrosis by intravenous liposomally entrapped glutathione. *Biochem. Pharmacol.* **1982**, *31*, 3601–3605. [CrossRef] [PubMed]
152. Knight, T.R.; Fariss, M.W.; Farhood, A.; Jaeschke, H. Role of lipid peroxidation as a mechanism of liver injury after acetaminophen overdose in mice. *Toxicol. Sci.* **2003**, *76*, 229–236. [CrossRef] [PubMed]
153. Younes, M.; Cornelius, S.; Siegers, C.P. Ferrous ion supported in vivo lipid peroxidation induced by paracetamol--its relation to hepatotoxicity. *Res. Commun. Chem. Pathol. Pharmacol.* **1986**, *51*, 89–99. [PubMed]
154. Albano, E.; Poli, G.; Chiarpotto, E.; Biasi, F.; Dianzani, M.U. Paracetamol-stimulated lipid peroxidation in isolated rat and mouse hepatocytes. *Chem. Biol. Interact.* **1983**, *47*, 249–263. [CrossRef] [PubMed]
155. Minamide, Y.; Horie, T.; Tomaru, A.; Awazu, S. Spontaneous chemiluminescence production, lipid peroxidation, and covalent binding in rat hepatocytes exposed to acetaminophen. *J. Pharm. Sci.* **1998**, *87*, 640–646. [CrossRef] [PubMed]
156. Wimborne, H.J.; Hu, J.; Takemoto, K.; Nguyen, N.T.; Jaeschke, H.; Lemasters, J.J.; Zhong, Z. Aldehyde dehydrogenase-2 activation decreases acetaminophen hepatotoxicity by prevention of mitochondrial depolarization. *Toxicol. Appl. Pharmacol.* **2020**, *396*, 114982. [CrossRef] [PubMed]
157. Chen, C.H.; Budas, G.R.; Churchill, E.N.; Disatnik, M.H.; Hurley, T.D.; Mochly-Rosen, D. Activation of aldehyde dehydrogenase-2 reduces ischemic damage to the heart. *Science* **2008**, *321*, 1493–1495. [CrossRef] [PubMed]

livers

MDPI

Review

Targeting Autophagy for Acetaminophen-Induced Liver Injury: An Update

Kaitlyn Hinz [1], Mengwei Niu [1], Hong-Min Ni [1] and Wen-Xing Ding [1,2,*]

[1] Department of Pharmacology, Toxicology and Therapeutics, University of Kansas Medical Center, Kansas City, KS 66160, USA; kgreenwood@kumc.edu (K.H.); mniu@kumc.edu (M.N.); hni@kumc.edu (H.-M.N.)
[2] Department of Internal Medicine, University of Kansas Medical Center, Kansas City, KS 66160, USA
* Correspondence: wxding@kumc.edu; Tel.: +1-913-588-9813

Abstract: Acetaminophen (APAP) overdose can induce hepatocyte necrosis and acute liver failure in experimental rodents and humans. APAP is mainly metabolized via hepatic cytochrome P450 enzymes to generate the highly reactive metabolite *N*-acetyl-*p*-benzoquinone imine (NAPQI), which forms acetaminophen protein adducts (APAP-adducts) and damages mitochondria, triggering necrosis. APAP-adducts and damaged mitochondria can be selectively removed by autophagy. Increasing evidence implies that the activation of autophagy may be beneficial for APAP-induced liver injury (AILI). In this minireview, we briefly summarize recent progress on autophagy, in particular, the pharmacological targeting of SQSTM1/p62 and TFEB in AILI.

Keywords: mitophagy; NRF2; p62/SQSTM1; TFEB

1. Introduction

Acetaminophen (APAP) is a widely used analgesic and antipyretic drug in the United States [1–3]. However, APAP overdose can lead to acute liver failure, which is responsible for nearly half of drug-induced liver injury cases and is a leading cause of liver failure in Western countries [4–7]. Currently, the most commonly used treatment for acetaminophen-induced liver injury (AILI) is N-acetylcysteine (NAC), which restores glutathione (GSH) levels in the liver. However, the time window for treatment with NAC is limited. Therefore, there is an urgent need to develop novel treatments for AILI [8].

Several distinctive phases of liver pathogenesis in AILI have been documented, including the early metabolic phase, injury phase, and liver repair/recovery phase [9]. In the early metabolic phase, APAP is mainly metabolized by conjugation with glucoronidate and sulfate in the liver via phase II enzymes, and only 5–9% of APAP is metabolized via cytochrome P450 enzymes, primarily, cytochrome P450 2E1 (CYP2E1) and CYP1A2, to form a highly reactive metabolite, *N*-acetyl-*p*-benzoquinone imine (NAPQI), which is detoxified by hepatic GSH. However, excessive NAPQI can covalently bind to intracellular proteins to form cytosolic and mitochondrial APAP protein adducts (APAP-adducts) leading to mitochondrial damage and increased oxidative stress, which are followed by the activation of c-Jun N-terminal kinase (JNK) and release of mitochondrial endonuclease G and an apoptosis-inducing factor to trigger DNA fragmentation and hepatocyte necrosis (necrotic injury phase) [10–14]. After the initial phase of necrotic injury, the liver undergoes several adaptive responses in the repair/recovery phase. These responses include the innate immune response and blood coagulation events, which can either worsen or alleviate AILI during the recovery phase [15–17]. Macrophages from the bloodstream can help resolve the injury by eliminating dead cells and inducing the death of neutrophils [18]. Recent evidence shows that during the late recovery phase of AILI, increased hepatic platelet aggregation can inhibit liver regeneration. This happens because of the increased secretion of the platelet adhesive protein, Von Willebrand factor (VWF), in the liver during AILI [19].

Autophagy, a lysosomal degradation pathway, removes APAP-adducts and damaged mitochondria as another line of adaptive protective response against AILI [20–23]. Autophagy can selectively remove protein aggregates and damaged/excess organelles, and is mediated by a group of proteins called autophagy receptor proteins, including SQSTM1/p62 (hereafter referred to as p62), optineurin, NDP52, NIX, BNIP3, FUNDC1, and prohibitin 2 [24–27]. As lysosomes sit at the end for the execution of autophagic degradation via lysosomal enzymes, the number and function of lysosomes are critical for completing the autophagy process. Increased lysosomal biogenesis is necessary to meet the need for the fusion with autophagosomes and subsequent autophagic degradation. The transcription regulation of lysosome biogenesis genes is mediated by transcription factor EB (TFEB), a basic helix–loop–helix leucine zipper transcription factor belonging to the coordinated lysosomal expression and regulation (CLEAR) gene network [28]. Notably, TFEB also regulates mitochondrial biogenesis by directly regulating the expression of PGC-1α, a key transcription coactivator in mitochondrial biogenesis [29,30]. The purpose of this review is to briefly summarize recent progress on manipulating p62 and TFEB in AILI, and hopefully stimulate more future studies to identify novel p62 and TFEB agonists to treat AILI.

2. Targeting p62 for AILI

p62 is a multidomain scaffold protein that plays a crucial role in various cellular processes, including signal transduction pathways for cell survival, cell death, and antioxidant stress responses [31–34].

At its N-terminus, the PB1 (Phox/Bemp1) domain of p62 is essential for its localization to the autophagosome formation site [35]. The PB1 domain mediates p62 self-oligomerization, and it also interacts with other PB1-containing proteins, such as atypical protein kinase Cζ (PKCζ) and neighbor of BRCA1 gene 1 (NBR1) [36,37]. Mitogen-activated protein kinase kinase kinase 3 (MEKK3) also contains a PB1 domain, which forms a heterodimer with the PB1 domain of p62 and binds to TRAF6, a lysine 63 (K63) E3 ligase, to trigger nuclear factor-κB (NF-κB) activation [38]. The PB1 domain is followed by a ZZ-type zinc finger (Znf) domain, which is required for efficient starvation-induced autophagy in mouse embryonic fibroblasts (MEF) [39], and it also binds to receptor interacting protein (RIP) to regulate NF-κB activation [40].

The N-end rule pathway is a proteolytic system in which single N-terminal amino acids serve as determinants of degrons called N-degrons [41]. This pathway helps to break down and dispose of certain proteins that are misfolded or otherwise damaged. N-degrons can be created by cutting the protein at the end and modifying the remaining N-terminal residues through reactions such as deamidation, oxidation, and arginylation. The main degron is Nt-Arg (N-terminal Arginine), which is created by adding L-Arg to Nt-Asp or Nt-Glu using Arginyl-tRNA-protein transferase 1. Proteins with Nt-Arg are recognized and bound by N-recognins, which contain a UBR box, and are then broken down into shorter peptides by the ubiquitin proteasome system (UPS). Recent evidence suggests that the ZZ domain of p62 is a structural and functional counterpart of the UBR box in N-recognins in the UPS-linked N-end rule pathway for autophagic degradation of Nt-arginylated substrates, including protein aggregates, and promotes mitophagy and ER-phagy [42–44].

Next to the ZZ domain is the TRAF binding (TB) domain, which also activates NF-κB via interacting with ubiquitin E3 ligase TRAF6 [33,45]. Additionally, p62 interacts with RAPTOR via the region between the ZZ and TB domains to activate the mechanistic targets of rapamycin complex 1 (mTORC1) [46].

p62 directly binds to LC3 through the LC3-interacting region (LIR), and thus acts as an autophagy receptor protein for selective autophagy [47,48]. Followed by the LIR domain is a Kelch-like ECH-associated protein 1 (KEAP1)-interacting region (KIR) that binds to KEAP1 and drives KEAP1 degradation by selective autophagy, resulting in nuclear factor erythroid 2-related factor 2 (*nfe2l2* or NRF2) activation via the noncanonical

KEAP1-NRF2 pathway [49–52]. p62 and KEAP1 positive aggregates have been observed in autophagy-deficient mouse livers, causing the persistent activation of NRF2 in the liver [53–55]. Finally, at the C-terminus of p62, the ubiquitin-associated (UBA) domain binds to ubiquitin-labeled proteins or damaged organelles and leads them into the autophagosome for degradation [33,56].

Recent studies demonstrate that autophagy, a lysosomal degradation pathway, protects against AILI by promoting the removal of APAP-adducts, damaged mitochondria, and stressed ER [20–23,44,57]. Several pieces of evidence support that autophagy may selectively remove APAP-adducts involving p62. First, the levels of hepatic APAP-adducts reach higher levels at the metabolic and injury phases but decline at the late recovery phase, suggesting the activation of an APAP-adduct removal mechanism at the late recovery phase. Interestingly, hepatic levels of p62 also increased after APAP treatment for 24 h, which is inversely correlated with the decreased hepatic levels of APAP-adducts [58]. Second, APAP-adducts colocalize with GFP-LC3 positive autophagosomes, and this colocalization is enhanced in the presence of a lysosomal inhibitor which raises lysosomal pH and blocks degradation [23]. Third, isolated autophagosomes and lysosomes from APAP-treated mouse livers contain APAP-adducts [23]. Fourth, APAP-AD are ubiquitin-positive and colocalized with a lysosomal marker LAMP1. Fifth, the levels of APAP-adducts increase in APAP-treated primary hepatocytes with p62 knockdown via an adenovirus shRNA treated with APAP, and in p62 whole body knockout (KO) mice at 24 h after APAP treatment [23,58]. Sixth, the pharmacological inhibition or activation of autophagy increases or decreases hepatic levels of APAP-adducts, respectively [20,23]. While the above evidence supports the role of p62 in the selective removal of APAP-adducts by autophagy, it remains unclear how p62 would be recruited to APAP-adducts. The UBA domain of p62 is likely critical as it can mediate its binding with ubiquitin-positive APAP-adducts. Indeed, in NAPQI-treated Hep3B cells, mutant p62 with UBA deletion failed to be recruited to the mitochondria, although its role in the removal of APAP-adducts was not determined [44]. Future studies to investigate the role of UBA-deleted p62 mutants in the removal of APAP-adducts are needed to test this hypothesis. Another important unanswered question is how APAP-adducts become ubiquitin-positive. Whether this would involve a specific E3 ligase remains to be determined.

As discussed earlier, the p62 ZZ domain interacts with Nt-Arg residues. p62 can serve as the N-recognin to facilitate p62 in complexes with cargoes, promoting selective autophagic cargo degradation [41–43]. Based on this principle, 3D structured modeling of p62 and screening a library of 540,000 compounds have led to identifying small molecules of p62 agonists that enhance its selective autophagic degradation [59,60].

Among these p62 agonists, YTK-2205 has been shown to protect against AILI in mice by promoting hepatic mitophagy, ER-phagy, and autophagy of ubiquitin protein aggregates without affecting the NRF2 pathway. While the YTK-2205 treatment offered marked protection against AILI based on the decreased serum alanine aminotransferase and hepatic necrotic areas in mice, the protection was lost when YTK-2205 was given 1.5 and 3.5 h post-APAP injection [44]. Therefore, the use of YTK-2205 for the clinical treatment of AILI patients will be limited. However, a combined treatment of YTK-2205 with NAC may offer better beneficial effects than NAC or YTK-2205 administration alone, which should be tested in animal models in the future. While YTK-2205 promotes the recruitment of p62 to ubiquitinated mitochondria and ER, it remains unclear how increased ubiquitinated mitochondria and ER would occur after APAP treatment [44]. We previously showed that APAP treatment increased mitochondrial PARKIN translocation and subsequently increased levels of mitochondrial ubiquitin and p62, and that both PARKIN and PINK1 are necessary for mitophagy in AILI [21,22]. Small molecule activators of PINK1 or PARKIN are currently under preclinical development [61]. It would be very interesting to test the beneficial therapeutic effects of the combination of PINK1 and PARKIN activators with YTK-2205 in AILI in the future.

In addition to its role in selective autophagy, p62 may also protect against AILI via its noncanonical NRF2 activation. As discussed earlier, p62 directly interacts with KEAP1 through KIR to activate NRF2 in a nontraditional way [50,52,62]. NRF2 activation then leads to the expression of genes that synthesize GSH and antioxidants as well as detoxifying enzymes, glutamate cysteine ligase (GCL), and NADPH quinone dehydrogenase 1 (NQO1), which protect against AILI [63,64]. In liver-specific Atg5 KO mice, the accumulation of p62 in the liver leads to persistent NRF2 activation, resulting in increased levels of NQO1 and better recovery of GSH, which in turn attenuates AILI [54].

In addition to its role in protecting against AILI, p62 also regulates the activation of other proteins, such as NF-κB and mTORC1, which may be involved in liver regeneration after an overdose of APAP, particularly, in the late recovery phase of AILI [33,37,65]. Indeed, APAP treatment activates mTORC1 at 24 h, which is associated with increased hepatic p62 and cell proliferation in mouse livers. In contrast, p62 KO mice showed decreased mTORC1 activation and cell proliferation with aggravated liver injury at 24 h after APAP treatment. While it appears that p62 is protective at the injury phase of AILI, p62 may halt the recovery phase of AILI as p62 KO mice recovered better than the wild-type mice at 48 h.

As mentioned earlier, increased hepatic VWF and platelet accumulation impair liver regeneration [19]. The p62 KO mice demonstrated a decrease in hepatic VWF and platelet aggregation, which are associated with increased cell proliferation and improved liver injury after 48 h of APAP treatment [58]. While it remains unclear how p62 would affect VWF and platelet recruitment to the liver, these observations clearly support a dual role of p62 in AILI in which p62 inhibits the injury phase of AILI by increasing the selective removal of APAP-adducts and damaged mitochondria through autophagy but impairs the recovery phase of AILI, likely by enhancing hepatic blood coagulation.

In summary, it appears that the role of p62 is very complex, and targeting p62 depends on the different stages of AILI. p62 protects against the early phase of AILI, likely by promoting the removal of APAP-adducts and damaged mitochondria as well as through NRF2 activation. However, p62 impairs the late phase of liver repair/regeneration by increasing hepatic coagulation in AILI (Figure 1). Since most AILI patients have already passed the injury phase, future studies for targeting p62-mediated blood coagulation activation in the late liver regeneration phase would be more clinically relevant.

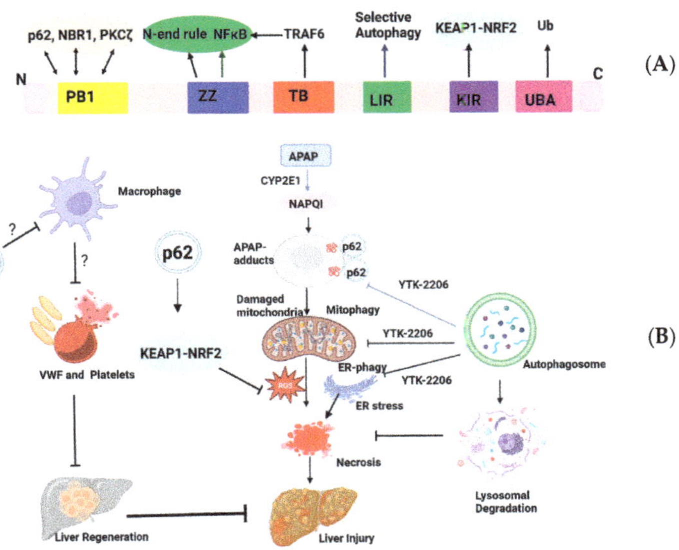

Figure 1. A proposed model for targeting p62 in acetaminophen-induced liver injury (AILI). (**A**) Schematic domain structure of sequestosome 1 (SQSTM1/p62). The Phox and Bem1 (PB1) domain sits near the N-terminus of p62 and interacts with PB1-containing proteins, including p62

itself, neighbor of *BRCA1* gene 1 (NBR1), and atypical protein kinase Cζ (PKCζ), to form homo-oligomers or hetero-oligomers. The ZZ-type zinc finger (ZZ) mediates NF-κB activation and N-end rule degradation. The tumor necrosis factor receptor-associated factor 6 (TRAF6)-binding domain (TB) interacts with TRAF6 for NF-κB activation. The LC3-interacting region (LIR) domain interacts with the microtubule light chain 3 (LC3) protein to trigger selective autophagy. The Kelch-like ECH-associated protein 1 (KEAP1)-interacting region (KIR) binds to KEAP1 for the noncanonical-nuclear factor erythroid 2-related factor 2 (NRF2) activation. The ubiquitin (UB)-associated (UBA) domain sits close to the C-terminus that binds to ubiquitinated proteins. (**B**) A proposed model for p62 in selective autophagy in AILI. APAP metabolism via cytochrome P450 2E1 (CYP2E1) generates NAPQI that forms APAP-adducts that are ubiquitinated by unknown mechanisms. APAP also induces mitochondria ubiquitination possibly via the PINK1-PARKIN pathway, and ER ubiquitination by mechanisms yet to be identified. p62 activates NRF2 to increase the expression of antioxidant genes, which helps to mitigate APAP-induced reactive oxygen species (ROS) production. YTK-2205 targets the ZZ domain and promotes the recruitment of p62 to the ubiquitinated mitochondria and ER as well as APAP-adducts for selective autophagy to remove APAP-adducts and damaged mitochondria and ER, resulting in decreased hepatocyte necrosis and liver injury. p62 inhibits hepatic macrophage activation by unknown mechanisms, which suppresses hepatic VWF and platelet activation, resulting in deceased liver regeneration in the late recovery phase of AILI. ?: mechanisms not known yet.

3. Targeting TFEB for AILI

Autophagic degradation relies on the lysosome, which is the terminal component of autophagy, containing more than 50 acid hydrolases. When autophagy is induced, increased lysosomal biogenesis is necessary to meet the need for fusion with autophagosomes and subsequent autophagic degradation. The transcription regulation of lysosome biogenesis genes is mediated by TFEB, which is a vital helix–loop–helix leucine zipper transcription factor belonging to the coordinated lysosomal expression and regulation (CLEAR) gene network [28,66]. Recent studies have shown that TFEB also regulates mitochondrial biogenesis by directly regulating the expression of peroxisome proliferator-activated receptor gamma coactivator-*1* alpha (PGC-1α), a key transcription coactivator for mitochondrial biogenesis [29,30]. TFEB is mainly regulated at its post-translational level via phosphorylation of specific amino acid residues. Several kinases, including the extracellular signal-regulated kinase 2 (ERK2), mTORC1, AKT, GSK3β, and protein kinase Cβ (PKCβ), phosphorylate TFEB at different sites [28,66–68]. TFEB is phosphorylated at Ser142 and Ser211 by mTORC1 and ERK2, which causes it to bind to the cytosolic chaperone 14-3-3 and inactivate in the cytosol [28,67]. Conversely, calcineurin dephosphorylates TFEB at Ser142 and Ser211, promoting its nuclear translocation in response to lysosomal Ca^{2+} release [69].

Our recent findings reveal a new autophagic flux scenario in mouse livers and pancreases after chronic plus binge alcohol treatment [29,70]. This scenario, which we have termed as insufficient autophagy, is characterized by impaired TFEB. Despite an increase in autophagic flux, insufficient autophagy conditions arise due to decreased TFEB-mediated lysosomal biogenesis. The limited number of lysosomes is not sufficient to fuse with all autophagosomes, resulting in a failure to reach full degradation capacity. The pharmacological or genetic activation of TFEB protects against alcohol-induced hepatitis and pancreatitis in mice [29,70]. Since the pharmacological activation of autophagy by mTORC1 inhibitors protects against AILI in the cotreatment and post-treatment of APAP mouse models [20,23] and inhibition of mTORC1 activates TFEB, it is conceivable to speculate that the activation of TFEB should also be beneficial for AILI.

We recently demonstrated that the hepatic levels of TFEB decreased in mouse livers at 6 and 24 h after APAP administration. Liver-specific deletion or overexpression of TFEB exacerbated or protected against AILI, respectively [71]. The activation of hepatic TFEB may protect against AILI via multiple mechanisms. First, the activation of TFEB increases lysosomal biogenesis, resulting in increased clearance of APAP-AD. Second, the overexpression of TFEB increases the hepatic expression of *Sqstm1*, leading to p62-mediated noncanonical NRF2 activation, and accelerates GSH resynthesis after an APAP overdose.

Third, the overexpression of TFEB increases PGC1α and mitochondrial transcription factor A (TFAM) as well as the expression of a group of mitochondrial genes, supporting the possible role of increased mitochondrial biogenesis in protecting against AILI [71].

AILI is often associated with hepatic JNK activation. Interestingly, it appears that p62-mediated selective autophagy may not be critical as p62 deficiency does not affect JNK activation [58]. On the other hand, the overexpression of TFEB inhibits APAP-induced JNK activation, suggesting that only the activation of selective autophagy is not required for inhibiting JNK activation [71]. Although there is currently no direct evidence available to explain why the overexpression of TFEB inhibits APAP-induced JNK activation, it is likely that increased mitochondria biogenesis to maintain a healthy pool of hepatic mitochondria may be involved. This is supported by the fact that TFEB also increases the expression of peroxisome proliferator-activated receptor-γ coactivator 1-α (PGC1α), a key transcription coactivator for mitochondria biogenesis.

While inhibiting mTORC1 can increase the activation of TFEB and autophagy, it may also hinder the synthesis of proteins and lipids, which are essential for cell proliferation. Therefore, inhibiting mTORC1 may not be an ideal approach for the late phase of AILI, which requires robust anabolic processes and hepatocyte proliferation. Studies have shown that mice with a genetic deletion of mTORC1 components do not show any protection against AILI due to impaired hepatocyte proliferation and liver regeneration [72]. Thus, it is crucial to search for activators of autophagy and TFEB that are independent of mTORC1 to address this issue. To identify more novel mTOR-independent TFEB agonists, we established a cell-based imaging, high-throughput screening for TFEB agonists using an FDA-approved library. We identified a group of TFEB agonists. Among them, we showed that the cotreatment of APAP with salinomycin, an antibacterial agent, activated TFEB and protected against AILI. Salinomycin treatment also markedly decreased both hepatic and serum APAP-AD and inhibited hepatic JNK activation without affecting mTORC1 activity. However, unpublished data from our lab showed that salinomycin lost its protection if it was given 2 h post-APAP administration, suggesting salinomycin may not be suitable for treating AILI patients. Moreover, as the protective effects of salinomycin against APAP were not validated in TFEB KO mice, it is also possible that other off-target mechanisms may contribute to the protective effects of salinomycin. Also, the mechanisms of how salinomycin activates TFEB remain to be determined in the future.

Narirutin (NR), a key bioactive component from a traditional Chinese medicinal herb, activates hepatic TFEB via enhanced calcineurin activity and protects against AILI in mice [73]. NR also significantly reduces hepatic levels of APAP-AD and oxidative stress but does not affect APAP-induced JNK activation. Importantly, NR exhibits protective effects against AILI even when administered 1 h after APAP injection in mice. The protective effects of NR are lost in liver-specific TFEB KO mice, suggesting that the protection against AILI with NR is mainly mediated by TFEB [73]. Overall, NR shows promise as an mTORC1-independent TFEB activator for treating AILI.

The inhibition of mTORC1 by a pharmacological inhibitor (Torin 1) induces TFEB activation resulting in increased autophagy and lysosomal biogenesis. Narirutin activates phosphatase calcineurin to increase TFEB dephosphorylation and activation. Salinomycin also activates TFEB by unknown mechanisms. TFEB activation increases lysosomal biogenesis and autophagy which help to remove APAP-adducts and damaged mitochondria, likely via p62, resulting in decreased mitochondrial ROS production and hepatocyte necrosis. The activation of TFEB also leads to increased PGC1α expression, resulting in increased mitochondrial biogenesis that may inhibit JNK activation. Therefore, the pharmacological activation of TFEB may be a promising approach for treating AILI (Figure 2).

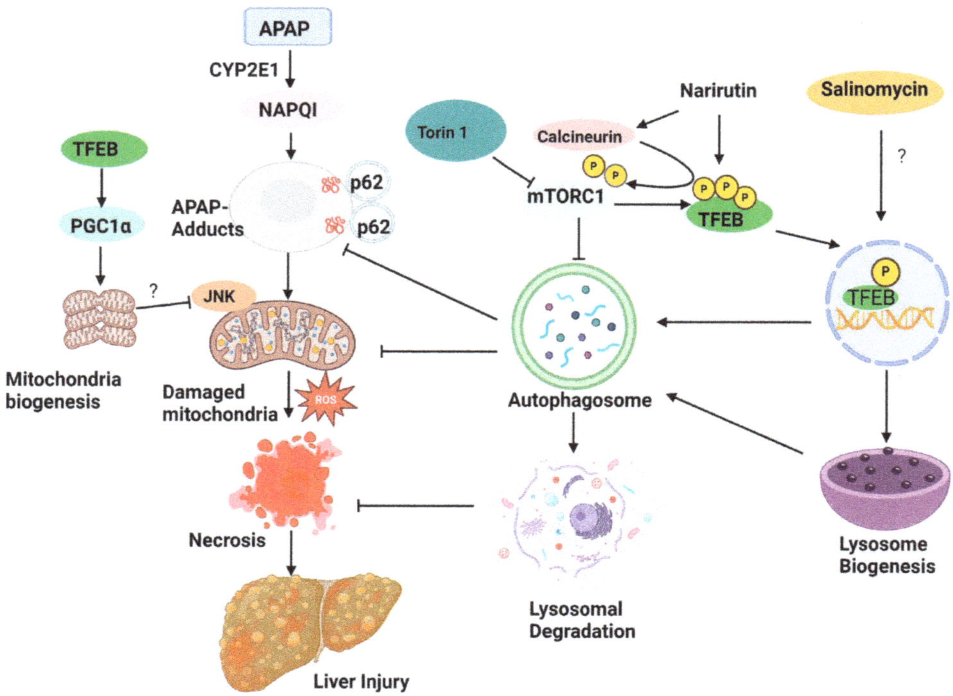

Figure 2. Induction of autophagy protects against acetaminophen-induced liver injury by removing APAP-adducts and damaged mitochondria. ?: mechanisms not known yet.

4. Conclusions and Future Perspectives

In summary, the evidence suggests that autophagy plays a crucial role in removing hepatic APAP-adducts and damaged mitochondria, which are key factors in APAP hepatotoxicity. Therefore, targeting autophagy machinery and lysosomal degradation shows promise for treating AILI. Emerging evidence supports that targeting p62-mediated selective autophagy and TFEB-mediated lysosomal biogenesis are potential therapeutic strategies for AILI. While the overexpression of both p62 and TFEB may be oncogenic, this may not be a concern for the acute liver failure of AILI patients. Further studies should be conducted to identify peptides that enhance p62 LIR-mediated selective autophagy for APAP-adducts and mitochondria, as well as to explore TFEB agonists independent of mTORC1 using high-throughput assays, either imaging-based or luciferase-based, for the TFEB promoter. In addition to the FDA-approved drug library, other small molecule/chemical libraries, including nature products and new synthetic chemicals, should be performed to identify more agonists for autophagy; p62 and TFEB can be tested in experimental AILI models. Moreover, more efforts should be put towards the late phase of liver repair/regeneration rather than the early injury phase when testing these p62 and TFEB agonists, which is more clinically relevant.

Author Contributions: H.-M.N. and W.-X.D. conceived the idea and drafted this manuscript. K.H. and M.N. read and revised this manuscript. All authors have read and agreed to the published version of the manuscript.

Funding: This study was supported in part by the National Institute of Health (NIH) funds R37 AA020518, R21 AA030617 (WXD), and R01DK134737 (HMN).

Institutional Review Board Statement: Not Applicable.

Informed Consent Statement: Not Applicable.

Data Availability Statement: No new data were created or analyzed in this study. Data sharing is not applicable to this article.

Conflicts of Interest: The authors declare that no conflicts of interest exist.

References

1. Mowry, J.B.; Spyker, D.A.; Brooks, D.E.; Zimmerman, A.; Schauben, J.L. 2015 Annual Report of the American Association of Poison Control Centers' National Poison Data System (NPDS): 33rd Annual Report. *Clin. Toxicol.* **2016**, *54*, 924–1109. [CrossRef]
2. Lee, W.M. Acetaminophen (APAP) hepatotoxicity—Isn't it time for APAP to go away? *J. Hepatol.* **2017**, *67*, 1324–1331. [CrossRef] [PubMed]
3. Larson, A.M. Acetaminophen hepatotoxicity. *Clin. Liver Dis.* **2007**, *11*, 525–548. [CrossRef]
4. Ostapowicz, G.; Fontana, R.J.; Schiødt, F.V.; Larson, A.; Davern, T.J.; Han, S.H.; McCashland, T.M.; Shakil, A.O.; Hay, J.E.; Hynan, L. Results of a prospective study of acute liver failure at 17 tertiary care centers in the United States. *Ann. Intern. Med.* **2002**, *137*, 947–954. [CrossRef]
5. Lee, W.M. Acetaminophen-related acute liver failure in the United States. *Hepatol. Res.* **2008**, *38*, S3–S8. [CrossRef]
6. Budnitz, D.S.; Lovegrove, M.C.; Crosby, A.E. Emergency department visits for overdoses of acetaminophen-containing products. *Am. J. Prev. Med.* **2011**, *40*, 585–592. [CrossRef]
7. Dart, R.C.; Mullins, M.E.; Matoushek, T.; Ruha, A.M.; Burns, M.M.; Simone, K.; Beuhler, M.C.; Heard, K.J.; Mazer-Amirshahi, M.; Stork, C.M.; et al. Management of Acetaminophen Poisoning in the US and Canada: A Consensus Statement. *JAMA Netw Open* **2023**, *6*, e2327739. [CrossRef]
8. Heard, K.J. Acetylcysteine for Acetaminophen Poisoning. *N. Engl. J. Med.* **2008**, *359*, 285–292. [CrossRef]
9. Bhushan, B.; Apte, U. Liver Regeneration after Acetaminophen Hepatotoxicity: Mechanisms and Therapeutic Opportunities. *Am. J. Pathol.* **2019**, *189*, 719–729. [CrossRef]
10. McGill, M.R.; Sharpe, M.R.; Williams, C.D.; Taha, M.; Curry, S.C.; Jaeschke, H. The mechanism underlying acetaminophen-induced hepatotoxicity in humans and mice involves mitochondrial damage and nuclear DNA fragmentation. *J. Clin. Investig.* **2012**, *122*, 1574–1583. [CrossRef]
11. Hinson, J.A.; Roberts, D.W.; James, L.P. Mechanisms of Acetaminophen-Induced Liver Necrosis. *Handb. Exp. Pharmacol.* **2010**, *196*, 369–405.
12. Yan, M.; Huo, Y.; Yin, S.; Hu, H. Mechanisms of acetaminophen-induced liver injury and its implications for therapeutic interventions. *Redox Biol.* **2018**, *17*, 274–283. [CrossRef]
13. Ramachandran, A.; Jaeschke, H. Acetaminophen Toxicity: Novel Insights Into Mechanisms and Future Perspectives. *Gene Expr.* **2018**, *18*, 19–30. [CrossRef]
14. Ramachandran, A.; Jaeschke, H. Acetaminophen hepatotoxicity: A mitochondrial perspective. *Adv. Pharmacol.* **2019**, *85*, 195–219.
15. Huebener, P.; Pradere, J.P.; Hernandez, C.; Gwak, G.Y.; Caviglia, J.M.; Mu, X.; Loike, J.D.; Schwabe, R.F. The HMGB1/RAGE axis triggers neutrophil-mediated injury amplification following necrosis. *J. Clin. Investig.* **2015**, *125*, 539–550. [CrossRef] [PubMed]
16. He, Y.; Feng, D.; Li, M.; Gao, Y.; Ramirez, T.; Cao, H.; Kim, S.J.; Yang, Y.; Cai, Y.; Ju, C.; et al. Hepatic mitochondrial DNA/Toll-like receptor 9/MicroRNA-223 forms a negative feedback loop to limit neutrophil overactivation and acetaminophen hepatotoxicity in mice. *Hepatology* **2017**, *66*, 220–234. [CrossRef] [PubMed]
17. Ganey, P.E.; Luyendyk, J.P.; Newport, S.W.; Eagle, T.M.; Maddox, J.F.; Mackman, N.; Roth, R.A. Role of the coagulation system in acetaminophen-induced hepatotoxicity in mice. *Hepatology* **2007**, *46*, 1177–1186. [CrossRef] [PubMed]
18. Holt, M.P.; Cheng, L.; Ju, C. Identification and characterization of infiltrating macrophages in acetaminophen-induced liver injury. *J. Leukoc. Biol.* **2008**, *84*, 1410–1421. [CrossRef]
19. Groeneveld, D.; Cline-Fedewa, H.; Baker, K.S.; Williams, K.J.; Roth, R.A.; Mittermeier, K.; Lisman, T.; Palumbo, J.S.; Luyendyk, J.P. Von Willebrand factor delays liver repair after acetaminophen-induced acute liver injury in mice. *J. Hepatol.* **2020**, *72*, 146–155. [CrossRef]
20. Ni, H.M.; Bockus, A.; Boggess, N.; Jaeschke, H.; Ding, W.X. Activation of autophagy protects against acetaminophen-induced hepatotoxicity. *Hepatology* **2012**, *55*, 222–232. [CrossRef]
21. Williams, J.A.; Ni, H.M.; Haynes, A.; Manley, S.; Li, Y.; Jaeschke, H.; Ding, W.X. Chronic Deletion and Acute Knockdown of Parkin Have Differential Responses to Acetaminophen-induced Mitophagy and Liver Injury in Mice. *J. Biol. Chem.* **2015**, *290*, 10934–10946. [CrossRef]
22. Wang, H.; Ni, H.M.; Chao, X.; Ma, X.; Rodriguez, Y.A.; Chavan, H.; Wang, S.; Krishnamurthy, P.; Dobrowsky, R.; Xu, D.X.; et al. Double deletion of PINK1 and Parkin impairs hepatic mitophagy and exacerbates acetaminophen-induced liver injury in mice. *Redox Biol.* **2019**, *22*, 101148. [CrossRef]

23. Ni, H.M.; McGill, M.R.; Chao, X.; Du, K.; Williams, J.A.; Xie, Y.; Jaeschke, H.; Ding, W.X. Removal of acetaminophen protein adducts by autophagy protects against acetaminophen-induced liver injury in mice. *J. Hepatol.* **2016**, *65*, 354–362. [CrossRef]
24. Kirkin, V.; Rogov, V.V. A Diversity of Selective Autophagy Receptors Determines the Specificity of the Autophagy Pathway. *Mol. Cell* **2019**, *76*, 268–285. [CrossRef]
25. Johansen, T.; Lamark, T. Selective Autophagy: ATG8 Family Proteins, LIR Motifs and Cargo Receptors. *J. Mol. Biol.* **2020**, *432*, 80–103. [CrossRef]
26. Ma, X.; McKeen, T.; Zhang, J.; Ding, W.X. Role and Mechanisms of Mitophagy in Liver Diseases. *Cells* **2020**, *9*, 837. [CrossRef] [PubMed]
27. Lamark, T.; Johansen, T. Mechanisms of Selective Autophagy. *Annu. Rev. Cell Dev. Biol.* **2021**, *37*, 143–169. [CrossRef]
28. Settembre, C.; Fraldi, A.; Medina, D.L.; Ballabio, A. Signals from the lysosome: A control centre for cellular clearance and energy metabolism. *Nat. Rev. Mol. Cell Biol.* **2013**, *14*, 283–296. [CrossRef]
29. Chao, X.; Wang, S.; Zhao, K.; Li, Y.; Williams, J.A.; Li, T.; Chavan, H.; Krishnamurthy, P.; He, X.C.; Li, L.; et al. Impaired TFEB-mediated Lysosome Biogenesis and Autophagy Promote Chronic Ethanol-induced Liver Injury and Steatosis in Mice. *Gastroenterology* **2018**, *155*, 865–879.e12. [CrossRef]
30. Settembre, C.; De Cegli, R.; Mansueto, G.; Saha, P.K.; Vetrini, F.; Visvikis, O.; Huynh, T.; Carissimo, A.; Palmer, D.; Klisch, T.J.; et al. TFEB controls cellular lipid metabolism through a starvation-induced autoregulatory loop. *Nat. Cell Biol.* **2013**, *15*, 647–658. [CrossRef]
31. Moscat, J.; Diaz-Meco, M.T. p62 at the crossroads of autophagy, apoptosis, and cancer. *Cell* **2009**, *137*, 1001–1004. [CrossRef]
32. Komatsu, M.; Kageyama, S.; Ichimura, Y. p62/SQSTM1/A170: Physiology and pathology. *Pharmacol. Res.* **2012**, *66*, 457–462. [CrossRef]
33. Manley, S.; Williams, J.A.; Ding, W.X. Role of p62/SQSTM1 in liver physiology and pathogenesis. *Exp. Biol. Med.* **2013**, *238*, 525–538. [CrossRef] [PubMed]
34. Qian, H.; Ding, W.X. SQSTM1/p62 and Hepatic Mallory-Denk Body Formation in Alcohol-Associated Liver Disease. *Am. J. Pathol.* **2023**, *193*, 1415–1426. [CrossRef]
35. Itakura, E.; Mizushima, N. p62 Targeting to the autophagosome formation site requires self-oligomerization but not LC3 binding. *J. Cell Biol.* **2011**, *192*, 17–27. [CrossRef]
36. Ren, J.; Wang, J.; Wang, Z.; Wu, J. Structural and biochemical insights into the homotypic PB1-PB1 complex between PKCζ and p62. *Sci. China Life Sci.* **2014**, *57*, 69–80. [CrossRef] [PubMed]
37. Sanchez-Martin, P.; Saito, T.; Komatsu, M. p62/SQSTM1: 'Jack of all trades' in health and cancer. *FEBS J.* **2019**, *286*, 8–23. [CrossRef]
38. Nakamura, K.; Kimple, A.J.; Siderovski, D.P.; Johnson, G.L. PB1 domain interaction of p62/sequestosome 1 and MEKK3 regulates NF-κB activation. *J. Biol. Chem.* **2010**, *285*, 2077–2089. [CrossRef] [PubMed]
39. Zhang, Y.; Mun, S.R.; Linares, J.F.; Ahn, J.; Towers, C.G.; Ji, C.H.; Fitzwalter, B.E.; Holden, M.R.; Mi, W.; Shi, X. ZZ-dependent regulation of p62/SQSTM1 in autophagy. *Nat. Commun.* **2018**, *9*, 4373. [CrossRef]
40. Sanz, L.; Sanchez, P.; Lallena, M.J.; Diaz-Meco, M.T.; Moscat, J. The interaction of p62 with RIP links the atypical PKCs to NF-kappaB activation. *EMBO J.* **1999**, *18*, 3044–3053. [CrossRef]
41. Varshavsky, A. N-degron and C-degron pathways of protein degradation. *Proc. Natl. Acad. Sci. USA* **2019**, *116*, 358–366. [CrossRef] [PubMed]
42. Cha-Molstad, H.; Sung, K.S.; Hwang, J.; Kim, K.A.; Yu, J.E.; Yoo, Y.D.; Jang, J.M.; Han, D.H.; Molstad, M.; Kim, J.G.; et al. Amino-terminal arginylation targets endoplasmic reticulum chaperone BiP for autophagy through p62 binding. *Nat. Cell Biol.* **2015**, *17*, 917–929. [CrossRef] [PubMed]
43. Cha-Molstad, H.; Lee, S.H.; Kim, J.G.; Sung, K.W.; Hwang, J.; Shim, S.M.; Ganipisetti, S.; McGuire, T.; Mook-Jung, I.; Ciechanover, A.; et al. Regulation of autophagic proteolysis by the N-recognin SQSTM1/p62 of the N-end rule pathway. *Autophagy* **2018**, *14*, 359–361. [CrossRef] [PubMed]
44. Kim, H.Y.; Yoon, H.S.; Heo, A.J.; Jung, E.J.; Ji, C.H.; Mun, S.R.; Lee, M.J.; Kwon, Y.T.; Park, J.W. Mitophagy and endoplasmic reticulum-phagy accelerated by a p62 ZZ ligand alleviates paracetamol-induced hepatotoxicity. *Br. J. Pharmacol.* **2023**, *180*, 1247–1266. [CrossRef] [PubMed]
45. Schimmack, G.; Schorpp, K.; Kutzner, K.; Gehring, T.; Brenke, J.K.; Hadian, K.; Krappmann, D. YOD1/TRAF6 association balances p62-dependent IL-1 signaling to NF-kappaB. *Elife* **2017**, *6*, e22416. [CrossRef] [PubMed]
46. Duran, A.; Amanchy, R.; Linares, J.F.; Joshi, J.; Abu-Baker, S.; Porollo, A.; Hansen, M.; Moscat, J.; Diaz-Meco, M.T. p62 is a key regulator of nutrient sensing in the mTORC1 pathway. *Mol. Cell* **2011**, *44*, 134–146. [CrossRef]
47. Ichimura, Y.; Kumanomidou, T.; Sou, Y.S.; Mizushima, T.; Ezaki, J.; Ueno, T.; Kominami, E.; Yamane, T.; Tanaka, K.; Komatsu, M. Structural basis for sorting mechanism of p62 in selective autophagy. *J. Biol. Chem.* **2008**, *283*, 22847–22857. [CrossRef] [PubMed]
48. Pankiv, S.; Clausen, T.H.; Lamark, T.; Brech, A.; Bruun, J.-A.; Outzen, H.; Øvervatn, A.; Bjørkøy, G.; Johansen, T. p62/SQSTM1 binds directly to Atg8/LC3 to facilitate degradation of ubiquitinated protein aggregates by autophagy. *J. Biol. Chem.* **2007**, *282*, 24131–24145. [CrossRef]

49. Katsuragi, Y.; Ichimura, Y.; Komatsu, M. Regulation of the Keap1–Nrf2 pathway by p62/SQSTM1. *Curr. Opin. Toxicol.* **2016**, *1*, 54–61. [CrossRef]
50. Komatsu, M.; Kurokawa, H.; Waguri, S.; Taguchi, K.; Kobayashi, A.; Ichimura, Y.; Sou, Y.S.; Ueno, I.; Sakamoto, A.; Tong, K.I.; et al. The selective autophagy substrate p62 activates the stress responsive transcription factor Nrf2 through inactivation of Keap1. *Nat. Cell Biol.* **2010**, *12*, 213–223. [CrossRef]
51. Ichimura, Y.; Waguri, S.; Sou, Y.S.; Kageyama, S.; Hasegawa, J.; Ishimura, R.; Saito, T.; Yang, Y.; Kouno, T.; Fukutomi, T.; et al. Phosphorylation of p62 activates the Keap1-Nrf2 pathway during selective autophagy. *Mol. Cell* **2013**, *51*, 618–631. [CrossRef] [PubMed]
52. Jain, A.; Lamark, T.; Sjottem, E.; Larsen, K.B.; Awuh, J.A.; Overvatn, A.; McMahon, M.; Hayes, J.D.; Johansen, T. p62/SQSTM1 is a target gene for transcription factor NRF2 and creates a positive feedback loop by inducing antioxidant response element-driven gene transcription. *J. Biol. Chem.* **2010**, *285*, 22576–22591. [CrossRef] [PubMed]
53. Inami, Y.; Waguri, S.; Sakamoto, A.; Kouno, T.; Nakada, K.; Hino, O.; Watanabe, S.; Ando, J.; Iwadate, M.; Yamamoto, M. Persistent activation of Nrf2 through p62 in hepatocellular carcinoma cells. *J. Cell Biol.* **2011**, *193*, 275–284. [CrossRef] [PubMed]
54. Ni, H.M.; Boggess, N.; McGill, M.R.; Lebofsky, M.; Borude, P.; Apte, U.; Jaeschke, H.; Ding, W.X. Liver-specific loss of Atg5 causes persistent activation of Nrf2 and protects against acetaminophen-induced liver injury. *Toxicol. Sci.* **2012**, *127*, 438–450. [CrossRef] [PubMed]
55. Ni, H.M.; Woolbright, B.L.; Williams, J.; Copple, B.; Cui, W.; Luyendyk, J.P.; Jaeschke, H.; Ding, W.X. Nrf2 promotes the development of fibrosis and tumorigenesis in mice with defective hepatic autophagy. *J. Hepatol.* **2014**, *61*, 617–625. [CrossRef] [PubMed]
56. Isogai, S.; Morimoto, D.; Arita, K.; Unzai, S.; Tenno, T.; Hasegawa, J.; Sou, Y.S.; Komatsu, M.; Tanaka, K.; Shirakawa, M.; et al. Crystal structure of the ubiquitin-associated (UBA) domain of p62 and its interaction with ubiquitin. *J. Biol. Chem.* **2011**, *286*, 31864–31874. [CrossRef] [PubMed]
57. Li, Y.; Ni, H.M.; Jaeschke, H.; Ding, W.X. Chlorpromazine protects against acetaminophen-induced liver injury in mice by modulating autophagy and c-Jun N-terminal kinase activation. *Liver Res.* **2019**, *3*, 65–74. [CrossRef] [PubMed]
58. Qian, H.; Bai, Q.; Yang, X.; Akakpo, J.Y.; Ji, L.; Yang, L.; Rulicke, T.; Zatloukal, K.; Jaeschke, H.; Ni, H.M.; et al. Dual roles of p62/SQSTM1 in the injury and recovery phases of acetaminophen-induced liver injury in mice. *Acta Pharm. Sin. B* **2021**, *11*, 3791–3805. [CrossRef]
59. Cha-Molstad, H.; Yu, J.E.; Feng, Z.W.; Lee, S.H.; Kim, J.G.; Yang, P.; Han, B.; Sung, K.W.; Yoo, Y.D.; Hwang, J.; et al. p62/SQSTM1/Sequestosome-1 is an N-recognin of the N-end rule pathway which modulates autophagosome biogenesis. *Nat. Commun.* **2017**, *8*, 102. [CrossRef]
60. Ji, C.H.; Kim, H.Y.; Heo, A.J.; Lee, S.H.; Lee, M.J.; Kim, S.B.; Srinivasrao, G.; Mun, S.R.; Cha-Molstad, H.; Ciechanover, A.; et al. The N-Degron Pathway Mediates ER-phagy. *Mol. Cell* **2019**, *75*, 1058–1072.e9. [CrossRef]
61. Miller, S.; Muqit, M.M.K. Therapeutic approaches to enhance PINK1/Parkin mediated mitophagy for the treatment of Parkinson's disease. *Neurosci. Lett.* **2019**, *705*, 7–13. [CrossRef] [PubMed]
62. Lau, A.; Wang, X.J.; Zhao, F.; Villeneuve, N.F.; Wu, T.; Jiang, T.; Sun, Z.; White, E.; Zhang, D.D. A noncanonical mechanism of Nrf2 activation by autophagy deficiency: Direct interaction between Keap1 and p62. *Mol. Cell. Biol.* **2010**, *30*, 3275–3285. [CrossRef] [PubMed]
63. Reisman, S.A.; Csanaky, I.L.; Aleksunes, L.M.; Klaassen, C.D. Altered disposition of acetaminophen in Nrf2-null and Keap1-knockdown mice. *Toxicol. Sci. Off. J. Soc. Toxicol.* **2009**, *109*, 31–40. [CrossRef]
64. Gum, S.I.; Cho, M.K. Recent updates on acetaminophen hepatotoxicity: The role of nrf2 in hepatoprotection. *Toxicol. Res.* **2013**, *29*, 165–172. [CrossRef]
65. Moscat, J.; Karin, M.; Diaz-Meco, M.T. p62 in Cancer: Signaling Adaptor Beyond Autophagy. *Cell* **2016**, *167*, 606–609. [CrossRef] [PubMed]
66. Napolitano, G.; Ballabio, A. TFEB at a glance. *J. Cell Sci.* **2016**, *129*, 2475–2481. [CrossRef] [PubMed]
67. Settembre, C.; Di Malta, C.; Polito, V.A.; Garcia Arencibia, M.; Vetrini, F.; Erdin, S.; Erdin, S.U.; Huynh, T.; Medina, D.; Colella, P.; et al. TFEB links autophagy to lysosomal biogenesis. *Science* **2011**, *332*, 1429–1433. [CrossRef] [PubMed]
68. Martina, J.A.; Diab, H.I.; Brady, O.A.; Puertollano, R. TFEB and TFE3 are novel components of the integrated stress response. *EMBO J.* **2016**, *35*, 479–495. [CrossRef] [PubMed]
69. Medina, D.L.; Di Paola, S.; Peluso, I.; Armani, A.; De Stefani, D.; Venditti, R.; Montefusco, S.; Scotto-Rosato, A.; Prezioso, C.; Forrester, A.; et al. Lysosomal calcium signalling regulates autophagy through calcineurin and TFEB. *Nat. Cell Biol.* **2015**, *17*, 288–299. [CrossRef]
70. Wang, S.; Ni, H.M.; Chao, X.; Ma, X.; Kolodecik, T.; De Lisle, R.; Ballabio, A.; Pacher, P.; Ding, W.X. Critical Role of TFEB-Mediated Lysosomal Biogenesis in Alcohol-Induced Pancreatitis in Mice and Humans. *Cell. Mol. Gastroenterol. Hepatol.* **2020**, *10*, 59–81. [CrossRef]
71. Chao, X.; Niu, M.; Wang, S.; Ma, X.; Yang, X.; Sun, H.; Hu, X.; Wang, H.; Zhang, L.; Huang, R.; et al. High-throughput screening of novel TFEB agonists in protecting against acetaminophen-induced liver injury in mice. *Acta Pharm. Sin. B* **2024**, *14*, 190–206. [CrossRef] [PubMed]

72. Sun, H.; Ni, H.-M.; McCracken, J.; Akakpo, J.Y.; Fulte, S.; Mckeen, T.; Jaeschke, H.; Wang, H.; Ding, W.X. Liver-specific deletion of mechanistic target of rapamycin does not protect against acetaminophen-induced liver injury in mice. *Liver Res.* **2021**, *5*, 79–87. [CrossRef] [PubMed]
73. Fang, Z.; Xu, Y.; Liu, G.; Shao, Q.; Niu, X.; Tai, W.; Shen, T.; Fan, M.; Chen, M.; Lei, L.; et al. Narirutin activates TFEB (transcription factor EB) to protect against Acetaminophen-induced liver injury by targeting PPP3/calcineurin. *Autophagy* **2023**, *19*, 2240–2256. [CrossRef] [PubMed]

livers

MDPI

Review

Acetylcysteine Treatment of Acetaminophen Overdose: Foundational and Clinical Development

Barry H. Rumack

Department of Emergency Medicine, University of Colorado School of Medicine, 12401 East 17th Avenue, Campus Box 215, Aurora, CO 80045, USA; barry.rumack@cuanschutz.edu

Abstract: N-acetyl para-aminophenol was suggested as a safer alternative to other drugs on the market for pain and fever in 1948. It was given the generic name "acetaminophen" in 1951 and the trade name "Tylenol" when it was put on the market in the USA in 1955 as a prescription drug to treat pediatric fever. It also received the generic name "paracetamol" in the UK where it was initially marketed in 1956 under the name "Panadol". Toxicity from overdose of acetaminophen was reported in 1966. Research at the US National Institutes of Health uncovered the mechanisms of toxicity and proposed a treatment in a foundational series of papers in 1973 and 1974. A nomogram was developed in 1973 and published in 1975 to guide estimation of patient risk of hepatic toxicity. Rapid development followed utilizing acetylcysteine given both orally and intravenously. Various protocols and methods of administration have been employed over time with the primary use today of acetylcysteine intravenously as the therapeutic method. The nomogram has been revised over time to the current version, published in 2023, which allows stratification of patients to a high-risk group over 300 mg/L at 4 h and standard risk above 150 mg/L at 4 h, except in the UK where the standard risk is defined very conservatively with a line above 100 mg/L at 4 h. Adjunct therapy with fomepizole in patients with massive ingestions, delay until arrival in a health care facility or renal injury has been proposed. The mortality rate with treatment has been substantially reduced and recovery from hepatic injury is achieved in almost all patients.

Keywords: acetaminophen; paracetamol; n-acetyl para-aminophenol; N-acetyl-para-amino benzoquinone imine; NAPQI; fomepizole; glutathione; glucuronide

1. Clinical Application of Acetaminophen (Paracetamol) for Fever and Pain

It has been 77 years since n-acetyl-p-aminophenol was suggested for clinical use in a publication "...that it may have distinct advantages over acetanilide and related as an analgesic". This publication by Bernard B. Brodie and Julius Axelrod in 1948 demonstrated in humans that when "...administered orally, it was not attended by the formation of methemoglobin" and should be considered as a less toxic alternative to acetophenetidin (phenacetin) [1].

Commercial development was considered a few years later. Robert Lincoln McNeil Jr. joined the family business, McNeil Laboratories, and decided he wanted to compete with aspirin (https://en.wikipedia.org/wiki/Robert_L._McNeil_Jr. (accessed on 21 April 2025)). He was aware of the work by Brodie and Axelrod and McNeil Laboratories began work to bring the analgesic and antipyretic to market in 1951. Robert McNeil coined the generic name "acetaminophen" (APAP) from the chemical name as a derivative N-***acet***yl-p-***aminophen***ol and a marketing colleague at the company also derived the brand name

"Tylenol" (N-ace***tyl***-p-aminoph***enol)*** from the chemical name. Tylenol was approved by the FDA as a prescription drug starting in 1955 for pediatric use as "Children's Tylenol Elixir" and became an over-the-counter drug, also marketed to adults, after the purchase of McNeil Laboratories in 1960 by Johnson and Johnson. It was introduced in the United Kingdom in 1956 by Frederick Stearns and Co, also initially as a prescription drug. They utilized the generic term "paracetamol" as a derivative from an alternative chemical name "***paraacet***yl-**am**ino-phen***ol*** with the trade name "Panadol".

2. Mechanisms of Toxicity of Acetaminophen (Paracetamol)

Within a few years following its introduction as an over-the-counter drug, cases of overdose were reported [2,3]. These reports were initially in the United Kingdom and then elsewhere. There were two key publications from Edinburgh in 1970 and 1971 describing the course of hepatic centrilobular necrosis from acetaminophen and the pharmacokinetics (Figure 1) without any known treatment [4,5].

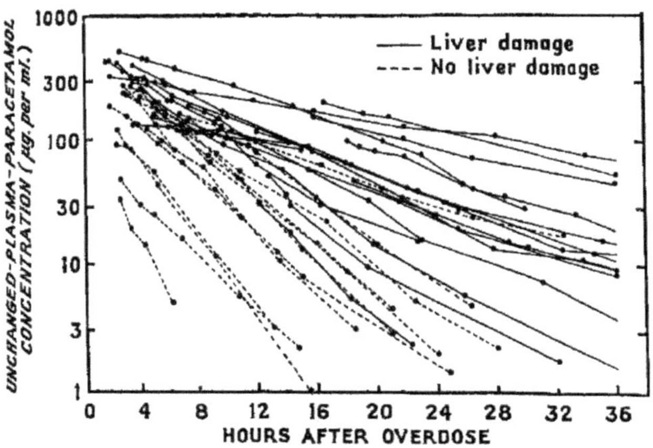

Figure 1. Plot of untreated patients from first acetaminophen level to 36 h post ingestion. Prescott LF, Roscoe P, Wright N, Brown SS. Plasma-paracetamol half-life and hepatic necrosis in patients with paracetamol overdosage. Lancet 1971;1(7698):519–22 [4].

During this time-period, Bernard Brodie at NIH was looking at carcinogenic compounds that were being activated to reactive species that were bound covalently to cellular macromolecules which produced toxicity. He postulated that this might occur with bromobenzene that also produced centrilobular necrosis in the liver. As part of this research, acetaminophen was used to block glucuronidation and sulfation of bromobenzene. His laboratory observed that acetaminophen control animals developed centrilobular necrosis *without* bromobenzene. Thus began an extraordinary research effort by Mitchell and colleagues at NIH focused on acetaminophen, which produced a landmark series of papers published in 1973 and 1974 [6–12]. These papers defined the mechanism of toxicity from acetaminophen and proposed a therapeutic approach. Further details from this time were recently published by one of the participants, David Jollow, in a comprehensive reminiscence [13].

Holtzman and colleagues had previously demonstrated that glutathione conjugated epoxides and further work by Calder had recently demonstrated such a metabolite from phenacetin [14,15]. The research in the Mitchell laboratory demonstrated that glutathione depletion and the administration of a surrogate could interfere with the toxic metabolite. They postulated a toxic intermediate which was then identified as N-acetyl-p-benzoquinone imine (NAPQI) as a highly electrophilic substance which could be conjugated by glutathione. Substantial additional work on NAPQI was carried out in the Nelson Laboratory at NIH and published in the 1980s [16,17]. A recent review discussed in detail that NAPQI covalently binds to different key mitochondrial enzymes, thus resulting in oxidative phosphorylation impairment and severe ATP depletion. As the number of overdoses producing hepatic toxicity increased and were reported clinically, there was substantial interest on the part of investigators in finding a treatment regimen which could be administered to these patients [18].

The author of this paper, Barry Rumack (BHR), had worked in the Holtzman laboratory at the National Institutes of Health from 1969 to 1971 on various aspects of hepatic metabolism. Toward the end of that time, there was discussion regarding the work being carried out in the Mitchell Laboratory on acetaminophen but none of the acetaminophen work was done in the Holtzman laboratory.

Barry Rumack was invited to do a clinical and research fellowship at the Royal Infirmary of Edinburgh Poisons Unit in 1973 with Henry Matthew who was Physician-in-Charge and Director of the Scottish Poisons Information Bureau. Two recently published papers provide historical information over 50 years of the clinical and research work, with a primary focus on the work carried out in Edinburgh and Denver [19,20].

The Royal Infirmary of Edinburgh Poisons Unit admitted patients with overdoses of acetaminophen during the time that Barry Rumack was in residence. The journal "Pediatrics" had asked Barry Rumack to write a paper regarding acetaminophen as there had been reports in the United States as well. As part of that paper, the journal requested a graphic representation of the risk from overdose rather than just the pharmacokinetic formulas. Rumack and Matthew wrote the paper together and utilized data from 30 cases from the paper published in 1971 and collected additional data from 34 cases and created a nomogram in 1973, which was published in 1975 [21]. This nomogram (Figure 2) permitted physicians to rapidly interpret levels of acetaminophen and provide a guide to the risk of hepatic toxicity. During that time, acetaminophen hepatic toxicity was defined with transaminase levels greater than 1000 IU/L. This was because the laboratory had to dilute samples and re-assay over this concentration in order to provide a transaminase measurement.

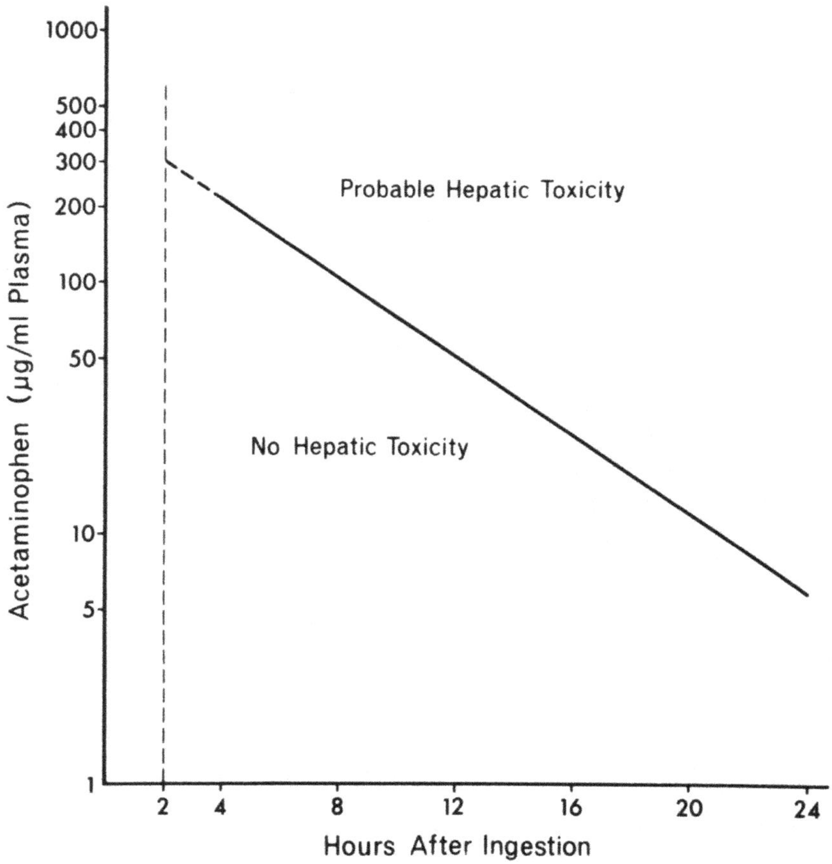

Figure 2. Original nomogram showing a dashed line from 2 to 4 h where there was insufficient data. The line was created from 64 patients and approximately 200 data points. Rumack BH, Matthew H. Acetaminophen poisoning and toxicity. Pediatrics. 1975 Jun;55(6):871–6. PMID: 1134886 [21].

3. Development of n-Acetylcysteine (NAC) Treatment of Acetaminophen Overdose

Mitchell et al. suggested the administration of cysteamine (4-mercaptoethanol) or other nucleophiles might provide a basis for treatment in humans [10]. This 1974 publication had elegantly demonstrated the production of metabolites following radioactively labeled acetaminophen being administered to human volunteers. Two human volunteers were given radioactive 3H-APAP 1200 mg with 100 microcuries (µc) and urine was collected at 12 h intervals for 48 h. The results were measured with 2.1% free APAP, 52.1% sulfate, 42% glucuronide and 3.8% mercapturic acid conjugate. Mercapturic acid, which is derived from glutathione catabolism, had previously been identified in animal studies because of the conversion of acetaminophen to an electrophilic molecule. These animal studies also demonstrated that mercapturic acid is proportional to an administered dose of acetaminophen [6–11]. Of the 12 volunteers, the remaining ten were given non-radioactive APAP doses 900, 1200 and 1800 mg, and 10 were given desipramine or metyrapone followed by APAP while 7 subjects received phenobarbital and then amobarbital prior to APAP. Phenobarbital and amobarbital increased mercapturic acid in 6 of 7 and desipramine decreased mercapturic acid in 4 of 10. The mouse studies in this paper demonstrated that pretreatment with cysteamine reduced the mortality rate and hepatic necrosis if given within 2 to 3 h. Dimercaprol also reduced necrosis but desipramine did not. Timing in mice is faster than humans and is longer than the murine 2 to 3 h, perhaps 6 to 8 or 10 in humans. The authors concluded, "cysteamine protects mice from arylation of hepatic macromolecules and glutathione may serve a similar protective role in humans" [10].

Based on this groundbreaking work by Mitchell et al. suggesting cysteamine, Prescott and colleagues at the Royal Infirmary of Edinburgh were able to treat a series of patients with cysteamine in early 1974. Cysteamine showed clinical success although with some significant side effects [22]. In fact, Prescott had to be admitted to his own poisons unit when he and a registrar suffered substantial toxicity after administering cysteamine to themselves to determine dosing [20]. This toxicity was primarily gastrointestinal and dehydration. Cysteamine administered to seven patients with severe acetaminophen overdosage treated within 4 to 10 h post ingestion resulted in no hepatic necrosis in five and mild transient hepatic injury in two. Eleven untreated patients all developed severe hepatic necrosis and two died [22]. This study was crucial to the understanding that a sulfhydryl containing medication could intervene to prevent toxicity from the toxic metabolite N-acetyl-p-benzoquinone imine (NAPQI) from acetaminophen in humans.

The medical director of McNeil Laboratoires, Thomas Gates, MD was aware in early 1974 of the paper by Rumack and Matthew which had not yet been published. In addition to the nomogram, the paper included epidemiologic information on 156 reported ingestions and two fatalities recorded in Denver from acetaminophen. There were a series of meetings and discussions and McNeil Laboratories, manufacturer of Tylenol, (a subsidiary of Johnson and Johnson at the time and now part of Kenvue) agreed to provide funding for further investigation of acetaminophen toxicity and potential treatments.

Cysteamine had been previously investigated as a radio protective agent by the US Army in the 1950s and was found to be too toxic for use in circumstances involving radioactive agents, primarily the atomic bomb tests being carried out at the time. Soldiers administered cysteamine developed gastrointestinal distress, nausea and vomiting. Rumack was aware of this toxicity from cysteamine and presented this information at meetings with several scientists including those from McNeil Laboratories regarding the development of a treatment for the increasing number of cases of acetaminophen overdose being seen by US poison centers.

Two investigators at McNeil Laboratories, Elliott Piperno and D.A. Berssenbruegge began examining all medications on the market which contained sulfhydryl groups in 1974. Agents investigated included methionine, cysteine, Dimercaprol (British Anti-Lewisite-BAL), penicillamine and Mucomyst (acetylcysteine) Working with Beagle dogs they determined that the most effective treatment with the least toxicity was acetylcysteine. The results of their work which were known starting in 1974 were eventually published [23,24]. Methionine, which was being investigated clinically at Guy's Hospital in London, was rejected for use in the United States as the survival rate in mice was decreased at higher dosages when administered at 1 or 4.5 h after acetaminophen [24]. Methionine continued to be utilized orally in some centers [25].

Rumack, Gates and colleagues then began working with the United States Food and Drug Administration (FDA) to develop an ANDA (Amended New Drug Application) to begin clinical trials in the United States of acetylcysteine (n-acetylcysteine, NAC, trade name Mucomyst).

The owner of the patent acetylcysteine (Mucomyst) was Mead Johnson (unrelated to Johnson and Johnson) and they declined to provide the work necessary to demonstrate that the orally administered sterile Mucomyst did not contain pyrogens so it could be administered intravenously. They did agree to allow access to the drug master file. During discussions with the FDA, it was made clear that the medication would only be approved for oral use. There was some consideration that oral acetylcysteine might be superior to intravenous acetylcysteine given its first-pass effect on the liver through the splanchnic circulation and absorption. It was clear from the primary use of acetylcysteine in patients with cystic fibrosis that oral administration would result in nausea and vomiting given the strong smell, despite being masked with various diluents [26].

Once the decision was made in early 1974 to use acetylcysteine, a dosing methodology was developed. A series of calculations were made and included in the submission to the FDA. The work of Mitchell et al. had shown that hepatic injury occurred in animals when glutathione was depleted by 70% and this was one of the bases for dosing calculations [10].

Calculation of acetaminophen ingestion that would produce hepatic toxicity or injury was based on 70% depletion of glutathione as demonstrated by experimental work [9,10].

The following assumptions were made:

(1) Normal human liver has approximately 4 mmoles of glutathione (GSH) per liter [10].
(2) Using the 1974 FDA standard 70 kg patient:
    a. The human liver in a 70 kg patient is about 1.5 L so ≅ 6 mmoles of GSH.
    b. Hepatic necrosis was reported in mice when there is 70% depletion of GSH.
    c. Seventy percent (0.70) × 6 mmoles = 4.2 mmoles depletion in a 70 kg patient to produce necrosis.
(3) APAP is 151.2 g/mole (151.2 mg/mmol)
    a. NAPQI production is 4% of an APAP absorbed dose.
    b. The measurement of 4.2 mmoles GSH is ≅ to 4.2 mmoles of NAPQI so roughly equivalent
    c. Four percent (0.04) × APAP dose = the amount of NAPQI produced.
    d. Solving the toxic dose of APAP to produce a 70% depletion of GSH:
        i. A measurement of 4.2 mmoles NAPQI/0.04 ≅ 105 mmols APAP.
        ii. A measurement of 105 mmoles APAP × 151.2 mg/mmol = 15,876 mg APAP.
    e. So, an absorbed dose of 15.9 g of APAP in a 70 kg human would be sufficient to deplete GSH by 70% and produce necrosis.
    f. Four percent of 15,876 mg of APAP would produce 635 mg of NAPQI.

Calculation of the initial acetylcysteine dosing regimen.

The assumption in 1974 was to match acetylcysteine administration with GSH depletion based on 4% of the 15.9 g dose producing 635 mg of NAPQI.

a. The 1.5 L liver contains ≅ 6 mmol of GSH.
b. Acetylcysteine is 163.2 g per mole or 163.2 mg/mmol and 1 g is 6.1 mmol.
c. Acetaminophen is 151.2 g per mole or 151.2 mg/mmol and 1 g is 6.6 mmol.
d. Acetylcysteine and acetaminophen are roughly equivalent on a molar basis.
e. GSH turnover was estimated to be 1.5 mmol/h and replacing 25% of the 4.2 mmol depletion was ≅1 mmol which resulted in a balance of ~2.5 mmol/h replacement per h.
f. Dividing 2.5 mmol/h by the 70 kg patient = 0.036 mmol/kg/hr.
g. A measurement of 0.036 mmol/kg × 163.2 mg/mmol acetylcysteine = 5.88 mg/kg/hr rounded to a 6 mg/kg/hr dose of acetylcysteine to replace the GSH turnover and binding to NAPQI.

Calculation of additional safety factors and accounting for 4 h dosing intervals.

(1) Initial protocol from the calculations gives the following:
    a. Administering 6 mg/kg/hr of acetylcysteine on a 4 h schedule resulted in 24 mg/kg/4 h.

   b. An initial loading dose of twice the maintenance dose was 48 mg/kg.
   c. The initial protocol was a loading dose followed by 11 maintenance doses over 48 h. However, this was changed to 60 h and 14 doses when in a correction to the first submission to be consistent with a 12 h half-life of APAP.

(2) We were fully aware that many patients consumed an overdose of greater than 15.9 g. Following several discussions with the FDA, the second resubmission of the protocol contained the following dosing methodology to account for higher doses and adding empirical safety factors, along with other changes:
   a. Loading dose of 140 mg/kg
   b. Seventeen maintenance doses every four hours of 70 mg/kg
   c. Acetylcysteine was administered for 72 h with a total dose of 1330 mg/kg.

4. Acetylcysteine Clinical Studies in Acetaminophen Overdose

A randomized controlled trial of acetylcysteine was an important part of the original submission to the FDA. The FDA was aware of the concerns that had been expressed about the ethics of a controlled trial in discussions held in 1974 and 1975. One concern was expressed at the conclusion of an article published in 1974 and the others were not published until 1976 [27–29]. Several letters were also received by the FDA questioning the ethics of a trial that would withhold acetylcysteine from the control group.

The FDA rejected the inclusion in our submission of a randomized controlled trial. Instead, the FDA required that it be re-written to treat all patients and use the historical patients from the Prescott et al. 1971 publication as the comparator [4]. This came as a great surprise to us as it was quite unusual for the FDA to require anything other than a randomized controlled trial. There has never been a placebo-controlled trial of acetylcysteine and no dose-response studies have ever been performed.

Further changes to our submission required that the nomogram developed in 1973 starting at 200 mg/L at 4 h have a new line with the same slope beginning at 150 mg/L at 4 h (the "treatment line") so that there would be a 25% safety factor. This "study design nomogram" also required a line at 300 mg/L at 4 h to see if there were differences with high-risk patients [30] (Figure 3). We added study lines at 400 mg/L and 500 mg/L to see if other risk levels could be determined. Other changes included the requirement that the acetylcysteine dosage in the protocol would have a loading dose and 17 additional doses over 72 h. The protocol also included the requirement that all samples of blood adhering to the protocol were to be shipped to the University of Colorado School of Medicine Drug Assay Laboratory by Federal Express. Thus, the concentrations could be compared as they were all analyzed by the same laboratory.

We had proposed in our submission that the study would be a United States National Multicenter Study (USNMS) where any physician in the United States could call a toll-free number at the Rocky Mountain Poison and Drug Center in Denver and after agreeing to the full protocol could administer acetylcysteine. Acetylcysteine was widely available in hospitals as Mucomyst. Patients were entered into the study based *only* on the history obtained by their physician. Very few hospitals were able to measure acetaminophen. This meant that many patients were treated but when acetaminophen levels were later obtained, they were below the treatment line. These patients were considered "acetylcysteine safety" patients as they received all 18 doses of acetylcysteine. The intent of the USNMS was to rapidly collect cases to figure out if acetylcysteine was a safe and effective treatment for an acetaminophen overdose in a large population.

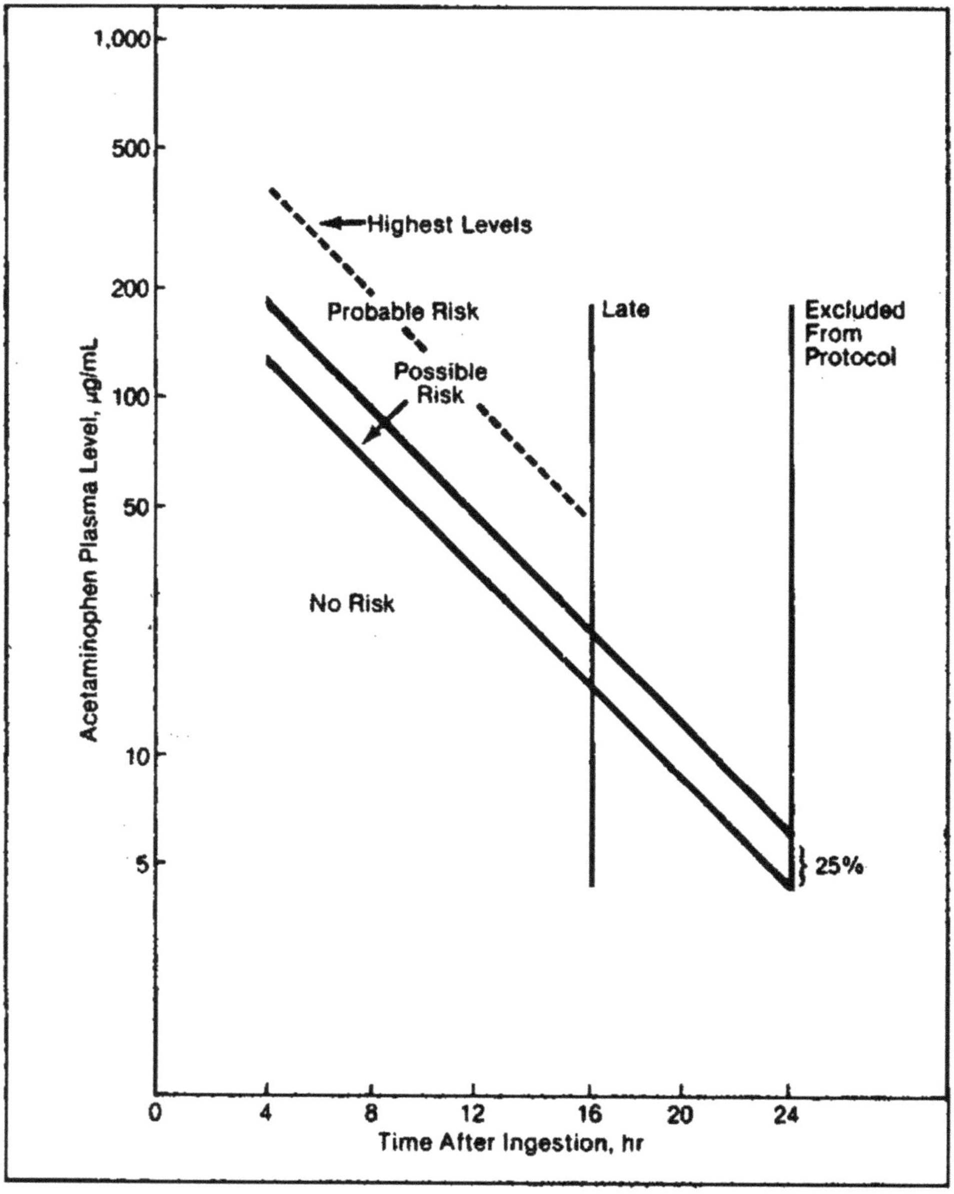

Figure 3. Study design nomogram showing the treatment line at 150 mg/L at 4 h and the high risk line at 300 mg/L at 4 h as well as the original nomogram line at 200 mg/L at 4 h. Rumack BH, Peterson RC, Koch GG, Amara IA. Acetaminophen overdose. Six hundred and sixty-two cases with evaluation of oral acetylcysteine treatment. Arch Intern Med. 1981 Feb 23;141(3 Spec No):380–5. doi: 10.1001/archinte.141.3.380. PMID: 7469629. [30].

The FDA approved the protocol incorporating several changes as described. The United States National Multicenter Study officially began accepting patients on 1 September 1976. The first patient treated with acetylcysteine for an acetaminophen overdose was reported in JAMA in 1977 [31]. Details of the approved protocol were presented at a symposium in New York City in November of 1977 and published in the proceedings in 1978 [32].

During this time the group in Edinburgh were also determining a protocol for intravenous administration of acetylcysteine as it was less toxic than cysteamine. The Edinburgh protocol was empirical but based on sound pharmacologic principles [33]. The UK was willing to permit acetylcysteine administration by the intravenous route. An intravenous regimen over 20.25 h was utilized and was published in 1979 [34]. Intravenous acetylcysteine was given as an initial dose of 150 mg/kg in 200 mL 5% dextrose over 15 min followed by 50 mg/kg in 500 mL 5% dextrose over four hours and 100 mg/kg in one liter 5% dextrose over the next 16 h. The total dose of the intravenous protocol was 300 mg/kg over 20.25 h as compared to the oral protocol with a total dose of 1330 mg/kg over 72 h. Intravenous acetylcysteine produced an anaphylactoid reaction along with some flushing, nausea and vomiting in some patients. These side effects have decreased with changes in the protocol extending the length of time over which the highest concentration is administered and decreasing the length of acetylcysteine administration in some cases [35,36].

The Guy's Hospital group of toxicologists in London investigated the use of methionine for acetaminophen overdose [37,38]. The publication from this group in 1981 reported that 132 cases of severe acetaminophen (paracetamol) poisoning were treated with oral methionine. Seven of 96 patients who received the antidote within ten hours of ingestion of the overdose had severe liver damage (aspartate transaminase level, greater than 1000 IU/L), but none of these patients died. Thirty-six patients received methionine between 10 and 24 h of ingestion; severe liver damage occurred in 47%, and two patients died. Despite some success in the treatment of acetaminophen overdose, methionine is no longer utilized.

The results of the first 100 patients treated with oral acetylcysteine in the USNMS were reported at a symposium held in New York City in November of 1977 [32]. Of the 49 patients treated within 10 h or less post overdose (by history), 17% (8) had transaminases of over 1000 IU/L and 45% (23) of those treated between 10 and 24 h developed transaminases over 1000 IU/L. For those patients who received the full acetylcysteine course but were later determined not to have acetaminophen levels above the nomogram line ("safety controls"), there were no abnormalities in any of the laboratory measurements. Acetylcysteine was therefore demonstrated to be effective when compared to the historical controls who, with supportive care, developed transaminases over 1000 IU/L in 55 to 71% of cases [39,40].

Prescott and colleagues published 100 cases of acetaminophen overdose treated with intravenous acetylcysteine in 1979 [34]. Of the 62 patients treated within 10 h or less post ingestion, only 2% (1) of patients developed a transaminase greater than 1000 IU/L. Of 38 patients treated between 10 and 24 h, 53% (20) of patients developed a transaminase greater than 1000 IU/L. There were 57 patients in this study that received supportive care only (controls) and 58% (33) developed a transaminase greater than 1000 IU/L. Further data were provided after stratifying patients into various risk groups. It was concluded that intravenous acetylcysteine was effective in protecting against hepatic toxicity when given within 8 to 10 h post ingestion.

The USNMS results were further detailed at a symposium in 1979 and published in 1981 [30]. The data utilized in this publication formed the basis for the submission to the FDA in support of the Abbreviated New Drug Application. The submission to the FDA was not required to provide historical controls as the data from the "safety" and untreated patients were considered sufficient. The FDA gave formal approval on 31 January 1985 for the oral use of acetylcysteine in the treatment of acetaminophen overdose. It carried the designation Mead Johnson 13–601 as that company owned the patent on Mucomyst.

The USNMS did not include children under the age of 13 but a parallel study was conducted at the same time. A paper looking at pharmacokinetics in children was published in 1978 and showed that based on half-life determinations, the metabolism is slower in the neonate but comparable to adults in both children and adolescents [41]. A previous pharmacokinetics paper after a dose of 10 mg/kg demonstrated that in children aged 9 and younger, sulfate conjugation was the primary route, but that at age 12 and above the "adult" glucuronide was predominant [42]. We were concerned that if sulfate conjugation was rate limiting, we might see higher levels of toxicity in children but in fact we saw lower levels of toxicity with similar acetaminophen concentrations. An initial publication in 1981 looking at 300 potential exposures reported that 17 had plasma levels measured with 5 above the 150 mg/L at the 4 h treatment line and 11 received acetylcysteine. The highest transaminase was 1660 IU/L and none of the remainder reached 1000 IU/L. There were 417 total cases of suspected exposure to an acetaminophen overdose collected in the parallel study to the USNMS and published in 1984 [43]. There were 55 patients with acetaminophen concentrations in the toxic range with the remaining either non-toxic or not interpretable. Of the 55 patients with potentially toxic levels, 43 were treated with acetylcysteine and 3 developed a transaminase of 1000 IU/L or greater. An additional 56 patients in the non-toxic group were treated with acetylcysteine without any laboratory abnormalities. The current recommendation is to treat children under the age of 13 in the same manner as adolescents and adults are treated, although the incidence of hepatic toxicity appears lower than that in patients aged 13 or greater.

The USNMS concluded in 1985 and a full analysis was published in 1988 in the New England Journal of Medicine [26]. There were 11,195 cases entered into the study, of which 2540 were treated with acetylcysteine and met inclusion criteria. There were 517 patients who received the full acetylcysteine treatment protocol but were later determined to be below the 150 mg/L line and were considered "acetylcysteine safety patients" as they did not meet inclusion criteria. The patients were stratified on a study nomogram utilizing lines beginning at 4 h and starting at 150 mg/L, 200 mg/L, 300 mg/L, 400 mg/L and 500 mg/L and further defined by delay to treatment. Those patients above the 300 mg/L line were characterized as "high risk". The 400 mg/L and 500 mg/L nomogram lines were not used in the final analysis. A standard nomogram simplified from the study design nomogram for assessing risk was in use from 1985 to 2023 (Figure 4).

As previously shown in smaller studies, those patients treated within the first 8 to 10 h post ingestion of acetaminophen (probable risk) had the lowest incidence of hepatic toxicity (transaminase greater than 1000 IU/L), which was 6.1% (32/527) in this study. The subset of those treated within the first 10 h whose concentrations were in the high-risk range had a higher incidence of hepatic toxicity, at 8.3% (17/206). There was a stepwise increase in hepatic toxicity related to longer time from ingestion to treatment between 10 and 24 h, with probable risk patients at 26.4% (247/935) and high-risk patients at 34.4% (199/578). Those patients between 16 and 24 h were all high risk with 41% (116/283) showing hepatic toxicity. These reports from the USNMS indicated that oral and intravenous acetylcysteine had a similar therapeutic benefit.

Because most hospitals could not measure acetaminophen concentrations, there were 517 patients treated based on history who did not have levels in excess of the 150 mg/L nomogram line. These patients had an incidence of 1.08% to 3.16% of transaminases greater than 1000 IU/L showing a non-zero risk of hepatotoxicity, possibly due to the inaccurate history of the time of ingestion of the overdose [44] (Figure 5).

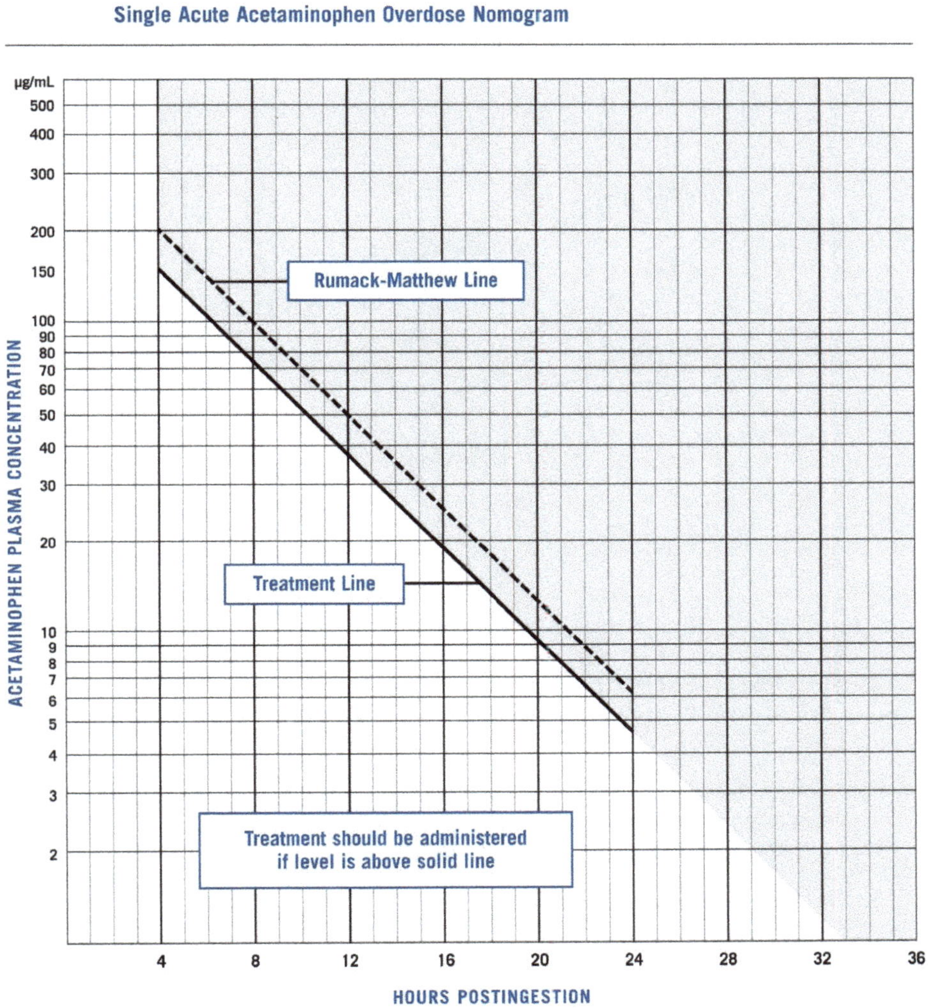

Figure 4. Simplified Rumack-Matthew nomogram adapted from the USNMS study design nomogram utilized from 1976 to 2023, when it was revised.

Intravenous acetylcysteine, following the protocol from Edinburgh, became the preferred method of administration. However, the UK regulatory authorities have required treatment based on a very conservative "100 mg/L at 4 h" post ingestion treatment line since 2012 [44].

Oral acetylcysteine remained the primary treatment for acetaminophen overdose in the United States until the intravenous version was approved by the FDA in January 2004. Intravenous acetylcysteine is now the most common method of treatment throughout the world. Oral acetylcysteine is still utilized occasionally although the smell, taste and resultant vomiting make it considerably less desirable.

A comparative study of intravenously treated patients compared to oral acetylcysteine-treated patients reported some may do better with the oral protocol [45]. This is not likely related to the route of administration but rather the total dose and duration of the acetylcysteine administered. The data comparison was between 1963 US patients treated orally and 2086 Canadian patients treated intravenously. The 20 h IV protocol was more effective when instituted early while the 72 h oral protocol was more effective when instituted in delayed patients. This is likely due to the 300 mg/kg total IV dose versus the 1330 mg/kg oral dose. Additional publications support this conclusion [26,33,45–48].

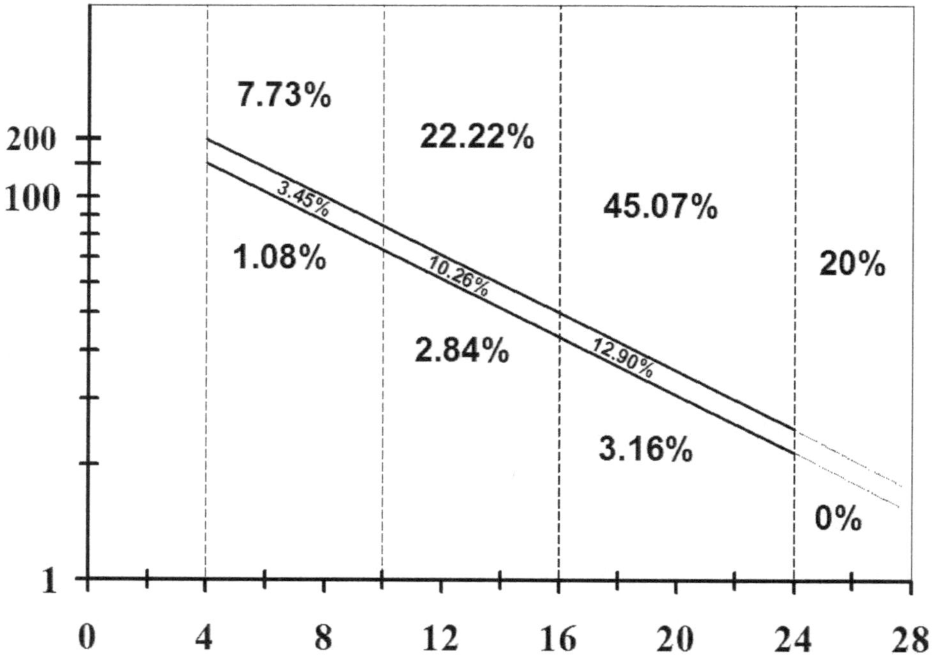

Figure 5. USNMS "Safety" patients who developed a transaminase of 1000 IU/L despite being below the 150 mg/L at 4 h protocol treatment line. Rumack BH. Acetaminophen hepatotoxicity: the first 35 years. J Toxicol Clin Toxicol. 2002;40(1):3–20. doi: 10.1081/clt-120002882. PMID: 11990202. [44].

5. Acetylcysteine in Pregnancy

There were 113 patients who were pregnant in the USNMS and 60 cases had full pregnancy outcome data [49]. There were 24 patients with acetaminophen levels above the treatment line of 150 mg/L. Of the ten treated with acetylcysteine within 10 h post-ingestion, eight delivered normal infants and two had elective abortions. Of ten patients treated 10–16 h post ingestion, five delivered viable infants, two had elective abortions, and three had spontaneous abortions. Of four treated within 16–24 h post ingestion, there was one spontaneous abortion, one stillbirth, one elective abortion, one delivery of a normal infant and one mother died. There was a statistically significant increase in the incidence of spontaneous abortion or fetal death when treatment was begun late. Acetylcysteine crosses the placenta and can be measured in the neonate [50]. Mean level of acetylcysteine in cord blood was 9.4 mcg/mL which is between the peak 13.9 mcg/mL and trough 5 mcg/mL levels previously reported [51]. The recommendation based on this small series is to treat as early as possible with acetylcysteine following normal protocols.

6. Acetylcysteine Failure in Renal Toxicity

Renal toxicity, while associated with fulminant hepatic failure in acetaminophen overdose, may also occur in patients with less severe cases of overdose. Acetylcysteine is ineffective in the treatment of renal toxicity and experimental work has uncovered the mechanism and provided an explanation [52]. While formation of APAP-CYS protein adducts occurs in the mitochondria of hepatocytes, these adducts are formed in the endoplasmic reticulum (ER) of proximal tubular cells of the kidney. The reactive metabolites trigger an ER stress-mediated activation of caspase-12 which results in apoptotic cell deaths in this area of the kidney. This contrasts with necrotic cell death in the liver. Acetylcysteine does not have any effect on this process in the kidney but fomepizole does prevent injury by attenuating renal cell death from apoptotic death in primary human kidney cells. Thus, based on the experimental evidence, fomepizole should be considered as an adjunct to acetylcysteine in patients with renal injury following acetaminophen overdose.

7. Acetylcysteine Administration, Stopping Criteria and Further Risk Analysis

Numerous one and two bag protocols have been devised to reduce the adverse effects of intravenous acetylcysteine, to reduce the complexity of the original three bag protocol and to shorten the time of hospitalization, especially in low-risk patients [35,36,53–60]. The Scottish and Newcastle anti-emetic pretreatment (SNAP) trial was quite rigorous and provides a methodology to stop treatment at 12 h [36]. An evaluation of adducts supports early cessation of acetylcysteine in appropriate circumstances [58].

Examples of acetylcysteine administration, as referenced above:

Oral—still utilized in some countries where intravenous use is not possible:

140 mg/kg loading dose followed by 17 doses 70 mg/kg every 4 h [26].

IV—original dose regimen: 150 mg/kg over 15 min, 50 mg/kg over 4 h and then 100 mg/kg over 16 h. Modified the initial infusion from 15 min to 1 h. No effect on anaphylactoid reactions, nausea or vomiting [34].

IV—one bag method: 30 g of NAC in one liter of IV fluid with a loading dose of 150 mg/kg over 1 h followed by a continuous infusion of 12.5 mg/kg/h [55].

IV—two bag 200 mg/kg over 4 h and 100 mg/kg over 16 h [56]

IV—SNAP Trial: 300 mg/kg over 12 h using a rapid infusion for 2 h (100 mg/kg) and a slower infusion for 10 h (200 mg/kg). Continue as needed [36].

IV—Hi-SNAP Trial: 300/kg, 450/kg and 600/kg study in progress [61].

Summary: At least 300 mg/kg during the first 20 to 24 h of treatment (except SNAP or Hi-SNAP).

The length of treatment with acetylcysteine is sufficient to decrease toxicity as part of the 20.25 h intravenous or 72 h oral protocol. However, providing criteria related to the status of the patient at the end of each protocol may be more appropriate [62]. Generally, there is no reason to administer acetylcysteine after there is no more acetaminophen to be converted to NAPQI and produce toxicity. However, there is experimental evidence that indicates continued administration of acetylcysteine may interfere with hepatic regeneration [63]. A recent consensus document for the United States and Canada makes specific recommendations in terms of stopping acetylcysteine [64]. This consensus publication also contains a revised nomogram showing only the 150 mg/L at 4 h and the 300 mg/L at the 4 h high-risk line. (Figure 6)

Acetylcysteine stopping criteria include the following:

- Acetaminophen concentration <10 μg/mL (mg/L);
- International normalized ratio (INR) <2.0;
- ALT/AST normal for patient, or if elevated have decreased from peak (25–50%);
- Patient is clinically well.

If acetylcysteine stopping criteria are NOT met then acetylcysteine should be administered at a rate of 6.25 mg/kg/hr or greater and transaminases, INR and APAP levels drawn at 12-to-24 h intervals until stopping criteria are met.

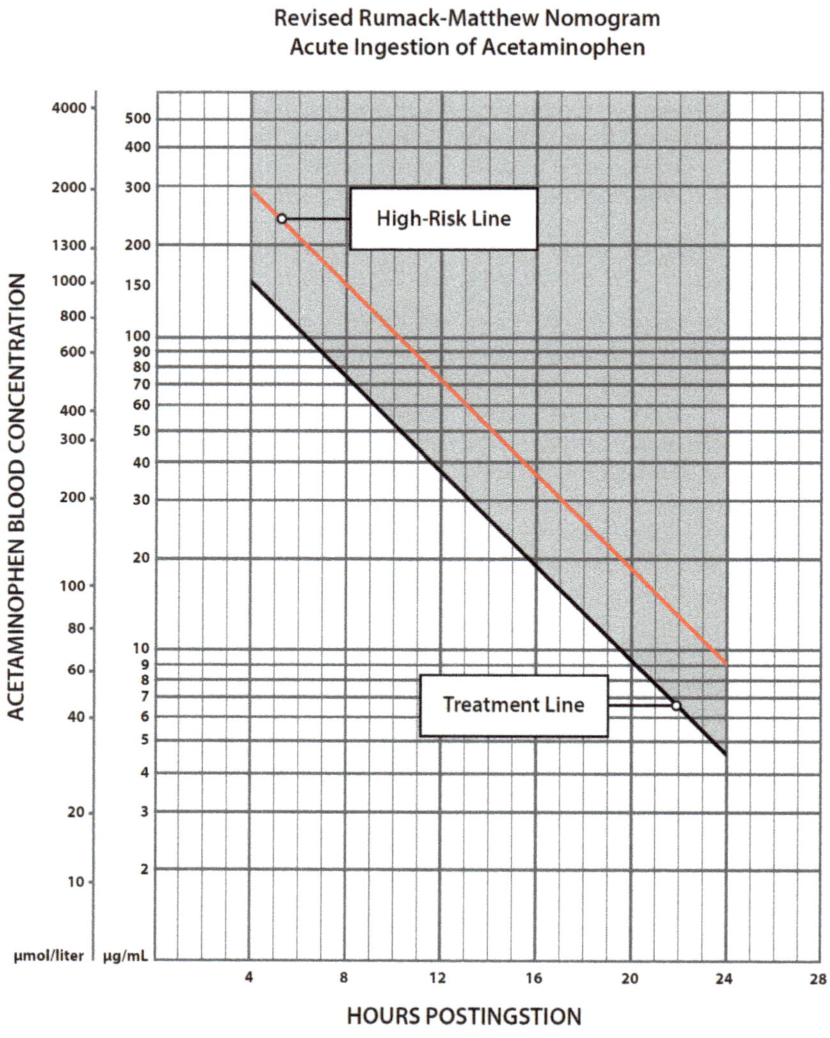

Figure 6. Revised consensus Rumack-Matthew nomogram with the standard 150 mg/L at 4 h treatment line and the "high risk" line at 300 mg/L at 4 h. Dart RC, Mullins ME, Matoushek T, Ruha AM, Burns MM, Simone K, Beuhler MC, Heard KJ, Mazer-Amirshahi M, Stork CM, Varney SM, Funk AR, Cantrell LF, Cole JB, Banner W, Stolbach AI, Hendrickson RG, Lucyk SN, Sivilotti MLA, Su MK, Nelson LS, Rumack BH. Management of Acetaminophen Poisoning in the US and Canada: A Consensus Statement. JAMA Netw Open. 2023 Aug 1;6(8):e2327739. doi: 10.1001/jamanetworkopen.2023.27739. Erratum in: JAMA Netw Open. 2023 Sep 5;6(9):e2337926. doi: 10.1001/jamanetworkopen.2023.37926. PMID: 37552484. [64].

The use of acetylcysteine in each patient is determined from a risk analysis by the treating physician. The use of the nomogram to plot the measured acetaminophen concentration versus time remains the primary method of risk determination where such laboratory analyses are rapidly available [64]. Several other methodologies have been developed to refine risk including a widely utilized multiplication product [65]. This simple calculation of the APAP concentration $\times$ ALT level provides a product estimating risk and is interpreted as follows:

Less than 1500 = low likelihood of hepatotoxicity with acetylcysteine-treatment (100% sensitivity and 100% specificity);

More than 10,000 = high likelihood of hepatotoxicity with acetylcysteine-treatment (sensitivity 80%, specificity 99.6%).

A more elegant approach to risk evaluation for use of acetylcysteine was developed known as the Psi parameter [66,67]. While the patient history of APAP dose ingested may be inaccurate, the Psi parameter utilizes the measured concentration to estimate the toxic metabolite (NAPQI) and estimate the quantity ingested during exposure using known pharmacokinetic principles.

Recently, an augmented method combining both the multiplication product and the Psi parameter was proposed [68]. This publication demonstrates that risk calculation from the acetaminophen concentration can be augmented with the inclusion of the timing of acetylcysteine treatment. Utilizing the proposed calculation, the authors were able to have both high sensitivity (96.5%) and high specificity (97.3%) based on an analysis of 421 case records. These authors previously provided a methodology for the evaluation of patients to receive acetylcysteine where the rapid availability of an acetaminophen level or transaminases is not possible [69]. This dose estimate method, using 150 mg/L as a cutoff, has a specificity of 55.3% when it is used, which results in 44.7% of patients being treated unnecessarily. The authors consider this acceptable in those circumstances where detailed rapid laboratory analysis is unavailable.

8. Acetylcysteine Adjunctive Treatment with Fomepizole and Other Therapies

The use of fomepizole as an adjunct to acetylcysteine should be considered especially in patients with delay until treatment, massive ingestions or renal injury. There is very solid experimental evidence for this adjunctive treatment [70]. Clinical use of fomepizole as an adjunct relies primarily on case reports and case series demonstrating use in humans [71,72]. It is hoped that current clinical trials underway will be able to answer the question as to use in a controlled setting. Fomepizole has been used for over 20 years effectively and safely with cases of methanol and ethylene glycol toxicity [73]. There is no known toxicity when utilized with acetylcysteine. There may be a place for adding fomepizole to acetylcysteine therapy to take advantage of its ability to inhibit CYP2E1 production of NAPQI and interfere further downstream with c-Jun N-terminal kinase [74,75]. Use of fomepizole in place of acetylcysteine is not recommended currently and although it is widely used, the results of clinical trials are yet to demonstrate absolute efficacy.

In addition to fomepizole, other therapies have been considered and some are under investigation. The following have been extensively reviewed in a recent publication [74].

- Calmangafodipir is a superoxide dismutase "mimetic" (manganese-dependent superoxide dismutase, Mn-SOD) 1. SOD is required in the cellular defense of reactive oxygen species and interferes with the formation of peroxynitrite, increases nitrotyrosine formation and hepatic toxicity. Mn-SOD mimetics, e.g., Mito-Tempo (mitochondria-targeted antioxidant) can enter mitochondria. Increasing Mn-SOD capacity can be effective in treating APAP toxicity. A phase IIb/III Albatross Trial of calmangafodipir for acetaminophen toxicity was to commence Q1 2024 but has not begun as of the writing of this article.
- Nrf2 binds to the ARE (antioxidant response element) and induces transcription of a large number of genes which all have protective roles in the APAP hepatotoxicity model. However, Nrf2 is activated by APAP and there may be no further benefit from further activation.

- Thrombopoietin Mimetic Peptide1 (PEG-TPOm) JNJ-26366821. PEG-TPO treatment appears to be beneficial when administered at 24 h after APAP overdose when NAC is ineffective. PEG-TPO arrests the progression of acetaminophen overdose-induced liver injury (AILI) and accelerates the onset of the proliferative response essential for liver recovery. Distinct from 4-MP which prevents injury but does not promote hepatocyte proliferation and liver recovery, PEG-TPO is a potential novel therapeutic for the enhancement of liver recovery after AILI1.
- Adenosine A2B receptor activators such as BAY 60-6583 decreased necrosis and enhanced infiltration of reparative macrophages when NAC would be ineffective. Clinical trials in cancer patients have begun.
- Whartons Jelly Mesenchymal Stem Cell (WJMSC) protected against liver injury at 6 h by preserving mitochondrial function despite JNK activation and its mitochondrial translocation accompanied by enhanced infiltration of macrophages with the reparative anti-inflammatory phenotype by 24 h. Clinical trials have begun.
- Lipid-nanoparticle-encapsulated mRNA of HGF (human grown factor) and EGF epidermal growth factor have been shown to be effective in the mouse model and may be further investigated.

9. Conclusions

Acetylcysteine has been the primary treatment for acetaminophen-overdose toxicity for over 50 years. Foundational research in the early 1970s played a critical role in the treatment of this overdose without which treatment could not have been devised. Acetylcysteine treatment, despite never having been part of a randomized controlled trial nor having a dose–response curve remains the successful treatment of choice to treat toxicity in most patients from this overdose. Standard intravenous treatment is 21 h and multiple methods of administration have been devised to reduce adverse reactions and deliver acetylcysteine safely. Patients with massive ingestions or delay in arrival in a health care facility may require longer treatment with acetylcysteine and/or at a higher dose. Individualized patient-focused treatment is considered the standard. Stopping criteria have been developed and these methods have been formalized in a recent consensus publication. Experimental work has shown that renal injury is based on a different mechanism and is characterized by apoptosis rather than necrosis as seen in the liver. Augmentation with fomepizole has been experimentally demonstrated and may be especially useful in patients with massive ingestions, delay until treatment or renal injury.

Funding: This research received no external funding.

Data Availability Statement: No new data were created or analyzed in this study. Data sharing is not applicable to this article.

Conflicts of Interest: The author declares no conflict of interest.

References

1. Brodie, B.B.; Axelrod, J. The estimation of acetanilide and its metabolic products, aniline, N-acetyl p-aminophenol and p-amino-phenol, free and total conjugated, in biological fluids and tissues. *J. Pharmacol. Exp. Ther.* **1948**, *94*, 22–28. [CrossRef] [PubMed]
2. Davidson, D.G.; Eastham, W.N. Acute liver necrosis following overdose of paracetamol. *Br. Med. J.* **1966**, *2*, 497–499. [CrossRef] [PubMed]
3. Thomson, J.S.; Prescott, L.F. Liver damage and impaired glucose tolerance after paracetamol overdosage. *Br. Med. J.* **1966**, *2*, 506–507. [CrossRef] [PubMed]
4. Prescott, L.F.; Roscoe, P.; Wright, N.; Brown, S.S. Plasma-paracetamol half-life and hepatic necrosis in patients with paracetamol overdosage. *Lancet* **1971**, *1*, 519–522. [CrossRef]
5. Proudfoot, A.T.; Wright, N. Acute paracetamol poisoning. *Br. Med. J.* **1970**, *3*, 557–558. [CrossRef]

6. Jollow, D.J.; Mitchell, J.R.; Potter, W.Z.; Davis, D.C.; Gillette, J.R.; Brodie, B.B. Acetaminophen-induced hepatic necrosis. II. Role of covalent binding in vivo. *J. Pharmacol. Exp. Ther.* **1973**, *187*, 195–202. [CrossRef]
7. Jollow, D.; Thorgeirsson, S.S.; Potter, W.Z.; Hashimoto, M.; Mitchell, J.R. Acetaminophen-induced hepatic necrosis. VI. Metabolic disposition of toxic and nontoxic doses of acetaminophen. *Pharmacology* **1974**, *12*, 251–271. [CrossRef]
8. Mitchell, J.R.; Jollow, D.J.; Potter, W.Z.; Davis, D.C.; Gillette, J.R.; Brodie, B.B. Acetaminophen-induced hepatic necrosis. I. Role of drug metabolism. *J. Pharmacol. Exp. Ther.* **1973**, *187*, 185–194.
9. Mitchell, J.R.; Jollow, D.J.; Potter, W.Z.; Gillette, J.R.; Brodie, B.B. Acetaminophen-induced hepatic necrosis. IV. Protective role of glutathione. *J. Pharmacol. Exp. Ther.* **1973**, *187*, 211–217. [CrossRef]
10. Mitchell, J.R.; Thorgeirsson, S.S.; Potter, W.Z.; Jollow, D.J.; Keiser, H. Acetaminophen-induced hepatic injury: Protective role of glutathione in man and rationale for therapy. *Clin. Pharmacol. Ther.* **1974**, *16*, 676–684. [CrossRef]
11. Potter, W.Z.; Davis, D.C.; Mitchell, J.R.; Jollow, D.J.; Gillette, J.R.; Brodie, B.B. Acetaminophen-induced hepatic necrosis. 3. Cytochrome P-450-mediated covalent binding in vitro. *J. Pharmacol. Exp. Ther.* **1973**, *187*, 203–210. [CrossRef] [PubMed]
12. Potter, W.Z.; Thorgeirsson, S.S.; Jollow, D.J.; Mitchell, J.R. Acetaminophen-induced hepatic necrosis. V. Correlation of hepatic necrosis, covalent binding and glutathione depletion in hamsters. *Pharmacology* **1974**, *12*, 129–143. [CrossRef] [PubMed]
13. Jollow, D. Acetaminophen-Induced Hepatic Necrosis: A Reminiscence. *Drug Metab. Dispos.* **2023**, *52*, 707–711. [CrossRef] [PubMed]
14. Calder, I.C.; Creek, M.J.; Williams, P.J. N-hydroxyphenacetinn as a precursor of 3-substituted 4-hydroxyacetanilide metabolites of phenacetin. *Chem. Biol. Interact.* **1974**, *8*, 87–90. [CrossRef]
15. Holtzman, J.L.; Gillette, J.R.; Milne, G.W. The incorporation of 18-O into naphthalene in the enzymatic formation of 1,2-dihydronaphthalene-1,2-diol. *J. Biol. Chem.* **1967**, *242*, 4386–4387. [CrossRef]
16. Dahlin, D.C.; Nelson, S.D. Synthesis, decomposition kinetics, and preliminary toxicological studies of pure N-acetyl-p-benzoquinone imine, a proposed toxic metabolite of acetaminophen. *J. Med. Chem.* **1982**, *25*, 885–886. [CrossRef] [PubMed]
17. Dahlin, D.C.; Miwa, G.T.; Lu, A.Y.; Nelson, S.D. N-acetyl-p-benzoquinone imine: A cytochrome P-450-mediated oxidation product of acetaminophen. *Proc. Natl. Acad. Sci. USA* **1984**, *81*, 1327–1331. [CrossRef] [PubMed] [PubMed Central]
18. Jaeschke, H.; Ramachandran, A. The multiple mechanisms and modes of cell death after acetaminophen overdose. *Explor. Dig. Dis.* **2025**, *4*, 100569. [CrossRef]
19. Bateman, D.N.; Dart, R.C.; Dear, J.W.; Prescott, L.F.; Rumack, B.H. Fifty years of paracetamol (acetaminophen) poisoning: The development of risk assessment and treatment 1973–2023 with particular focus on contributions published from Edinburgh and Denver. *Clin. Toxicol.* **2023**, *61*, 1020–1031. [CrossRef]
20. Prescott, L.F. Paracetamol (acetaminophen) poisoning: The early years. *Br. J. Clin. Pharmacol.* **2024**, *90*, 127–134. [CrossRef]
21. Rumack, B.H.; Matthew, H. Acetaminophen poisoning and toxicity. *Pediatrics* **1975**, *55*, 871–876. [CrossRef] [PubMed]
22. Prescott, L.F.; Swainson, C.P.; Forrest, A.R.W.; Newton, R.W.; Wright, N.; Matthew, H. Successful treatment of severe paracetamol overdosage with cysteamine. *Lancet* **1974**, *1*, 588–592. [CrossRef] [PubMed]
23. Piperno, E.; Berssenbruegge, D.A. Reversal of experimental paracetamol toxicosis with N-acetylcysteine. *Lancet* **1976**, *2*, 738–739. [CrossRef] [PubMed]
24. Piperno, E.; Mosher, A.H.; Berssenbruegge, D.A.; Winkler, J.D.; Smith, R.B. Pathophysiology of acetaminophen overdosage toxicity: Implications for management. *Pediatrics* **1978**, *62 Pt 2* (Suppl. S5), 880–889.
25. Meredith, T.J.; Goulding, R. Paracetamol. *Postgrad. Med. J.* **1980**, *56*, 459–473. [CrossRef]
26. Smilkstein, M.J.; Knapp, G.L.; Kulig, K.W.; Rumack, B.H. Efficacy of oral N-acetylcysteine in the treatment of acetaminophen overdose. Analysis of the national multicenter study (1976 to 1985) [see comments]. *N. Engl. J. Med.* **1988**, *319*, 1557–1562. [CrossRef]
27. Hughes, R.D.; Trewby, P.; Williams, R. Letter: Cysteamine for paracetamol poisoning. *Lancet* **1976**, *1*, 536.
28. Koch-Weser, J. Drug therapy. *Acetaminophen. N. Engl. J. Med.* **1976**, *295*, 1297–1300. [CrossRef]
29. Prescott, L.F.; Matthew, H. Cysteamine for Paracetamol Overdosage. *Lancet* **1974**, *303*, 998. [CrossRef]
30. Rumack, B.H.; Peterson, R.C.; Koch, G.G.; Amara, I.A. Acetaminophen overdose. 662 cases with evaluation of oral acetylcysteine treatment. *Arch. Intern. Med.* **1981**, *141*, 380–385. [CrossRef]
31. Peterson, R.G.; Rumack, B.H. Treating acute acetaminophen poisoning with acetylcysteine. *JAMA* **1977**, *237*, 2406–2407. [CrossRef] [PubMed]
32. Rumack, B.H.; Peterson, R.G. Acetaminophen overdose: Incidence, diagnosis, and management in 416 patients. *Pediatrics* **1978**, *62 Pt 2* (Suppl. S5), 898–903. [CrossRef] [PubMed]
33. Rumack, B.H.; Bateman, D.N. Acetaminophen and acetylcysteine dose and duration: Past, present and future. *Clin. Toxicol.* **2012**, *50*, 91–98. [CrossRef] [PubMed]
34. Prescott, L.F.; Illingworth, R.N.; Critchley, J.A.; Stewart, M.J.; Adam, R.D.; Proudfoot, A.T. Intravenous N-acetylcystine: The treatment of choice for paracetamol poisoning. *Br. Med. J.* **1979**, *2*, 1097–1100. [CrossRef]

35. Bateman, D.N.; Dear, J.W.; Thanacoody, H.R.; Thomas, S.H.; Eddleston, M.; Sandilands, E.A.; Coyle, J.; Cooper, J.G.; Rodriguez, A.; Butcher, I.; et al. Reduction of adverse effects from intravenous acetylcysteine treatment for paracetamol poisoning: A randomised controlled trial. *Lancet* **2014**, *383*, 697–704. [CrossRef]
36. Pettie, J.M.; Caparrotta, T.M.; Hunter, R.W.; Morrison, E.E.; Wood, D.M.; Dargan, P.I.; Thanacoody, R.H.; Thomas, S.H.L.; Elamin, M.E.M.O.; Francis, B.; et al. Safety and Efficacy of the SNAP 12-hour Acetylcysteine Regimen for the Treatment of Paracetamol Overdose. *EClinicalMedicine* **2019**, *11*, 11–17. [CrossRef]
37. Crome, P.; Volans, G.N.; Vale, J.A.; Widdop, B.; Goulding, R. Oral methionine in the treatment of severe paracetamol (Acetaminophen) overdose. *Lancet* **1976**, *2*, 829–830. [CrossRef]
38. Vale, J.A.; Meredith, T.J.; Goulding, R. Treatment of acetaminophen poisoning. The use of oral methionine. *Arch. Intern. Med.* **1981**, *141*, 394–396. [CrossRef]
39. Douglas, A.P.; Hamlyn, A.N.; James, O. Controlled trial of cysteamine in treatment of acute paracetamol (acetaminophen) poisoning. *Lancet* **1976**, *1*, 111–115. [CrossRef]
40. Prescott, L.F.; Sutherland, G.R.; Park, J.; Smith, I.J.; Proudfoot, A.T. Cysteamine, methionine, and penicillamine in the treatment of paracetamol poisoning. *Lancet* **1976**, *2*, 109–113. [CrossRef]
41. Peterson, R.G.; Rumack, B.H. Pharmacokinetics of acetaminophen in children. *Pediatrics* **1978**, *62 Pt 2* (Suppl. S5), 877–879. [CrossRef] [PubMed]
42. Miller, R.P.; Roberts, R.J.; Fischer, L.J. Acetaminophen elimination kinetics in neonates, children, and adults. *Clin. Pharmacol. Ther.* **1976**, *19*, 284–294. [CrossRef] [PubMed]
43. Rumack, B.H. Acetaminophen overdose in young children. Treatment and effects of alcohol and other additional ingestants in 417 cases. *Am. J. Dis. Child.* **1984**, *138*, 428–433. [CrossRef] [PubMed]
44. Rumack, B.H. Acetaminophen hepatotoxicity: The first 35 years. *J. Toxicol. Clin. Toxicol.* **2002**, *40*, 3–20. [CrossRef]
45. Yarema, M.C.; Johnson, D.W.; Berlin, R.J.; Sivilotti, M.L.; Nettel-Aguirre, A.; Brant, R.F.; Spyker, D.A.; Bailey, B.; Chalut, D.; Lee, J.S.; et al. Comparison of the 20-hour intravenous and 72-hour oral acetylcysteine protocols for the treatment of acute acetaminophen poisoning. *Ann. Emerg. Med.* **2009**, *54*, 606–614. [CrossRef]
46. Cairney, D.G.; Beckwith, H.K.; Al-Hourani, K.; Eddleston, M.; Bateman, D.N.; Dear, J.W. Plasma paracetamol concentration at hospital presentation has a dose-dependent relationship with liver injury despite prompt treatment with intravenous acetylcysteine. *Clin. Toxicol.* **2016**, *54*, 405–410. [CrossRef]
47. Hendrickson, R.G. What is the most appropriate dose of N-acetylcysteine after massive acetaminophen overdose? *Clin. Toxicol.* **2019**, *57*, 686–691. [CrossRef]
48. Marks, D.J.; Dargan, P.I.; Archer, J.R.; Davies, C.L.; Dines, A.M.; Wood, D.M.; Greene, S.L. Outcomes from massive paracetamol overdose: A retrospective observational study. *Br. J. Clin. Pharmacol.* **2017**, *83*, 1263–1272. [CrossRef]
49. Riggs, B.S.; Bronstein, A.C.; Kulig, K.; Archer, P.G.; Rumack, B.H. Acute acetaminophen overdose during pregnancy. *Obstet. Gynecol.* **1989**, *74*, 247–253.
50. Horowitz, R.S.; Dart, R.C.; Jarvie, D.R.; Bearer, C.F.; Gupta, U. Placental transfer of N-acetylcysteine following human maternal acetaminophen toxicity. *J. Toxicol. Clin. Toxicol.* **1997**, *35*, 447–451. [CrossRef]
51. North, D.S.; Peterson, R.G.; Krenzelok, E.P. Effect of activated charcoal administration on acetylcysteine serum levels in humans. *Am. J. Hosp. Pharm.* **1981**, *38*, 1022–1024. [CrossRef] [PubMed]
52. Akakpo, J.Y.; Ramachandran, A.; Rumack, B.H.; Wallace, D.P.; Jaeschke, H. Lack of mitochondrial Cyp2E1 drives acetaminophen-induced ER stress-mediated apoptosis in mouse and human kidneys: Inhibition by 4-methylpyrazole but not N-acetylcysteine. *Toxicology* **2023**, *500*, 153692. [CrossRef] [PubMed]
53. Chiew, A.L.; Gluud, C.; Brok, J.; Buckley, N.A. Interventions for paracetamol (acetaminophen) overdose. *Cochrane Database Syst. Rev.* **2018**, *2*, CD003328. [CrossRef] [PubMed]
54. Hoyte, C.; Dart, R.C. Transition to two-bag intravenous acetylcysteine for acetaminophen overdose: A poison center's experience. *Clin. Toxicol.* **2019**, *57*, 217–218. [CrossRef]
55. Johnson, M.T.; McCammon, C.A.; Mullins, M.E.; Halcomb, S.E. Evaluation of a simplified N-acetylcysteine dosing regimen for the treatment of acetaminophen toxicity. *Ann. Pharmacother.* **2011**, *45*, 713–720. [CrossRef]
56. O'Callaghan, C.; Graudins, A.; Wong, A. A two-bag acetylcysteine regimen is associated with shorter delays and interruptions in the treatment of paracetamol overdose. *Clin. Toxicol.* **2022**, *60*, 319–323. [CrossRef]
57. Sandilands, E.A.; Bateman, D.N. Adverse reactions associated with acetylcysteine. *Clin. Toxicol.* **2009**, *47*, 81–88. [CrossRef]
58. Wong, A.; Heard, K.; Graudins, A.; Dart, R.; Sivilotti, M.L. Adducts Post Acetaminophen Overdose Treated with a 12-Hour vs 20-Hour Acetylcysteine Infusion. *J. Med. Toxicol.* **2020**, *16*, 188–194. [CrossRef]
59. Wong, A.; Isbister, G.; McNulty, R.; Isoardi, K.; Harris, K.; Chiew, A.; Greene, S.; Gunja, N.; Buckley, N.; Page, C.; et al. Efficacy of a two bag acetylcysteine regimen to treat paracetamol overdose (2NAC study). *EClinicalMedicine* **2020**, *20*, 100288. [CrossRef]

60. Wong, A.; McNulty, R.; Taylor, D.; Sivilotti, M.; Greene, S.; Gunja, N.; Koutsogiannis, Z.; Graudins, A. The NACSTOP Trial: A Multicenter, Cluster-Controlled Trial of Early Cessation of Acetylcysteine in Acetaminophen Overdose. *Hepatology* **2019**, *69*, 774–784. [CrossRef]
61. Humphries, C.; Clarke, E.; Eddleston, M.; Gillings, M.; Irvine, S.; Keating, L.; Miell, A.; Milne, L.; Muir, L.; O'Brien, R.; et al. HiSNAP trial-a multicentre, randomised, open-label, blinded end point, safety and efficacy trial of conventional (300 mg/kg) versus higher doses of acetylcysteine (450 mg/kg and 600 mg/kg) in patients with paracetamol overdose in the UK: Study protocol. *BMJ Open.* **2025**, *15*, e097432. [CrossRef] [PubMed] [PubMed Central]
62. Dart, R.C.; Rumack, B.H. Patient-tailored acetylcysteine administration. *Ann. Emerg. Med.* **2007**, *50*, 280–281. [CrossRef] [PubMed]
63. Akakpo, J.Y.; Jaeschke, M.W.; Ramachandran, A.; Curry, S.C.; Rumack, B.H.; Jaeschke, H. Delayed administration of N-acetylcysteine blunts recovery after an acetaminophen overdose unlike 4-methylpyrazole. *Arch. Toxicol.* **2021**, *95*, 3377–3391. [CrossRef] [PubMed]
64. Dart, R.C.; Mullins, M.E.; Matoushek, T.; Ruha, A.M.; Burns, M.M.; Simone, K.; Beuhler, M.C.; Heard, K.J.; Mazer-Amirshahi, M.; Stork, C.M.; et al. Management of Acetaminophen Poisoning in the US and Canada: A Consensus Statement. *JAMA Netw. Open* **2023**, *6*, e2327739. [CrossRef]
65. Wong, A.; Sivilotti, M.L.; Gunja, N.; McNulty, R.; Graudins, A. Accuracy of the paracetamol-aminotransferase product to predict hepatotoxicity in paracetamol overdose treated with a 2-bag acetylcysteine regimen. *Clin. Toxicol.* **2018**, *56*, 182–188. [CrossRef]
66. Chomchai, S.; Chomchai, C.; Anusornsuwan, T. Acetaminophen psi parameter: A useful tool to quantify hepatotoxicity risk in acute acetaminophen overdose. *Clin. Toxicol.* **2011**, *49*, 664–667. [CrossRef]
67. Sivilotti, M.L.; Yarema, M.C.; Juurlink, D.N.; Good, A.M.; Johnson, D.W. A risk quantification instrument for acute acetaminophen overdose patients treated with N-acetylcysteine. *Ann. Emerg. Med.* **2005**, *46*, 263–271. [CrossRef]
68. Chomchai, S.; Mekavuthikul, P.; Phuditshinnapatra, J.; Chomchai, C. Augmenting the sensitivity for hepatotoxicity prediction in acute paracetamol overdose: Combining psi (psi) parameter and paracetamol concentration aminotransferase activity multiplication product. *Clin. Toxicol.* **2024**, *62*, 714–725. [CrossRef]
69. Chomchai, S.; Mekavuthikul, P.; Phuditshinnapatra, J.; Chomchai, C. Sensitivity of dose-estimations for acute acetaminophen overdose in predicting hepatotoxicity risk using the Rumack-Matthew Nomogram. *Pharmacol. Res. Perspect.* **2022**, *10*, e00920. [CrossRef]
70. Akakpo, J.Y.; Ramachandran, A.; Duan, L.; Schaich, M.A.; Jaeschke, M.W.; Freudenthal, B.D.; Ding, W.-X.; Rumack, B.H.; Jaeschke, H. Delayed Treatment With 4-Methylpyrazole Protects Against Acetaminophen Hepatotoxicity in Mice by Inhibition of c-Jun n-Terminal Kinase. *Toxicol. Sci.* **2019**, *170*, 57–68. [CrossRef]
71. Link, S.L.; Rampon, G.; Osmon, S.; Scalzo, A.J.; Rumack, B.H. Fomepizole as an adjunct in acetylcysteine treated acetaminophen overdose patients: A case series. *Clin. Toxicol.* **2022**, *60*, 472–477. [CrossRef] [PubMed]
72. Shah, K.R.; Fox, C.; Geib, A.J.; Murphy, C.; Kopec, K.; Kerns II, W.; Dulaney, A.; Beuhler, M.C. Fomepizole as an adjunctive treatment in severe acetaminophen ingestions: A case series. *Clin. Toxicol.* **2021**, *59*, 71–72. [CrossRef] [PubMed]
73. Rasamison, R.; Besson, H.; Berleur, M.P.; Schicchi, A.; Mégarbane, B. Analysis of fomepizole safety based on a 16-year post-marketing experience in France. *Clin. Toxicol.* **2020**, *58*, 742–747. [CrossRef] [PubMed]
74. Ramachandran, A.; Akakpo, J.Y.; Curry, S.C.; Rumack, B.H.; Jaeschke, H. Clinically relevant therapeutic approaches against acetaminophen hepatotoxicity and acute liver failure. *Biochem. Pharmacol.* **2024**, *228*, 116056. [CrossRef]
75. Akakpo, J.Y.; Ramachandran, A.; Curry, S.C.; Rumack, B.H.; Jaeschke, H. Comparing N-acetylcysteine and 4-methylpyrazole as antidotes for acetaminophen overdose. *Arch. Toxicol.* **2022**, *96*, 453–465. [CrossRef]

MDPI AG
Grosspeteranlage 5
4052 Basel
Switzerland
Tel.: +41 61 683 77 34

Livers Editorial Office
E-mail: livers@mdpi.com
www.mdpi.com/journal/livers

www.ingramcontent.com/pod-product-compliance
Lightning Source LLC
Chambersburg PA
CBHW062041220926
51850CB00010B/2628
* 9 7 8 3 7 2 5 8 5 5 3 9 1 *